Learning Disability Nursing

Dedication

We would like to dedicate this book to all the people with learning disabilities, their families, learning disability nurses and other professionals we have had the privilege of working alongside and learning from.

To order, or for details of our bulk discounts, please go to our website www.criticalpublishing.com or contact our distributor, Ingram Publisher Services (IPS UK), 10 Thornbury Road, Plymouth PL6 7PP, telephone 01752 202301 or email IPSUK.orders@ingramcontent.com.

Learning Disability Nursing

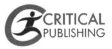
CRITICAL
PUBLISHING

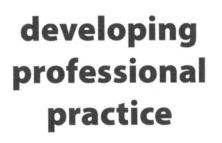

developing professional practice

Ruth Northway and Paula Hopes

First published in 2022 by Critical Publishing Ltd

British Library Cataloguing in Publication Data
A CIP record for this book is available from the British Library

ISBN: 978-1-914171-35-2

This book is also available in the following e-book formats:
EPUB ISBN: 978-1-914171-36-9
Adobe e-book ISBN: 978-1-914171-37-6

Cover design by Out of House Limited
Text design by Greensplash
Project management by Newgen Publishing UK
Printed and bound in Great Britain by 4edge, Essex

Critical Publishing
3 Connaught Road
St Albans
AL3 5RX

www.criticalpublishing.com

Printed on FSC accredited paper

Contents

About the authors

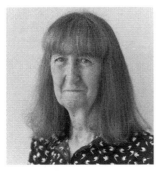

Ruth Northway

Ruth Northway is Professor of Learning Disability Nursing at the University of South Wales and has over 30 years' experience of working in nurse education. During this time she has been involved in curriculum development, and module and course delivery at both undergraduate and postgraduate levels. Her current role continues to see her directly involved in the education of learning disability nurses as well as in developing learning disability research and involvement in wider professional groups and networks. She was a member of the Thought Leadership Group that developed the Standards of Proficiency for Registered Nurses (NMC, 2018a).

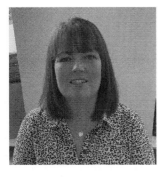

Paula Hopes

Paula Hopes has worked as a senior lecturer in two universities, educating future nurses and other aspirant health professionals in meeting the health and well-being needs of people with learning disabilities. She is an external examiner at Limerick University and has worked in universities in England and Wales, so she has a knowledge of the varied drivers, policies and influences on nurse education as well as the experience of people with learning disabilities and their families. She has taught at pre- and post-registration level and has supervised the academic work of students and registrants. She is the Welsh representative at the Learning Disability Professional Senate and co-chair of the UK Learning Disability Nurse Consultant Network.

Introduction

Registered learning disability nurses in the United Kingdom (UK) comprise one of the smaller fields of nursing and, over the years, there have been many challenges to the continued existence of this field of practice. However, there have also been many positive developments and learning disability nurses continue to play a key role in promoting the health and well-being of people with learning disabilities. Their roles have diversified, and the profession continues to develop to meet the changing needs of those it works alongside, and the changing context within which they work. This requires a questioning approach and critical thinking, it requires flexibility and creativity, and it requires a commitment to continuous professional development (CPD). This book aims to promote such professional attributes.

Whether you are a student or a registered nurse, we believe that this book will provide you with an important resource to facilitate your professional development. It is innovative in the approach taken which brings together theory and practice relevant to the development of learning disability nurses and nursing. This is achieved through exploration of a range of topics, the use of case studies and encouraging critical thinking through reflective activities. At the beginning of each chapter, specific links are made to the outcomes required within the NMC Standards for Nurse Education (2018a) and the NMC Code of Conduct (NMC, 2018b). This enables you to make direct links to the requirements of undergraduate nursing courses in the UK and to key areas required of registered nurses when seeking revalidation.

While aimed primarily at learning disability students and registered nurses in the UK, the material covered in this volume is also relevant to nurses who specialise in providing support for people with learning/intellectual disabilities in other countries. The terminology used in this book is 'learning disability' since this is the terminology applied in the UK to this field of practice. However, for international readers the terms learning disability and intellectual disability should be taken as meaning the same. It also has relevance for nurses working in other fields of nursing who wish to develop their practice to enhance the care and support they provide for children, young people, adults and older adults with learning/intellectual disabilities.

Each chapter can be accessed as a free-standing resource but many of the topics explored are interrelated and therefore you will be cross-referred to other chapters and sections where appropriate. We hope that this will assist you to integrate and use the knowledge effectively. The book is organised in three sections which each build upon each other.

SECTION 1: THE FOUNDATIONS OF LEARNING DISABILITY NURSING

As the title of this section suggests, its focus is on key areas upon which learning disability nursing has developed: the foundations of learning disability nursing.

Chapter 1 takes a historical view to explore the development of learning disability nursing from the nineteenth century to the current day. It does this in the context of how societal attitudes towards, and models of care and support for, people with learning disabilities have developed. It also briefly looks at international developments relating to nursing care for people with learning disabilities.

Chapter 2 highlights the importance of a strong value base within learning disability nursing and some of the legal and ethical dilemmas that learning disability nurses may encounter. It also seeks to provide you with tools to assist you in responding to these challenges and dilemmas.

Communication is central to learning disability nursing and therefore Chapter 3 brings together practical and evidence-based approaches to developing communication with people with learning disabilities and their families. Examples for augmenting and developing communication skills are given in line with best practice models. There is also identification of the skills needed to effectively communicate with other professionals, recognising barriers to communication and providing structured methods for imparting and receiving information.

Chapter 4 clarifies the importance of evidence-based practice and identifies the issues that need to be addressed when seeking to promote such an approach. It also explores the need to further develop the evidence base for learning disability nursing recognising the challenges that may be encountered.

SECTION 2: KEY DIMENSIONS OF CONTEMPORARY PRACTICE

Within Section 2, the focus moves to explore several key elements of learning disability nursing practice. The importance of working across the lifespan to identify challenges to health and well-being and strategies to prevent or the impact of such challenges are explored.

Chapter 5 focuses on assessing need. There is exploration of the importance of holistic assessment and the contribution that registered learning disability nurses make to this. The chapter recognises the skills, knowledge and understanding of the Registered Nurse Learning Disabilities (RNLD) and the processes that support professionals in making their assessments. Discussion on skills required to undertake assessments in partnership and identification of specific tools and structures connects the chapter directly to the practical application to professional practice.

Chapter 6 focuses on planning and delivering care in partnership with others. It explores person-centred planning and other approaches to planning and delivering care and support. Care planning frameworks are introduced and there is detailed discussion on the various areas where you will develop care plans.

A key feature of learning disability nursing is that it takes a lifespan approach. Chapter 7, therefore, explores the contribution of learning disability nurses at key life stages – children, young people, adults and older adults. The role of the learning disability nurse at different stages is identified with practical examples of the ways that nurses will work together with people and their families across the lifespan.

Chapter 8 explores the importance of learning disability nurses understanding and adopting a public health approach. It introduces you to key public health concepts and considers some of the challenges in adopting a public health approach to addressing the health inequalities experienced by people with learning disabilities. It also explores how you can use such an approach to inform your practice.

Chapter 9 focuses on supporting those whose behaviour challenges. It identifies the role of the learning disability nurse in understanding behaviours that challenge and working in partnership to support well-being using approaches such as positive behavioural support. Some influences on behavioural presentation, including sensory and environmental factors as well as the quality of life issues, are described.

SECTION 3: ADVANCING LEARNING DISABILITY NURSING PRACTICE

As noted above, it is important that learning disability nursing, as a profession, continues to develop its practice. Section 3 of the book therefore focuses on enabling you to develop strategies which will enable you to contribute to such professional development.

Chapter 10 explores innovation in practice. Its emphasis is on recognising the need for learning disability nurses to adopt a creative and innovative approach to practice. There are examples of change in language, concepts, models and demonstration of the roles learning disability nurses have in identifying areas for change. The chapter goes on to describe tips for increasing your confidence in leading on innovation, managing change and evaluating impact, as well as advice for sustaining change in practice.

Effective leadership is central to advancing professional practice and Chapter 11 therefore explores the need for leadership within learning disability nursing. Different leadership approaches and the importance of organisational culture are considered as well as the negative impact of poor leadership. It also encourages you to consider your own development as a leader.

Chapter 12 is the final chapter and focuses on both the wider development of learning disability nursing and your own professional development. Links are made to the revalidation requirements that all registered nurses need to meet and a 'tool kit' to support your development is offered.

USING THIS BOOK

We hope that you will find this book both useful and interesting. To gain maximum benefit, we would encourage you to complete the critical reflection activities either individually or with colleagues. We have also provided details of additional resources at the end of each chapter should you wish to read further.

Section 1

The foundations for practice

1 The development of learning disability nursing

Chapter aims

This chapter provides a context for this book through an examination of how the profession of learning disability nursing has developed. It explores developments from the beginnings of institutional care in the 1800s through to the current day. Since this is inextricably linked with the development of care and support provided for people with learning disabilities, a brief overview of patterns of care and support is first explored. Finally, consideration is given to nursing care of people with intellectual disabilities in other countries.

In achieving these aims, it is necessary, at times, to use terminology that is not acceptable to use today to refer to people with learning disabilities. Terminology has changed over time and what is not acceptable now would, at the time, have been viewed as being appropriate. Indeed, the terminology we use today will likely be viewed negatively in the future. It is also important to recognise that change does not happen overnight and therefore differing terminology may be used at the same time: the new is introduced while the old gradually wanes.

Professional standards and expectations

In the Standards of Proficiency for Registered Nurses, the NMC (2018a) notes the necessity of regularly reviewing such standards to ensure that they remain contemporary and fit for purpose. Accordingly, in developing the current standards, changes in society and healthcare, their implications for nursing practice, and the knowledge and skills required of nurses now and in the future were all considered (NMC, 2018a). This suggests two things. First, there is a professional expectation that nursing, as a profession, needs to keep its practice constantly under review to ensure that it remains relevant to the needs of individuals, communities and society. Second, that to achieve this, nurses and nursing need to have an awareness of the relationship between their practice and wider society. The latter also requires that we understand not only the present but also that we are able to place developments in a historical context.

THE RELEVANCE OF HISTORY

You might be wondering why this book, which focuses on professional development within learning disability nursing, commences with a chapter that looks back and takes a historical perspective. The rationale for including this chapter is that to understand where we are today as a profession, and to build for the future, we need to understand where we have been, what has changed and why such changes occurred. Mitchell (2019) suggests that studying the history of learning disability nursing both provides us with perspective and helps to identify a body of professional work we can use to develop future practice and education. He also questions how subsequent generations of learning disability nurses will view today's practice (Mitchell, 2019).

Critical reflection 1.1

Imagine you are describing current learning disability nursing to a future generation of learning disability nurses.

- What are the key features you would mention?
- What do you think they would make of your description?

Of course, no profession develops in isolation, and this is certainly true of learning disability nursing. As has been noted above, the history of this field of nursing practice is inextricably linked with the history of those for whom it provides care and support, and the varying policies and legislation that have shaped service provision. This, in turn, has been shaped by wider societal beliefs and attitudes. However, another key influence on the history of learning disability nursing is the wider development of the nursing profession and (as will be seen later in the chapter) tensions have often been evident as to whether learning disability nursing should be viewed as part of the wider profession of nursing (Mitchell, 2000). Figure 1.1 illustrates this range of influences on the development of learning disability nursing.

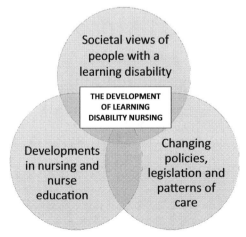

Figure 1.1 Influences on the developing role of the learning disability nurse

Before exploring how learning disability nursing developed and has evolved, this chapter, therefore, first briefly considers changing views of people with intellectual disabilities and the differing historical patterns of care and support provided in the context of such views.

PEOPLE WITH LEARNING DISABILITIES IN THE UK: A BRIEF OVERVIEW OF HISTORY AND CHANGING MODELS OF CARE

Ryan and Thomas (1987), in a key text documenting how people with learning disabilities have been viewed and supported by society over time, argue that:

> The changing definitions of difference constitute the history of mentally handicapped people. These definitions have always been conceived of by others, never are they the expression of a group of people finding their identity, their own history. The assertion of difference between people is seldom neutral ... The differences between mentally handicapped people and others have mostly been seen negatively, making them a problem to themselves and others.
>
> (Ryan and Thomas, 1987, p 13)

The terminology of 'mentally handicapped' was viewed as appropriate at the time Ryan and Thomas were writing and since that time both the terminology and the extent to which people with learning disabilities themselves have found a 'voice' in asserting their own identity have changed. However, a look at history reveals how this group of people have been viewed in different ways at different points in time and how this, in turn, has shaped public and policy perceptions about how their differences should be addressed and support provided.

People with learning disabilities have always existed within society, but since this chapter focuses on the development of learning disability nursing, it starts by examining their history from the nineteenth century onwards, given this is where the origins of nursing lie.

Critical reflection 1.2

Think about how people with learning disabilities are viewed within current society.

- How does this reflect current patterns of care and support?

The development of educational institutions

Ryan and Thomas (1987) note that the beginning of the nineteenth century saw the development for the first time of educational provision of those termed (at that time) as 'idiots'. Building on the work of people such as Seguin, educational institutions started to develop whose aim was to provide education for 'idiots' with a view to improving their situation through a programme of instruction, occupation and leisure aimed at returning them to their families and communities. However, the number of people within institutions grew with Ryan and Thomas (1987) noting that in 1864 there were approximately 400, rising to about 2000 in 1914 housed in six asylums. Many more were housed within workhouses and institutions for the 'insane' (psychiatric).

As conditions within institutions began to deteriorate, the focus shifted from education to containment and control, and management shifted to the medical profession (Ryan and Thomas, 1987). However, the 'failure' of the educational approach was *attributed to the hopeless nature of the idiots*' rather than to a failure to take account of wider societal factors that were leading to a more general move towards institutionalisation, and which were making it more difficult for those considered 'idiots' to survive in the community (Ryan and Thomas, 1987).

With growing numbers within the institutions, those living there increasingly became seen by wider society as 'different' with this difference being viewed as meaning they were perceived as being less than human and a risk to society. They were physically segregated from wider society, and this reinforced the sense of difference and being a danger to others. As Ryan and Thomas (1987, p 107) observe, '*An indeterminant linking of mental deficiency with all kinds of social problems became commonplace*'. Coupled with a growing interest in genetics and eugenic fears, there was pressure to 'control' those considered 'idiots' and, in particular, to prevent them from reproducing.

The National Association for the Care and Control of the Feebleminded was established in 1896. As the name suggests, a key area of focus was on ensuring 'control' and they campaigned for lifelong segregation of those considered to be mentally defective. The 1908 Radnor Commission examined this issue and sought to make recommendations for the development of new legislation. The Commission concluded that mental defectiveness was inherited and that the appropriate solution was to prevent them from having children through lifelong segregation and supervision in institutions for '*as long as may be necessary*' (Radnor Commission, 1908, cited in Ryan and Thomas, 1987, p 107).

The resulting 1913 Mental Deficiency Act classified people as 'idiots', 'imbeciles', 'feeble-minded' and 'moral imbeciles' with those considered to be 'idiots' as having the greatest support needs. Inclusion of the category of 'moral imbeciles' made it possible for women with illegitimate children who were in receipt of poor relief to be institutionalised (Open University, 2022). Implementation of this Act was slow and in 1929 the Wood Committee reported that people considered to be mentally defective continued to be a threat to society (Ryan and Thomas, 1987). This committee concluded that:

> If we are to prevent the racial disaster of mental deficiency we must deal with not only the mentally defective person, but the whole subnormal group from which the majority of them come.
>
> (Wood Committee, 1929, cited in Ryan and Thomas, 1987, p 108)

A medical model of care

The number of institutions and the numbers living within them continued to grow reaching 32,000 by 1939 (Ryan and Thomas, 1987). In 1948 when the National Health Service was established, the institutions became part of this service and became long-stay hospitals. The medical model of care thus was firmly established. However, in 1959 the Mental Health Act removed the need for compulsory detention in such hospitals by introducing the category of informal patients who (in theory at least) were free to leave the hospital. This legislation also enabled the development by local authorities of community-based services although little progress was made in this area.

During the 1960s, research began to question whether institutional long-term care was appropriate. For example, studies undertaken by Tizard and colleagues in the early 1960s examined provision for children in long-stay hospitals. They concluded that smaller residential units were preferable but that reducing the size of such units alone was insufficient to ensure child-oriented care: attention to changing the pattern of care was also required and this required action in relation to both staffing levels and the training of staff (King et al, 1971).

In 1967, however, an expose in the News of the World Sunday newspaper revealed poor standards of care in Ely Hospital, Cardiff. A staff member had tried to raise concerns within the hospital and the health authority, but these had not been acted upon and hence they alerted the media. As a result of this, an enquiry into standards of care was established and this was reported in 1969. The report highlighted a range of issues relating to care, abuse, staffing and management and made several recommendations.

Publication of the Ely Hospital Enquiry Report shone a light on conditions within such hospitals and prompted a desire for reform. In 1971 the Government published the White Paper *Better Services for the Mentally Handicapped*. Described at the time as making proposals that were '*both simple and sweeping*' (Jones, 1972), this document set several targets for reducing the number of long-stay hospital beds and the development of community-based services such as residential homes and arrangements for fostering. Change was to occur over a 15–20-year period and would see hospitals focusing on those who, due to their needs, required constant nursing care while local authorities would develop services and support the greater integration of mentally handicapped people into mainstream social, educational and health services (Jones, 1972).

Movement towards community-based care and support

Progress towards achievement of the targets set in *Better Services* was, however, slow. The numbers living within long-stay institutions did not significantly decline and conditions in the hospitals (often old buildings not specifically designed for their current purpose) failed to improve. Indeed, other inquiries followed such as those in Normansfield Hospital (1977) and Leavesden Hospital (1978).

In 1983, the Welsh Office noted this lack of progress towards the 1971 targets arguing that 80 per cent of the funding for services for people with a mental handicap was being spent on the 20 per cent of people living in the long-stay hospitals while only 20 per cent was being used to fund the development of services for the majority (80 per cent) living with their families in the community (Welsh Office, 1983). To effect change they ring fenced additional funding for the development of community-based support in Wales. The provision of funding, however, was contingent on proposed developments complying with three key principles, namely that they would support the right of people with a mental handicap to be treated as individuals, to normal patterns of life in the community, and to receive support from their communities and from professionals.

These principles echoed those set out in the Jay Report (1979) (see below) and reflected the philosophy of normalisation that was beginning to influence thinking in relation to services for people with a mental handicap in the UK. Normalisation had its origins in Scandinavia with the Danish Mental Retardation Act stating in 1959 that services should create support for people with a mental handicap that enabled them to live lives 'as close to normal living conditions as normal' (Bank-Mikkelson, 1980, p 56). This was expanded on by Nirje (1980) to encompass elements such as a normal pattern to the day, a normal rhythm to the week, progression through the stages of the lifecycle and equal access to economic standards in relation to either welfare benefits or paid employment.

However, in the UK more generally, it was the North American version of normalisation promoted by Wolf Wolfensberger that was adopted. Later becoming known as social role valorisation (Wolfensberger, 1984), this approach argued that people with a mental handicap are cast into devalued roles by wider society and that this influences how they are viewed and treated. To change such negative treatment, therefore, what was required was for services and support to promote positive social roles using culturally valued means.

Against this backdrop, there was a renewed focus on the development of community-based services (to prevent the need for admission to hospital), resettlement of those currently living within long-stay hospitals and eventual closure of such establishments. However, wider reforms were also taking place in relation to the development of community-based services across service user groups. A report by the Audit Commission (1986) called for radical change to address both the slow and uneven progress being made and the lack of organisational co-ordination between health and social care.

In 1989 the Department of Health (1989a) published the White Paper *Community Care in the Next Decade and Beyond*, which set out arrangements for the provision of community-based care. Alongside this, another White Paper *Working for Patients* (Department of Health, 1989b) set out future plans for the provision of health services. Taken together, these policies sought to make a clear distinction between healthcare (provided by health services) and social care (provided by local authorities) while recognising that they needed to work together. Community care was to be based on the assessment of need through a care management system; a move to a mixed economy of care in which independent service providers play a key role was also advocated.

The 1990s saw further development of community services and the closure of many long-stay hospitals. At the end of the 1990s, there was a move to devolution with health and social care becoming the responsibility of devolved governments in the different countries of the UK. While the general trend of policy development in relation to services and support for people with learning disabilities remained the same in each country, there were also some variations with countries publishing their own policy documents. It is these policies that shape current patterns of care and support for people with learning disabilities.

THE DEVELOPMENT OF LEARNING DISABILITY NURSING

Many books on the history of nursing make little or no reference to learning disability nursing. As Mitchell and Smith (2003) observe, learning disability nursing has often been viewed as being *'on the margins of nursing'*. Its history is different from that of adult nursing and has been shaped by different factors (see Figure 1.1). However, it is also a history in which learning disability nurses themselves have increasingly shaped and led the development of their profession. This section therefore explores developments in learning disability nursing, broader nursing developments and nurse education since each of these has (and continue to) exert an influence. It will trace the history starting with the origins of the profession – the expansion of institutional care in the late nineteenth century. The terminology used to refer to the group of nurses will reflect that used at a particular point in history from Mental Deficiency (until 1940s), to Mental Subnormality (until 1970s), to Mental Handicap from the 1970s to the current terminology of 'learning disability'.

The rise of institutions

As noted above, the latter part of the nineteenth century saw the expansion of institutions as numbers within them grew and their focus moved away from the provision of education to containment. The workforce within these institutions was referred to as attendants. The 1913 Mental Deficiency Act, overseen by the Board of Control, led to the expansion of the institutions which required a suitable workforce. Mitchell (2001) argues that nursing was seen as the answer to this problem being viewed as useful by both the Board of Control and the Royal Medico-Psychological Association (RMPA) since as a profession it was *'cheap, efficient and pliable'*. Such characteristics were seen as ideal to support the development of institutional care (Mitchell, 2001).

The RMPA had previously provided a training scheme and qualification which allowed flexibility to allow for adaptation to the needs of individual institutions (Mitchell, 2000). However, the introduction of the 1913 Mental Deficiency Act led the RMPA to develop a separate, specific qualification for mental deficiency nurses. Prior to this, they would have been awarded an asylum nurse certificate which was the qualification for those working in the asylums primarily caring for those with mental illness. The first national certificates for mental deficiency nursing were issued by the RMPA in 1919 (Mitchell, 2019).

Alongside this, however, the General Nursing Council was also being established with a remit to develop and maintain a nursing register. There was considerable debate as to whether nurses working in the long-stay institutions should be considered nurses and included in such a register. Nursing was generally viewed within the context of a sickness focused, medical model its aim being to assist with 'curing' those experiencing ill health. Mental deficiency nursing (as it was then called) did not conform to this model and thus did not seem to be a suitable fit for the proposed register.

Eventually, mental deficiency nursing was included as a subsidiary section of the mental nursing supplementary register in 1920. Mitchell (2000) argues that this 'secondary' status laid the foundation for the 'constant challenge' faced by nurses working in this specialism to be recognised as part of the nursing profession. Indeed, as will be seen below, the debate as to their place in the profession has been a recurring theme throughout the decades.

The GNC introduced examinations for mental deficiency nurses in 1926. However, opportunities for training in this specialism remained limited. By 1936, of the 67 institutions with over 100 residents, only 30 were recognised by the RMPA for the provision of training and only ten of these were also recognised by the GNC (Board of Control cited in Mitchell, 2001). The RMPA produced a textbook (The Manual for Mental Deficiency Nurses) which became known as 'the green book' in 1931 (Stephenson, 2019) and, until the 1950s, psychiatrists (via the RMPA) maintained significant control over the examination of mental deficiency nurses (Mitchell, 2019). Many nurses in this specialism chose to register with the RMPA rather than the GNC until after the Second World War (Mitchell, 2000).

Institutions become hospitals

When institutions became hospitals and part of the NHS in 1948, the central role of nurses within this model of provision was confirmed. The RMPA register was closed, and all Mental Deficiency Nurses registered with the General Nursing Council. However, the Mental Deficiency Nursing qualification was not viewed as being equal to other nursing qualifications even within the context of long-stay hospitals specifically focused on providing care for people deemed to have a mental deficiency. Nurses working in such institutions were often encouraged to undertake an additional (general) nursing qualification in order 'to be recognised as nurses' by the wider nursing profession (Parrish and Sines, 1997, p 1123). The recruitment of nurses who were dually qualified (mental deficiency and general) was also encouraged for senior leadership roles (Mitchell, 2001).

As noted earlier in this chapter, the Ely Hospital Enquiry (DHSS, 1969) drew public attention to the poor conditions and abusive practices existing within such settings. Given that nurses formed the largest professional group within the hospital it is perhaps to be expected that their practice should be a key area of focus for the enquiry. However, in the report of the enquiry an entire chapter was devoted to nursing practice. The report notes that many of the nursing staff were having to work in poor conditions, with poor staffing levels, and that they were working hard to deliver care 'by their own standards' (DHSS, 1969). Nonetheless, the committee also noted that standards of nursing care fell short 'not merely of the ideal which is attainable in the 1960s but of a standard which is obtainable and practical even in the hospital as it stands today' (DHSS, 1969, Sect 227). Key areas of concern related to the use of seclusion, inadequate standards of personal care for residents, standards relating to management of deaths, insufficient medical supervision for practices such as suturing, the use of residents to undertake domestic work on the wards, a casual approach to reporting of incidents, arrangements for handovers and poor ward management.

It was noted that when the qualifications of the nursing staff at Ely were examined, some had gained them via years of experience (rather than by studying for a nursing qualification) while most others were qualified in either mental health or general nursing. Most staff were unqualified nursing assistants and standards of induction and in service training were insufficient. Taken together, these factors were felt to contribute to the existence of a nursing workforce that was isolated and not up to date with modern standards of care for the mentally subnormal. It was concluded that '*Lax and old-fashioned standards of nursing, reminiscent in too many ways of the old era of "custodial care", have been accepted*' (DHSS, 1969). Unsurprisingly, a range of recommendations were made including those relating to the training and management of nursing staff. Of wider concern was that the publication of a nationwide survey of long-stay hospitals (Morris, 1969) revealed that the findings at Ely Hospital were not confined to that institution with similar problems existing elsewhere (Brown, 1992).

Adapting to changing philosophies and the move to community-based care and support

The nursing syllabus for nurses training to become Registered Nurses for the Mentally Subnormal was again revised in 1970 and it covered four broad areas:

I.   *A systematic study of the human individual.*

II. *Concepts of mental subnormality and the nursing, teaching, training, and treatment of the mentally handicapped including the legal and administrative aspects.*

III. *Fundamentals of community care.*

IV. *The nursing of bodily disorders commonly associated with the mentally handicapped.*

(The General Nursing Council of England and Wales, 1970, p 2)

There are few aspects of these areas of study that require comment. First, terminology is beginning to change from 'mental subnormality' to 'mental handicap'. This mixing of terminology in the document was a recognition of imminent legal and policy changes but the terminology at the time the document was issued officially remained that of 'subnormality'. Second, while the provision of care and support at that time was almost entirely based within the long-stay hospitals, a key area of the syllabus was focused on the '*fundamentals of community care*' again signalling a move for mental subnormality/handicap nurses to encompass community-based care and support. Indeed, the syllabus stated that both the theoretical and practical elements of the course should focus on preparation of the nurse for work in both the hospital and the community. Third, the educational role of the nurse remained a key element recognising the original educational functions of institutions. However, there was also a focus on understanding nursing care in relation to the health problems commonly experienced by people with a mental handicap.

When detailing the curriculum content in relation to supporting people in community settings, reference is also made to the 'consultative role' of the mental handicap nurse noting the need for co-operation with other professionals such as social workers, as well as with families (GNC, 1970). In this respect, the elements we recognise today as working in partnership and interdisciplinary working were beginning to emerge.

Critical reflection 1.3

- Look at the areas covered in the 1970 nursing syllabus detailed above. How do they compare to the current Standards (NMC, 2018a)?

Nurse training in the 1970s involved a three-year course within which there were 120–140 study days (30 days of these forming an initial six-week introductory study block) (GNC, 1970). The remaining time was spent undertaking clinical placements in a range of settings. The training was provided by schools of nursing based in, or attached to, long-stay hospitals and student nurses were employees of the health authority receiving a wage from them. While undertaking clinical placements, they were thus considered employees and counted in the staffing establishment. Award of the qualification and entry to the register was determined by a final three-hour examination that was centrally set and marked by the GNC.

The Better Services for the Mentally Handicapped White Paper (DHSS,1971) proposed reforms to patterns of care and support for people with a mental handicap and a greater focus on the development of community-based supports. In the context of changing models of care, and questions being posed regarding the appropriateness of long-stay hospital provision, it is perhaps unsurprising that the future of mental subnormality nursing was questioned. In 1972 the Briggs Report recommended that this field of nursing should no longer be a part of the nursing profession and that a new professional group should emerge (Mitchell, 2003).

In February 1975, the government announced an enquiry into 'mental handicap nursing and care' to be chaired by Peggy Jay. The outcomes of this enquiry subsequently became the Jay Report (DHSS, 1979). However, the report noted that there were challenges in relation to the remit of the enquiry since while they included the broad brief of focusing on mental handicap nursing and care it also moved to consider the roles, aims and skills of professional staff providing residential care for people with a mental handicap in the context of current and developing policies. The Committee gathered evidence via a variety of methods and considered this in the context of three key principles.

a) *Mentally handicapped people have a right to enjoy normal patterns of life in the community.*

b) *Mentally handicapped people have a right to be treated as individuals.*

c) *Mentally handicapped people will require additional help from the communities in which they live and from professional services if they are to develop to their maximum potential as individuals.*

(DHSS, 1979, paragraph 89)

They proposed a model of care based on these principles and used this to determine the workforce requirements to deliver this. They concluded that there was a need for a common training for staff working in residential care and that what was required was more in line with the training provided by the Central Council for the Training and Education in Social Work (CCETSW), namely the Certificate in Social Services (CSS) than the nursing qualification provided by the GNC. The formation of a group to develop the CSS was thus recommended along with the need for CCETSW and the GNC to collaborate to develop post-qualifying courses for general, psychiatric and children's nurses to provide care for 'very severely handicapped residents'.

The Committee argued that for mental handicap nurses what would be required was more than a different approach to their role and required a 'new professional identity' (par 339). They felt that many would be willing to take on a new identity as a residential care worker seeing the benefits this would bring to those for whom they provided care. However, they also recognised that some may choose to remain within the nursing profession and to move away from working with people with a mental handicap. The following recommendation was therefore also made:

> *Any mental handicap nurse who prefers to remain in nursing should be offered a place on one of the shortened courses for nurses wishing to transfer from one part of the Register or Roll to another.*
>
> (DHSS, 1979, Recommendation 44)

This was not the first time it had been suggested that the profession of mental subnormality/handicap nursing should not continue. However, the Jay Report received a 'barrage' of criticism from nurses working in this field of practice who (while welcoming discussions of changing philosophies and additional resources) were opposed to the transfer of training to CCETSW wanting to remain as nurses working with people with a mental handicap (Mitchell, 2003). Of course, views of the motivations underpinning such opposition vary, and Ryan and Thomas (1987) suggest that nurses reacted defensively being motivated by self-interest and failed to critically reflect on the need for change within the systems in which they worked. However, Mitchell (2003) argues that the Jay Committee '*completely failed to foresee*' the extent to which nurses working in this specialism could and would transform itself and suggests that the Jay Report may have provided the impetus for such transformation.

One response was to review the syllabus of training for nurses wishing to specialise in the care and support of people with a mental handicap. The '*Syllabus of Training Professional Register – Part 5. Registered Nurses for the Mentally Handicapped 1982*' (National Boards for England and Wales, 1985) was developed and subsequently implemented. This not only changed the terminology to 'mental handicap' but also signalled a move from training based on a medical model to one that encompassed a social model of care. Significantly, the explicit principles upon which the syllabus was based are those that informed the Jay Committee (see above). Table 1.1 details the sections included in this syllabus and provides you with an overview of the key areas of knowledge and skills required.

Table 1.1 The sections of the 1982 Mental Handicap Nursing Syllabus

Section number	Focus
1	The nursing process
2	The skills of communication and alternative methods of communication
3	Education and mentally handicapped people
4	The sociology of organisations
5	Normalisation and human rights
6	Management
7	Principles of development
8	Causation, nature and effects of mental handicap
9	Partnership with families
10	Developing care and training programmes
11	Maintenance of the living environment
12	Children
13	Adolescents
14	Adults
15	The elderly person
16	People with multiple handicaps
17	Facilitating integration and rehabilitation into the community
18	Maintaining optimum health
19	Professional development

(National Boards of England and Wales, 1985)

Mental handicap nursing thus continued to be a distinct field of nursing practice and nurses started to move from hospital-based posts to working in community settings, often within multidisciplinary teams (MDTs). However, debates regarding continuation of the specialism had not gone away. At the end of the 1980s wider developments and reforms in relation to community care (see earlier in the chapter) once again gave rise to consideration regarding future options for the profession. Changes also occurred in nurse education and, more broadly, in relation to the regulation of the nursing profession.

In 1983, the United Kingdom Central Council for Nursing and Midwifery (UKCC) was established and replaced the General Nursing Council. This new body was expected to maintain the nursing and midwifery registers, provide guidance to the professions and to handle any complaints arising from professional misconduct. Alongside this new body, four national boards (one in each country of the UK) were set up to monitor nursing and midwifery education and to maintain records of training in relation to students. A key development was the publication in 1983 of a *'Code of Professional Conduct for the Nurse, Midwife and Health Visitor'* which was soon superseded by the publication of a second edition in 1984 (UKCC, 1984). For the first time in the UK, this Code provided a clear set of standards to guide the professional behaviour of nurses and against which their behaviour could be assessed should it be brought into question. It stressed a range of requirements including that all nurses were accountable for their practice and the exercise of professional accountability, that they were required to promote and safeguard the well-being and interests of those they support, that they needed to maintain and improve their professional knowledge and competence and that they needed to have regard to the environment of care and to make known to appropriate persons where this environment presented a risk to the provision of safe care (UKCC, 1984).

The Project 2000 reforms of nurse education began to be implemented in 1989 and learning disability nursing (as it was becoming) remained within this curriculum as a distinct field of nursing. However, in contrast to previous curricula, which had seen each of the fields educated separately, Project 2000 introduced an 18-month 'common core' which was studied by all fields together followed by an 18-month 'branch' programme. Concerns were expressed by learning disability nurses and other specialist areas of nursing that this change would lead to dilution of their skills (Brown, 1992).

This new curriculum sought to place more emphasis on health promotion, the prevention of ill health and community-based care (National Audit Office, 1992) and it could perhaps be suggested that this change within nurse education overall reflected changes that had already been adopted within learning disability nurse education (see discussion above). However, it did mean that learning disability student nurses gained experience learning alongside students from other fields of practice and undertook clinical placements outside of learning disability settings. It also meant that all students, regardless of their field of practice, started to receive education (and sometimes clinical placements) in relation to care and support of people with learning disabilities. Given growing awareness of the health needs of people with learning disabilities and the fact that they often had negative experiences of healthcare, this was an important development.

Another key difference with Project 2000 was that nurse education moved away from hospital schools of nursing into higher education establishments. Student nurses were no longer employed by health services and instead were university-based students who received a bursary. This meant that, except for a period of rostered service later in their course, they were supernumerary while on placement. The level of education was also raised to diploma level study as a minimum.

In 1990, the four Chief Nursing Officers of the UK asked Professor Chris Cullen to chair a working group focused on the skills of mental handicap nurses in the context of changing patterns of care and tasked with considering options for future development. The resulting report set out several potential options, namely:

○   *mental handicap nurses as the core-direct care providers;*

○   *the creation of a new caring profession;*

○   *wait and see;*

○   *planned run-down of the profession nurses;*

○   *promotion of the healthcare role of mental handicap nurses.*

(Cullen, 1991, pp 9–17)

These options were assessed against a range of criteria including feasibility, coherence with values and policy, professionalism, the extent to which they offered a secure starting point for development and the extent to which they differed from current practice and the healthcare needs of people with a mental handicap. Having undertaken such an assessment, it was felt that the best option was to promote the healthcare role of the mental handicap nurse. However, it recognised that health and social care are *'inextricably linked'* and that such a role would require working alongside other healthcare professionals within the context of community care. It also stressed that the skills possessed by mental handicap nurses are *'facility-independent'* meaning that they can be transferred and used within whichever settings people with mental handicap are located: the knowledge and skills of mental handicap nurses are not dependent on the existence of long-stay hospitals.

It was recognised that while this option avoided radical change it required an evolutionary approach and that this, in turn, required leadership and the provision of educational support at both pre-qualifying and post-registration levels. The report noted that the new 'Project 2000' nursing curriculum offered nursing students a 'first rate education' that would prepare the future workforce (Cullen, 1991).

Interestingly, following the publication of the Cullen Report (1991) the Royal College of Nursing (RCN, 1992) published a report of a working group charged with reviewing a 1985 document examining the role and function of community learning disability nurses. The introduction to this report notes that people with a learning disability should have access to the knowledge and skills wherever they reside, thus echoing the view of the Cullen Report (1991). Among other elements of the role, this report also stressed that community learning disability nurses have a key focus on meeting health-related needs through health promotion, providing support in relation to both physical and mental health problems, health monitoring and working in partnership with other health professionals.

As community care reforms advanced, it was felt that there remained a lack of awareness regarding the contribution of the learning disability nurse. Indeed, the RCN (1992) noted that confusion regarding the role of the community learning disability nurse remained. Hence, in 1994 the *Learning Disability Nursing Project* was established by the Department of Health. This sought to provide information to a wide range of stakeholders to ensure that the skills of learning disability nurses were used in the most appropriate way to meet identified needs. For example, one publication was aimed at those who had responsibility for commissioning health and social care services (Department of Health, 1995). This identified the purpose of learning disability nursing as being to work in partnership with individuals to enhance their autonomy by seeking to:

- *mitigate the effects of disability;*
- *achieve optimum health;*
- *facilitate access to and encourage involvement in local communities;*
- *increase personal competence;*
- *maximise choice;*
- *enhance the contribution of others either formally or informally involved in supporting the individual.*

(Department of Health, 1995, p 7)

While acknowledging that learning disability nurses occupy a range of roles, the document argued that the distinct contribution they make is through their focus on influencing behaviours and lifestyles to achieve optimum health. It highlighted their contribution in relation to nutrition, management of epilepsy, promotion of continence, injury prevention, medication monitoring and alleviation of behavioural difficulties (Department of Health, 1995).

In 1998, the UKCC published specific guidelines for nurses working with people with mental health problems or learning disabilities (UKCC, 1998). While recognising that the needs of individuals in these two groups differ, it also noted that significant changes had occurred in the models of care in recent years and that consequently nurses working in these fields had felt the need for the provision of additional guidance. It noted the challenges of ethical decision-making (see Chapter 2 for further discussion) and sought to provide guidance to inform such decision-making and critical reflection rather than setting out a '*rule book*'. It was also stressed that this document should be read alongside other UKCC publications, in particular, the Code. Table 1.2 provides an overview of the areas covered in this document.

Table 1.2 Guidelines for mental health and learning disabilities nursing

Focus of guidance	Key principles
Accountability	Integral to professional practice requires weighing the interests of patients/service users and using professional judgement to make decisions for which you are professionally accountable. This requires that knowledge and skills are kept up to date.
Consent	Three overriding professional responsibilities – acting in the patient/service user's best interests and obtaining consent before providing treatment or care, demonstrating transparency and professional accountability in the process of establishing consent and accurately recording discussions and decisions relating to consent.
Interdisciplinary working	Complex service user/patient needs require a team response which may be interprofessional and interagency. This necessitates a shared understanding, co-operation and respect.
Evidence-based practice	Service users/patients should be able to assume that the care they receive is based on sound evidence.

→

Focus of guidance	Key principles
Advocacy	Nurses should promote and safeguard the interests of service users/patients and not assume that only they know what is best for the service user.
Autonomy	There is a professional responsibility to promote service user/patient independence and autonomy. The service user/patient should be involved in decision-making wherever possible.
Relationships	Nurses must be aware of the power imbalance that exists between their role and their patients/service users. Their power and influence should be directed to meeting patient/service user needs.
Confidentiality	Confidentiality is central to a therapeutic relationship and should only be broken under exceptional circumstances and after careful consideration.
Risk management	Risk management involves assessment of risk based on knowledge, skills and competence. Nurses are accountable for both actions and omissions and should be aware that there may be conflicts between professional accountability and service user autonomy.

(UKCC, 1998)

Case study 1.1

Paul O'Donnell started his 'Mental Subnormality' nurse training in 1978 at a school of nursing attached to a group of long-stay hospitals for people referred to at that time as having a 'mental handicap'. His training consisted of short study blocks in the school of nursing and longer extended placements working on various wards within the long-stay hospitals. He also undertook placements in a special school and in the recreation department within the hospital. Locally there was a new development where a few nurses had started to work outside of the hospital in the community. While he was training, the Jay Report was published and there were concerns about whether 'mental subnormality' nursing would continue. However, when he qualified, he secured a staff nurse post on one of the wards in a hospital which cared for 35 men with severe and profound 'mental handicap' (this terminology was starting to be used when he qualified).

As a staff nurse and then as a charge nurse in the same hospital, Paul was responsible for supporting student nurses undertaking placements on his ward. However, things were beginning to change. First, nurse training was changed following publication of a new syllabus and there was much more of a focus on a social model of care. Second, there were moves to close the long-stay hospitals and to 'resettle' people in the community. In the mid-1980s as resettlement gathered pace, Paul decided to apply for a community charge nurse post in the growing community nursing team. After working for a while as a community charge nurse, Paul was promoted to the post of senior nurse in the community team. He also took the opportunity to gain his community nursing qualification.

One aspect of his role that Paul had always enjoyed was supporting student nurses and in the 1990s, when nurse education moved from hospital schools of nursing to universities, he decided that he would like to work as a nursing lecturer. Moving to this role was a big change and he needed to undertake further study both to gain a teaching qualification and then, later, to gain a master's level qualification. He had never envisaged going to university let alone working in one.

Although Paul really enjoyed his role in the university, he also liked new challenges. When a nurse consultant post in learning disability nursing was advertised, he decided to apply as he felt this would enable him to not only retain his teaching role but also to work in clinical practice and take on a leadership role.

Recently a student undertaking a placement with him asked Paul what advice he would give to a student at the start of their career. Having thought for a minute he replied that learning disability nursing offers great opportunities for career development even if other people try to tell you they are not there, and even if you cannot envisage them at present (he did not ever envisage working as a consultant nurse or gaining a master's degree as these opportunities were not available when he was training). Opportunities both present themselves and can be created – be open to identifying and taking them.

Moving forward in a new century

At the beginning of the 2000s, reforms were again seen in relation to nurse education. A Commission was established (UKCC, 1999) since concerns were being voiced regarding the ability of the Project 2000 courses to prepare practitioners who were 'fit for practice' at the point of registration and calls from the government for nurse education to be more oriented to clinical practice (Bradshaw, 2000). A key area of criticism was a perceived lack of skills training (Grundy, 2001). The Commission's recommendations sought to recognise both the strengths of the theoretical preparation that nurses were now receiving while also emphasising the importance of clinical preparation and the need for stronger links between universities and healthcare providers. It advocated a move to a competency-based approach to nurse education and competency-based statements that had to be achieved for entry to the nursing register were subsequently developed (Grundy, 2001). However, Bradshaw (2000) notes that the practice of specialisation at a pre-registration level was also identified as an area requiring further consideration in terms of whether it should be brought in line with the generic model of nurse education adopted in other countries.

It could have been that this latter recommendation again led to debates regarding the future role of the learning disability nurse. However, in practice the changes introduced meant that the common foundation programme was reduced in length from 18 months to 12 and that the branch programme was extended to two years (Lord, 2002). Learning disability students thus moved to spending longer studying in their chosen field and less time studying alongside students from other branches studying the generic elements of the course.

In 2002, the UKCC and the four national boards were replaced by the Nursing and Midwifery Council. The functions of this new body were to regulate the profession through setting and monitoring standards for professional behaviour and education, to maintain the professional register and to investigate concerns regarding professional behaviour. Its work was to be overseen by a Council which initially comprised members appointed by the government. This transitional Council, however, was subsequently replaced by a Council comprising both appointed and elected members (NMC, 2003).

During the early years of the twenty-first century, learning disability nurses started to diversify their roles and the locations in which they worked as the long-stay hospitals closed and new patterns of service provision emerged. Increasingly independent providers took responsibility for service provision and many nurses worked outside of the health service. However, in 2011 a BBC Panorama programme was televised that provided evidence of abuse of patients with learning disabilities in one such independent hospital.

Winterbourne View, an independent hospital in Bristol, provided care for 24 adults with learning disabilities or autism. Many of those placed there were 'out of area' placements meaning that they were often placed at a distance from their families. Concerns regarding standards of care had been raised by a nurse working within the hospital but these had not been addressed either by the hospital management or by the Care Quality Commission (CQC). Echoing the Ely Hospital scandal in 1967, the member of staff had then gone to the media and evidence was gathered by the BBC using covert filming in Winterbourne View.

The subsequent serious care review report (Flynn, 2012) notes the abuse, punishment, and inappropriate use of restraint that residents were subjected to, and that physical healthcare was poor. A lack of appropriate management, adequate safeguarding procedures and staff education and development were also identified. Eventually, 11 members of staff, including two registered nurses, were convicted of abuse and wilful neglect. Once again there were calls for changes to be made to patterns of care and once again learning disability nurses were implicated both directly (through the nurses at Winterbourne) and through association with existing patterns of care.

In 2012, under the auspices of the four Chief Nursing Officers of the UK, the report of the Modernising Learning Disability Nursing Project was published. Titled 'Strengthening the Commitment' (Scottish Government et al, 2012), this document aimed to provide direction to learning disability nursing across the UK and to ensure the right nurses, with the right knowledge and skills, were in the right place at the right time to meet the changing needs of people with learning disabilities. It set out a clear value base for learning disability nursing (see Chapter 2 for further discussion) and focused on strengthening capacity, capability, quality and the profession. In total, 17 recommendations were made with actions required from individual practitioners, service providers, educators and policymakers. Many of these recommendations will be referred to at various points during this book (eg Chapters 2 and 11).

What was different between this report and previous ones was that there was a clear structure to oversee implementation. A UK wide Steering Group was established, this was informed by implementation groups in each of the four countries of the UK who, in turn, were informed by local implementation groups. In addition, the UK Learning Disability Consultant Nurse Network and the Learning and Intellectual Disability Nursing Academic Network (LIDNAN) played a key role.

The original intention was for the implementation period to run for three years. However, in 2015 progress was reviewed and while there was evidence of developments in some areas it was also recognised that more needed to be done. Accordingly, a new phase of '*Living the Commitment*' (Scottish Government et al, 2015) was launched to continue this work for a further three years. The priority areas for development over the coming three years were identified as:

o   strengthening the unique role and contribution of learning disability nurses;

o   strengthening leadership among learning disability nurses;

o   regulation, revalidation, workforce and the professional development of learning disability nurses;

o   quality improvement, impact and assurance.

The implementation structure for this additional three-year period remained largely as it had been for the original three years of the programme. A final report '*Sustaining the Commitment*' (Scottish Government et al, 2018) was then produced. This provided an overview of achievements (such as strengthening leadership, the development of professional networks and raising the profile of learning disability nursing) and set out future direction for the development of learning disability nursing in each of the countries of the UK. While recognising the challenges that remained in terms of health inequalities and workforce issues, it signalled the end of the coordinated programme of development across the UK but stressed the importance of all countries continuing to work together to address such challenges.

It would be a mistake, however, to assume that all developments during this period were positive. Unfortunately, in 2019 BBC Panorama once again exposed abusive care at Whorlton Hall, an independent hospital (Plomin, 2019). In common with previous inquiries, bullying, abuse and a negative culture of care were evident. Nine members of staff were subsequently charged with ill treatment or wilful neglect including three registered nurses who were suspended from the register pending investigation. They all pleaded not guilty and are due to stand trial in 2023 (Kennedy and Huntley, 2021).

In 2018, pre-registration nurse education was again revised with the introduction of the Standards of Proficiency for Registered Nurses (NMC, 2018a). In a departure from the previous competency-based approach, this new system moved to a focus on outcomes.

Another key difference was that rather than setting different outcomes for each of the four fields of nursing practice common outcomes were set. The rationale for this was

> *because registered nurses must be able to meet the person-centred, holistic care needs of the people they encounter in their practice who may be at any stage of life and who may have a range of mental, physical, cognitive or behavioural health challenges*

(NMC, 2018a)

However, it is also stressed that nurses need to be able to '*demonstrate a greater depth of knowledge and the additional more advanced skills required to meet the specific care needs of people in their chosen field of practice*' (NMC, 2018a). Since students following courses based on these standards are yet to qualify, it is not possible to assess the impact of this most recent change on the preparation of registered learning disability nurses. However, what is evident is that, despite the move to generic statements of outcomes, learning disability nursing remains a distinct field of practice in the UK.

Critical reflection 1.4

Imagine that you have been asked to put together a case as to why learning disability nursing should continue as a field of nursing practice in the UK.

- What arguments would you put forward?
- What evidence would you cite?

Recurring themes

As can be seen from the preceding discussion, the position of learning disability nursing within the nursing profession in the UK has been, and continues to be, a recurring theme within the development of the profession. Stephenson (2019) goes as far as to say that the story of learning disability nursing '*is one of survival against the odds*' in the context of '*attempts to do away with it altogether*'. If you are a learning disability nurse it is almost certain that, at some point, you have faced the question 'Are you a proper/real nurse?'. Underpinning this question is a narrow view of nursing as being focused on working in acute care hospitals with people who are ill.

Since few learning disability nurses work in acute hospitals, and tend to focus more on assisting people to achieve health and well-being than on treatment of those who are acutely ill, it can easily be seen that we do not conform to this widely held perception of nursing. However, when the NMC Standards (2018a) are examined, it would be fair to say that what is required has long been part of the practice of learning disability nurses – providing care across the lifespan, across diverse settings and a focus on promoting and maintaining health. In this respect, perhaps learning disability nurses and nursing have been ahead of developments in other fields of nursing. Indeed, Mitchell (2004) has argued that the lack of a clear definition of learning disability nursing has been an advantage rather than a hindrance since it has enabled us to adapt to the changing needs of those we support.

INTERNATIONAL DEVELOPMENTS

While the focus in this chapter has been on the development of learning disability nursing within the UK, it is important to place this in an international context. At present, the only other country to offer a specific pre-qualifying course preparing students to become registered nurses in the field of learning disability is the Republic of Ireland. Here a four-year undergraduate course enables students to become Registered Nurses (Intellectual Disability). The fourth year of the course comprises an internship where the students work in clinical practice and prepare for becoming a registered practitioner.

Intellectual disability nursing in Ireland has shared many similar challenges in relation to marginalisation within the nursing profession as in the UK but it does have a somewhat different history (Sweeney and Mitchell, 2009). It was not recognised as a specialism within nursing until 1959 when the first two schools of nursing were established by the Daughters of Charity at St Joseph's, Clonsilla, Dublin and Brothers of Charity at St John of God, Drumcar, County Louth (Doody et al, 2012). As can be seen, therefore, its origins lie in the provision of services by religious orders.

In common with the UK, the 1980s saw the beginnings of a shift in philosophies of care and this impacted on the preparation of intellectual disability nurses. In 1992, An Bord Altranais (ABA), the Irish Nursing Council, revised the requirements for the nursing curriculum indicating that the following broad areas needed to be covered (discussed in Doody et al, 2012, p 10):

o *Nursing and professional development.*

o *Person-centred care.*

o *Health sciences and applied nursing principles.*

o *Nursing, sociology, law and environment.*

The move to university-based, degree-level education occurred in 2002 and the four-year programme in existence today commenced.

While there has been a move away from long-stay institutional care provision in Ireland some segregated, congregate settings remain. In common with the UK, debates have taken place regarding the future role of RNIDs in the context of this changing pattern of service provision and in 2018 the report *Shaping the Future of Intellectual Disability Nursing in Ireland* (McCarron et al, 2018) was published.

Based on data gathered from a range of sources, this report identified four key themes:

1 *person-centredness and person-centred planning;*

2 *supporting individuals with an intellectual disability with their health, well-being and social care;*

3 *developing nursing capacity, capability and professional leadership;*

4 *improving the experience and outcomes for individual with an intellectual disability.*

(McCarron et al, 2018, p 61)

The role of the RNID across the lifespan and across settings was stressed and 32 recommendations were made for the development of practice, education, leadership and research to ensure that the role remains relevant to the changing needs of people with intellectual disabilities and the changing policy context. These recommendations were proposed as the basis for an action plan to be achieved within five years.

Other countries have previously trained specialist nurses to support people with learning disabilities but have moved away from this to a generic training. In Australia, the move towards deinstitutionalisation from the 1960s onwards led to an examination of the role of the nurse specialising in the care of those with intellectual disabilities. While such examination reflects that which also occurred in the UK it had a different outcome in Australia and led to the discontinuation of specialist intellectual disability nursing (Wilson et al, 2022). However, despite this lack of specialist education there remain nurses who specialise in providing care and support for people with intellectual disabilities in Australia (Wilson et al, 2022).

The Professional Association of Nurses in Developmental Disabilities Australia (PANDDA) recently produced a second edition of their *Standards for Nursing Practice* to guide nurses working with people with intellectual disabilities and their families. The eight standards are organised in four domains:

1   *a central dyadic relationship;*

2   *fundamental knowledge and skills relevant to intellectual and developmental disability;*

3   *professional relationships, cognisant of ethical, legal, and research-based practice relevant to intellectual and developmental disability;*

4   *intellectual and developmental disability nursing as a specialty area of practice.*
(PANDDA, 2020, p 5)

In the United States of America (US), the pre-registration nursing course is a generic one with no specialisation. However, some nurses do subsequently specialise in caring for people with intellectual and developmental disabilities. The Developmental Disabilities Nurses Association (DDNA) provides certification for registered nurses and licensed practical/vocational nurses as well as ongoing education for its members. It has developed Practice Standards for Developmental Disability Nurses (DDNA, 2020) which encompass the following areas:

○   *establishing a therapeutic relationship;*

○   *role of the DD nurse in the interprofessional team;*

○   *data collection;*

○   *identification of healthcare needs;*

○   *planning, implementation, evaluation;*

   ○   *role of the DD nurse in quality assurance;*

   ○   *role of the DD nurse as an advocate;*

   ○   *role of the DD nurse as an educator;*

   ○   *role of the DD nurse in social and community inclusion;*

   ○   *continued competence.*

(DDNA, 2020)

Perhaps because different countries take different approaches to the provision of nursing care for people with learning disabilities, few international/multi-country research studies exist. However, a recent online survey in the context of the Covid-19 pandemic received a total of 369 responses from nurses working in the field of learning/intellectual disabilities from the US, Canada, UK, Ireland, and New Zealand (Desroches et al, 2022). The respondents to this mixed methods survey were primarily from the US and no comparison between countries was undertaken. However, several key challenges facing nurses working in the field of nursing practice in the context of the pandemic were identified, namely supporting the socialisation of service users, interpreting and helping others to understand Covid-19 guidelines, access to and continuity of care and the impact of Covid fatigue over time. While undertaken in a specific context and at a specific time, this study perhaps opens the possibility of future international collaborative research which will enable us to compare the impact of different approaches to learning/intellectual disability nursing.

Critical reflection 1.5

Look at the information provided above regarding nursing care of people with learning disabilities in other countries. Choose one country and compare this with the current Standards in the UK (NMC, 2018a).

- What do you feel are the implications of any similarities and differences in terms of the nursing support provided for people with learning disabilities?

Chapter summary

This chapter has explored the history of learning disability nursing in the UK from the late 1800s to the current day. Legislation, policy and changing approaches to nurse education have also been considered since these have shaped professional development. It has provided a context within which the rest of the book can be considered as the focus moves to the future development of learning disability nursing practice.

FURTHER READING

Atkinson, D, Jackson, M and Walmsley, J (1997) *Forgotten Lives. Exploring the History of Learning Disability*. Plymouth: BILD Publications.

This book provides an overview of the use of oral history to develop our understanding of historical approaches to care. It also includes a personal life story of a woman who spent many years living in an institution.

Gates, B, Griffiths, C, Atherton, H L, McAnelly, S, Keenan, P, Fleming, S, Doyle, C, Cleary, M and Sutton, P (2020) *Intellectual Disability Nursing. An Oral History Project*. Bingley: Emerald Publishing.

This book reports on an oral history project of learning/intellectual disability nurses in both the UK and Ireland. It also provides information regarding the development of nursing in these countries.

RESOURCES

Hidden Now Heard, the Voice of Learning Disability in Wales: www.peoplescollection.wales/users/15475 (accessed 21 June 2022).

This is the website for the archive developed from the Mencap Cymru 'Hidden Now Heard' oral history project. Here you can access a range of images and oral histories contributed by both people with learning disabilities and staff who lived or worked in long-stay institutions across Wales.

Timeline of Disability History: www.open.ac.uk/health-and-social-care/research/shld/time line-learning-disability-history (accessed 21 June 2022).

This is a link to a timeline of learning disability history developed by the Open University Social History of Learning Disability Group.

The importance of values, law and ethics

Chapter aims

The aim of this chapter is to explore how values, the law and ethics are key foundations for learning disability nursing and their importance in supporting ethical decision-making in practice. It explores what each of these areas encompasses, how they relate to each other and considers their relevance to the development of professional learning disability nursing practice.

Professional standards and expectations

The NMC Standards (NMC, 2018a) indicate that, at the point of registration, nurses must be able to:

> *1.1 understand and act in accordance with the Code: Professional standards of practice and behaviour for nurses, midwives, and nursing associates, and fulfil all registration requirements*

As will be seen later in this chapter, the Code (NMC, 2018b) places several responsibilities on nurses to maintain professional values, act ethically and work within legal frameworks. Accordingly, to ensure that student nurses are prepared to take on such responsibilities, the NMC Standards (2018a) include the following statement of proficiency:

> *1.2 understand and apply relevant legal, regulatory and governance requirements, policies, and ethical frameworks, including any mandatory reporting duties, to all areas of practice, differentiating where appropriate between the devolved legislatures of the United Kingdom*

This chapter supports development in this area of professional practice.

VALUES

Strengthening the Commitment (Scottish Government et al, 2012) highlighted the strength of the value base within learning disability nursing, arguing that it '*remains the key element underpinning practice*'. The specific values that report identified as being key to learning disability nursing are explored below, but first it is important to consider what we mean by 'values' and how our personal and professional values are shaped and inform our day to day lives. Before reading on, take some time to complete Critical reflection 2.1.

Critical reflection 2.1

Take a few moments to reflect on your personal understanding of 'values'. Some areas to explore are as follows.

- How would you define 'values'?
- Which values do you feel are important to you?
- What do you feel has influenced your value base?
- How did your values influence your decision to be a learning disability nurse?
- How do your values influence your nursing practice?

The nature of values, their development and impact

In everyday language, we often refer to (for example) 'valued' friends and colleagues, the 'value' of our savings and whether we feel 'valued' by others. We also talk about a loss of value, such as decline in the value of property or 'changing' values in society. If something is valued, then it is held in esteem and desired, and a loss of value means that these qualities are reduced or lost. In relation to people with learning disabilities both history and current times provide evidence that their lives are often viewed by wider society as being less valued than others and they are therefore referred to as a 'devalued' group (see Chapter 1) – something which learning disability nursing practice seeks to challenge and change.

In the specific context of this discussion, 'values' refers to those principles and qualities that we as individuals hold in esteem. Those you noted down in Critical reflection 2.1 might have included things such as honesty, person-centredness, equality, fairness and justice. These are the principles and qualities that are important to us, which guide our own behaviours, and also influence our expectations of the behaviour of others.

Our personal values are shaped by several different influences such as our family, our friends, our religion, our culture and our education. They do, however, sometimes change over time and what was important to us at one point in our lives (what we value) may not be so important at a later stage. You might want to look back to the answers you gave to Critical reflection 2.1 and think about whether your values have changed over time and what influenced any such changes.

You bring your personal values to your nursing practice – indeed it may be because of these values that you decided to become a learning disability nurse. For example, if you value justice and equality you might have chosen to be a learning disability nurse as you are aware that people with learning disabilities often experience injustice and inequality and you wish to make a difference.

However, when you start to pursue your chosen career path you learn that there are other values that also impact upon your practice as set out in Figure 2.1.

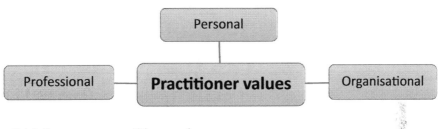

Figure 2.1 Influences on practitioner values

Very early in your nursing career, you will be made aware that there are key professional values that you will be expected to uphold. These are evident in the Standards (NMC, 2018a) that set out the knowledge, skills and attitudes you need to demonstrate in order to become a registered nurse, and also in the NMC Code (2018b). Indeed, in the introduction to the Code (NMC, 2018b) it states that '*The values and principles set out in the Code can be applied in a range of different practice settings, but they are not negotiable or discretionary*'. It is essential, therefore, that you are aware of the values and principles that are identified within the Code and that you always uphold them. To assist you with this, take some time to complete Critical reflection 2.2.

Critical reflection 2.2

Read through the Code (NMC, 2018b) and:

- note down what you feel are the key principles and values that are mentioned in this document;

- reflect on what you feel it means to demonstrate these principles in learning disability nursing practice.

In reviewing the Code (NMC, 2018b), you will hopefully have identified and noted down key values that include kindness, compassion, respect, partnership, privacy, honesty, safety, protection, integrity and confidentiality. In addition, you will have noted that nurses are required to practice in a person-centred way, to challenge discrimination and to advocate for those they support.

As well as being required to uphold professional values, you will also encounter organisational values in the various settings within which you work. Sometimes these values are made explicit in mission statements or charters but even where such documents are not available it is usually possible to determine how a service views (or values) those who use it and those who work within it. This is often experienced as organisational culture and the problems that can arise from poor cultures of care have been widely noted (see, for example, CQC (2020) and also Chapter 11).

Often our personal, professional and organisational values will be in accordance with each other since we tend to choose a profession that reflects our personal values and seek employment in organisations that promote such values. However, it is also important to recognise that there can be times when tensions between different values are experienced. For example, at a personal level the value of honesty may be very important to you, but you find yourself in a situation where you are asked to withhold information from an adult with learning disabilities you are supporting by a member of their family who says that the individual will not be able to cope with that information. Alternatively, you may be asked to undertake a placement working in a forensic service but are concerned since you recognise the importance of behaving professionally, but also know that you may find this difficult because the offences committed by some of those who use the service are in opposition to values which are important to you. Mee (2012) describes the personal and professional conflict a nurse caring for an individual who has committed offences may experience where their thoughts about the service user can be both valuing and devaluing.

The potential impact on the way we treat those we care for means it is essential that we are all self-aware and recognise our own values so that we can anticipate when we might experience such conflicts and take steps to manage such situations. This is also emphasised in the NMC Code (2018b) where it states we need to ensure that we don't express our personal beliefs to others in an inappropriate way (Clause 20.7).

The importance of values in nursing practice

The Cambridge Online Dictionary (2021) define 'values' as '*the principles that help you to decide what is right and wrong, and how to act in various situations*'. This highlights two important elements that are important when you consider the relationship between values and professional practice:

○   values act as a guide to our professional decision-making;

○   values provide a basis for action (practice).

It also raises the question of who decides what is 'right' or 'wrong' and this is an issue that will be explored further in this chapter when you read about ethics. It is evident that professional values are an integral component of nursing whatever the field of practice. In relation to learning disability nursing, however, as was noted above, the *Strengthening the Commitment* report (Scottish Government et al, 2012, p 7) stressed that the value base for learning disability nursing is 'strong' and that it *'remains the key element underpinning practice'*. Figure 2.2 sets out those values identified in the report as providing the basis for learning disability nursing.

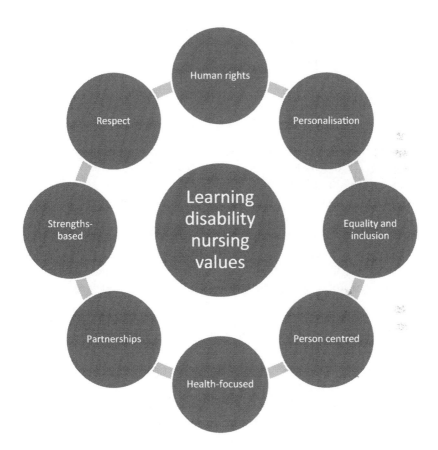

Figure 2.2 The principles underpinning the value base of learning disability nursing practice
(Adapted from Scottish Government et al, 2012)

These values are identified separately here but, in practice, they are very much interrelated. For example, if your practice is *person-centred* then your starting point will be the wishes and desires of the individuals you support which should lead to *personalisation* of such support. This will require you to work in *partnership* with the individual, their family, and carers, and with other professionals and agencies. By seeking to build upon their *strengths* you will be treating individuals with *respect.*

Human rights are those rights which apply to everyone regardless of age, gender or disability. Many relate to values discussed above such as the right to be treated with respect and the right to *equality and inclusion*. These rights are set out in law (discussed later in this chapter). It is recognised, however, that disabled people are at particular risk of having their rights infringed or denied and therefore the United Nations (2006) developed the *Convention on the Rights of Persons with Disabilities*. Article 25 of this document relates to the right of disabled persons '*to enjoy the highest attainable standard of health without discrimination on the grounds of disability*'. Given the evidence that people with learning disabilities experience significant inequalities and inequities in health (explored in Chapter 8), it can be seen why as a learning disability nurse being *health-focused* is central to your role in seeking to protect the right of people with learning disabilities to their highest attainable standard of health.

LAW

Griffith and Tengnah (2020, p 29) define law as '*a rule of human conduct imposed upon and enforced among the members of a given state*'. They further highlight that such rules are 'positive' in that they require us to do (or not do) something and that a sanction may be imposed if we do not comply (we break the law). However, there are also 'normative' rules which set out what a person 'should' (rather than must) do. There is an expectation that individuals will behave in a particular way but if they choose not to then formal legal sanctions are not applied. There is, therefore, a link between the values discussed earlier in this chapter and the content and function of law. It reflects societal values and seeks to ensure that these are upheld through positive rules and seeks to shape values and behaviour through normative rules.

In the context of healthcare, both positive and normative 'rules' and laws are evident (Griffith and Tengnah, 2020). As learning disability nurses, we need to ensure that we comply (for example) with legislation relating to the capacity of individuals to make their own decisions. However, there is also an expectation that, during our practice, we demonstrate respect for those we are supporting and treat them with dignity. While formal legal sanctions may be applied if we fail to adhere to legislation, it is important to remember that professional sanctions may be applied if we fail to follow the normative rules of our profession as detailed in our professional code (NMC, 2018b).

In the UK, we have quite a complex situation in relation to legislation. For example, the Equality Act (Gov.uk, 2010), which drew together all previous anti-discriminatory legislation, applies across Great Britain but not within Northern Ireland. Historically Scotland has always had a different legal system while England and Wales have been closely linked. However, since devolution within the UK responsibility for the development of key areas of legislation (including health and social care) has been devolved to the various administrations. For this reason, the NMC (2018a, 2018b) remind us of the importance of practising within the legal framework of the country within which we are working.

It is beyond the scope of this chapter to set out all the key legislation in each of the four UK countries (although examples are provided). First, however, it explores why it is important for learning disability nurses to understand the law and explores some key areas of relevance to your practice.

Why do learning disability nurses need an understanding of the law?

There are many reasons why, as a learning disability nurse, you need to understand the law. First, nursing as a profession is regulated by the law. In addition, our day-to-day work takes place within a legal context which determines how we practice. Consider, for example, requirements relating to health and safety, safe storage of data and laws relating to negligence. However, a key reason why learning disability nurses need to understand the law is that the lives of those we support are often impacted in many ways by legal considerations. To help you think about this read through James Stephens' case study below and try to identify points in his life when various laws have impacted on his life and what those laws might be.

Case study 2.1

James Stephens

James is 36 years old and currently lives in a supported living house along with one other man of a similar age. He likes football and enjoys attending matches when he can. He also enjoys listening to music and often spends a lot of time in his bedroom with his headphones on.

When he was at school James was assessed as having mild to moderate learning disabilities and therefore attended a special school. When he left school, he attended a local FE college for a while but did not enjoy it and therefore 'dropped out' of his course. He then spent all his time at home and did not have any contact with adult learning disability services. His father had died while he was at school and so he continued to live with his mother but over time her health deteriorated, and James became her primary carer. Unfortunately, she died two years ago and following her death James continued to live alone for some months.

About five months after his mother died James' neighbours contacted social services as they were concerned that they had not seen James for some time but they had seen what they described as 'very shifty' characters visiting his house

→

on a regular basis. When social services followed this up, it became apparent that James had been targeted by a group of local youths who had convinced him that they were his friends, who had used his house for various illegal activities such as drug dealing, and who had taken money from him. This group of youths were deemed to have committed 'mate crime' and were dealt with by the police. However, James was found to be in a poor physical and mental state. He was malnourished not having had sufficient money to buy food, and he was severely depressed both due to the death of his mother and due to the stress of more recent events.

Despite being in poor physical and mental health, James said that he did not want to receive support. However, he was deemed at that time not to have the capacity to make that decision and to be a risk to himself. He was, therefore, sectioned and admitted to a local assessment and treatment unit. Once there he was assessed, made good progress and a detailed plan of care and support was put in place in readiness for his discharge. At that point he moved to where he is currently living.

In reading through this case study, you will hopefully have identified a several key points where legislation has impacted on James' life. This includes:

o   his schooling (being assessed as having special educational needs);

o   when he was subjected to mate crime and financial abuse (safeguarding legislation);

o   when he was admitted to the assessment and treatment unit (capacity and mental health legislation); and

o   when he was discharged (legislation linked to care and support planning and legislation concerning eligibility for welfare benefits).

It is, therefore, essential that as a learning disability nurse you understand key legal requirements so that you are aware of the rights of those you support and what they are entitled to (for example) in terms of services and financial support. You can then use this knowledge either to provide support for an individual to advocate for themselves or to advocate on their behalf. One such scenario might involve seeking to ensure that an individual has access to healthcare that meets their needs. Changes may be needed to the way in which services are provided for an individual you support but an argument for this to happen will be strengthened by an awareness that the Equality Act (2010) places a duty on services to make reasonable adjustments. Similarly, while you will recognise if an individual or group is being subjected to poor treatment you will be able to challenge this more effectively if you can argue that degrading and inhuman treatment are contrary to the Human Rights Act (1998).

Key legislation informing your practice

As mentioned above, there are many aspects of legislation that impact on the lives of people with learning disabilities. It is not possible here to explore them all so several key areas are explored, namely human rights, equality, mental capacity, mental health and safeguarding. The relevant legislation that applies in the different nations of the UK is set out in Table 2.1 to assist you with identifying that which applies in the country within which you are practising. Remember, however, that legislation is constantly being revised and developed and hence it is important that you regularly check for any such developments so that you ensure your practice is within current legal frameworks.

Table 2.1 Key legislation relating to the lives of people with learning disabilities in the UK

	England	**Wales**	**Scotland**	**Northern Ireland**
Human rights	Human Rights Act 1998	Human Rights Act 1998	Human Rights Act 1998	Human Rights Act 1998
Equality	Equality Act 2010	Equality Act 2010	Equality Act 2010	There is no single piece of equalities legislation in Northern Ireland. In relation to disability discrimination this is covered by the Disability Discrimination Act (1995) (used to apply across the UK). The Northern Ireland Act 1998 also places a statutory obligation on public authorities to carry out their functions with due regard to the need to promote equality (including in relation to disability)
Mental capacity	Mental Capacity Act 2005	Mental Capacity Act 2005	Adults with Incapacity (Scotland) Act 2000	Mental Capacity Act (Northern Ireland) 2016
Mental health	Mental Health Act 1983	Mental Health Act 1983	Mental Health (Care and Treatment) (Scotland) Act 2005 as amended by Mental Health (Scotland) Act 2015	Mental Health (Northern Ireland) Order 2011
Safeguarding	The Care Act 2014	Social Services and Well-being (Wales) Act 2014	Adult Support and Protection (Scotland) Act 2007	Safeguarding Board (Northern Ireland) Act 2011

Human rights

The importance of human rights as a basis for learning disability nursing practice has been noted earlier in this chapter (Scottish Government et al, 2012). However, it is important to recognise that in the UK, the Human Rights Act (1998) provides a legal framework which seeks to protect the rights of all citizens including those of people with a learning disability. A number of rights are included within this Act including the right to life, the right to freedom from torture and inhuman or degrading treatment, the right to education and the right to protection from discrimination (Equality and Human Rights Commission, 2018). However, despite this legal protection a report by the House of Lords and House of Commons Joint Committee on Human Rights (2008) reported that people with learning disabilities remained at increased risk of their rights not being upheld and called for action to be taken to address this. Learning disability nurses play a key role in promoting such rights and in recognising and acting where they are infringed.

Equality

The Equality Act (Gov.uk, 2010) applies in England, Wales and Scotland and brought together a range of pre-existing equalities legislation into one Act. This Act seeks to challenge discrimination and disadvantage for those identified as having specified 'protected characteristics' of which disability is one. However, other characteristics include age, sex and race and it is also important to remember that people with learning disabilities may be discriminated against based on these characteristics as well as dis-ability. For example, an individual with a learning disability could be subjected to hate crime based on their race as well as on the basis of their disability. The Equality Act (Gov.uk, 2010) is also the legislation that places a duty on service providers to make reasonable adjustments to ensure that disabled people are able to access goods and services on a level equal to that experienced by non-disabled persons. This legal require-ment is one that, as a learning disability nurse you are likely to be familiar with, and it is an area where the knowledge and skills of the learning disability nurse, working in partnership with others, can promote improved access to healthcare for people with learning disabilities.

Mental capacity

Mental capacity relates to the ability to make decisions, and for such decisions to be informed an individual needs to understand and retain relevant information and be able to use this information to reach a decision. However, some people may lack the capacity to make informed decisions and, in such circumstances, it is important that there is legislation in place to protect their interests. Mental capacity legislation differs across the countries of the UK but there are certain principles that are shared which include promoting the rights of those who lack capacity and creating mechanisms to allow for substitute decision-making (Wilson, 2017). Key areas where such legislation may need to be applied are where financial decisions need to be made, where decisions are required regarding welfare and where decisions are required in relation to med-ical treatment (Wilson, 2017). While each of these areas may be a focus of concern for learning disability nurses, it is perhaps the area relating to medical treatment that is of relevance to practice. The Confidential Inquiry into Premature Deaths of People with Learning Disabilities (CIPOLD (Heslop et al, 2013) identified significant concerns regarding the level of understanding of mental capacity legislation and the impact this can have on mortality. It is essential, therefore, that as a learning disability nurse you have a good understanding of mental capacity legislation so that you can advocate for those you support and so that you can educate others.

Mental health

As with mental capacity legislation, mental health legislation also varies across the UK. In general, however, it seeks to protect individuals who are a danger to themselves or others due to mental health disorders, makes provisions for compulsory detention in hospital for assessment and treatment and sets out requirements for review of such provisions. Where someone with a learning disability is experiencing a mental health disorder, and they are presenting a danger to themselves or other people, then they may be subject to the relevant mental health legislation and therefore it is important that learning disability nurses have a good understanding of this legal framework and how it should be used in practice.

It was noted above that it is important to keep up to date with legislation as it is subject to review and change. Mental health legislation in England and Wales is a good example of this since (at the time of writing) a consultation is underway regarding reform of this legislation (DHSC, 2021). It is also important to note that the Covid-19 pandemic also led to temporary changes to the existing mental health legislation being made.

Safeguarding

The final area of legislation noted in Table 2.1 is that relating to safeguarding. This is an interesting area since while safeguarding children has operated within a legal frame-work for many years it is a relatively recent development for adult safeguarding to have a legal basis. Scotland was the first country in the UK to introduce such legislation with the Adult Support and Protection (Scotland) Act in 2007. As with other areas of law there are differences between the countries of the UK, but all the legislation is concerned with defining abuse, identifying those at risk of harm and abuse, setting out measures/powers to assess allegations, actions required and systems for managing and monitoring safeguarding at a national level.

One further thing it is important to note in relation to legislation is that while the law itself usually sets out the key principles, further information may be required to under-stand how these should be implemented in practice. In many instances, therefore, there are accompanying codes of practice that set out how the legislation should be used (see, for example, the Mental Health Act 1983 Code of Practice; Department of Health, 1983).

ETHICS

There are many available definitions of ethics, and Ellis (2020) suggests that this term can mean both different things to different people, and also different things for one individual either at different points in their life or when they are confronted with different situations. Despite this challenge, however, it is important to try and clarify what we mean by the term.

Barker (2013) states that ethics is a set of principles that determine what we should do, or what is considered to be the 'right' conduct in a given situation. He also argues that it is a system of moral values which guide why believe that something is the right thing to do. Ethics thus requires us to consider both the 'what' (in terms of our decisions and behaviours) and the 'why' (we feel this is the right decision and action).

There are several different approaches to ethics which Watkinson (2015) categorises as:

o   descriptive – concerned with describing people's beliefs about values and what is considered right and wrong;

o   normative – focuses on the criteria which determine how people 'should' act and which inform the development of rules by which people are expected to live – this is reflected in (for example) the laws within a particular country;

o   metaethics – concerned with examining moral thought and moral language and how this compares to other approaches to speaking and writing;

o   applied ethics – focuses on how we use morals and values in our day-to-day lives and practice.

While each of these approaches has relevance to nursing, the focus in this chapter is on applied ethics which Thompson et al (2006) argue is concerned with both how we can act in an appropriate, effective manner and with being able to provide a justification for our actions by referring to commonly held or accepted principles. Such principles include our professional code (NMC, 2018b), values and legislation as discussed in earlier sections of this chapter. As you will see below, drawing upon these principles can assist in making professional decisions that are ethical, further reinforcing the importance of nurses having an awareness of both values and legislation. First, however, it is important to understand the importance of ethics in the context of learning disability nursing practice.

Ethics and learning disability nursing

The NMC Standards (2018a) make it explicit that all registered nurses need to understand and apply relevant ethical frameworks in their practice. In relation to supporting people with learning disabilities, however, there can be particular ethical issues that need to be considered and addressed. Indeed Kay (1994) observed that while working to support people with learning disabilities is a privilege it can also be a 'minefield' of moral and ethical dilemmas. Nonetheless, despite this being written in 1994, and despite the diverse range of ethical issues encountered when supporting people with learning disabilities, there has been relatively little written that specifically explores ethical aspects of learning disability nursing.

Often when people think about ethical issues, there is a tendency to recall what might be termed 'major' incidents such as safeguarding issues or discriminatory withholding of treatment. However, ethical considerations also arise in our day-to-day practice in situations such as making sure that those we support have access to appropriate and timely information to assist their decision-making, and in ensuring that they can exercise choice in relation to (for example) their daily activities. This means that if you are to identify ethical issues and respond in an ethical manner it is essential that you develop what is referred to as 'ethical sensitivity'. Noting that this is an attribute essential within nursing, Esmaelzadeh et al (2017, p 5) studied nurse leaders and identified five key areas of ethical sensitivity.

1. Sensitivity to care – a focus on promoting care that is sensitive to patient needs and on monitoring standards.

2. Sensitivity to errors – being sensitive to the potential for errors, seeking to avoid errors and taking appropriate action when errors occur.

3. Sensitivity to communication – ensuring appropriate communication with both patients and colleagues.

4. Sensitivity in decision-making – making ethical decisions and educating others regarding ethical decision-making.

5. Sensitivity to ethical care – being sensitive to ethical principles and values, and adhering to these in practice.

While this study was undertaken in a different country and in a different field of practice, these areas appear transferable to the context of learning disability nursing. They alert us to the areas of practice where ethical issues can arise and raise our awareness of the range of professional knowledge, skills and behaviours we need to develop if we are to provide ethical care for those we support.

As noted above, there is limited literature relating to ethical practice in the context of learning disability nursing, and research on this topic is even more scarce. However, Solvoll et al (2015) undertook a study in Norway to identify the ethical challenges faced by healthcare workers in residential facilities for people with learning disabilities. Through analysis of what are described as 'focused conversations', four key themes emerged. The first related to a feeling of being squeezed between conflicting actions and values. An example of this is noted as being a situation where staff were seeking to support an individual to make their own decisions, but the individual chose to smoke excessively which had a negative impact on their health. The staff concerned felt conflicted between supporting the right of the individual to make their own decisions (about smoking) and their duty to promote the health of the individual. A second challenge was identified as relating to their role in speaking up or advocating for those they support. This was felt to be particularly difficult when, for example, the wishes of the individual they are supporting do not accord with family wishes. In such circumstances, staff reported that they were often left feeling that they should do more. The third area of concern was identified as 'searching shared responsibility' and this related to the burden of responsibility staff felt for decision-making and their need to speak with others about this and to share the responsibility. The final theme related to the desire to have 'immediate and fixed' solutions to ethical challenges. In practice, while discussion with others can help to clarify then nature of ethical issues and to explore possible solutions such solutions are, however, seldom fixed since situations change and there is a need to constantly review and adjust as necessary. While this study was again undertaken in a different country and involved a range of healthcare professionals, the issues identified are relevant to the practice of learning disability nurses and you are likely to recognise them from your experience.

It can, therefore, be common for learning disability nurses to encounter what are often described as ethical 'dilemmas' where there are different potential courses of action but the 'right' course of action is not always obvious, and we are not sure what to do (Ellis, 2020). In some instances, there may be two possible ways forward that both appear positive but a decision still needs to be made. In other situations, the options may all seem to be negative, but a choice needs to be made as to which option is the least negative. As Solvoll et al (2015) report, we may also feel 'squeezed' between actions that conflict with each other.

Such situations can arise, for example, where you must decide about how best to use fixed resources such as your time. One example would be when two people you are supporting both need your input at the same time, but it is not possible for you to meet both their needs simultaneously. Who should you support? Alternatively, an individual may ask you to advocate for them but to do so it would mean that you must risk ruining professional relationships that have taken time to establish and that, if lost, would limit your ability to effectively support other people with learning disabilities. You can probably add some examples of your own here.

Solvoll et al (2015) argue that standing up for what you believe is right requires courage particularly in situations where your beliefs are not popular with others. However, they also argue that courage can be learnt through a continual process of self-development. A key element of this learning is to develop the skills of ethical decision-making so that we can both make sound ethical decisions and communicate the rationale for such decisions. Developing an understanding of key ethical theories and principles is an integral part of this process.

Ethical theories and principles

If you have had an eye test, you will be familiar with the process through which you are asked to say whether adding different lenses in different combinations helps you to see more, or less, clearly. This analogy can help with understanding the role different ethical theories and principles play in assisting us to make decisions regarding how we should act in each situation. They can provide us with different 'lenses' through which we can explore issues and dilemmas. They encourage us to consider different perspectives or ways of looking at a situation and provide us with different questions we can use to guide our thinking. There are several different theoretical approaches to ethics but here four are considered – consequentialism, deontology, virtue ethics and relational ethics.

Consequentialism

Consequentialism is an approach to ethics in which the rightness or appropriateness of a decision or course of action is determined by its consequences, the aim being to achieve a positive outcome (Ellis, 2020). In this context, it is important to understand that consequences (both negative and positive) can arise both taking a course of action and from deciding not to act; both therefore need to be considered. For example, you may be concerned that administering a particular medication could lead to an individual experiencing side effects, but it would also be essential that the consequences of the medication not being administered are carefully considered. Similarly, you may be asked to withhold information regarding a bereavement from an individual you are supporting by a member of their family because of fears that the individual may become upset. Here it is important to understand that while the individual may (understandably) be upset, other (and perhaps more serious) negative consequences may be experienced if the information is withheld. One common example of a consequentialist approach is utilitarianism in which a good action is viewed as one which achieves the maximum benefit for the greatest number of people.

Deontology

Deontology is an ethical approach which holds that all humans have value and must be treated with respect (Watkinson, 2015). In contrast to consequentialism (that judges actions by their outcomes), deontology judges actions by whether or not they are made in accordance with moral rules which we have a duty to follow. Such an approach is commonly referred to in nursing when we refer to our duty of care but Ellis (2020) notes that one difficulty with deontology is that in some situations there can be conflicting rules and it can be difficult to determine which should be followed. This was highlighted in the earlier example provided by Solvoll et al (2015) where the participant felt there was a conflict between their duty to respect the autonomy of an individual (to smoke excessively) and their duty to protect the health of that individual.

Virtue ethics

A further approach to ethics is what is referred to as *virtue ethics*. Here the basis for decision-making is moral character – as Ellis (2020, p 77) states '*The virtuous person does what is right and in the right way because that is what a virtuous person does*'. Such virtues include care, compassion, empathy and courage (Avery, 2013) but you might wish here to also think back to the values explored earlier in the chapter. Whereas consequentialism considers outcomes of decisions, and deontology focuses on the rules or duties that guide decisions and actions, virtue ethics focuses on what motivates people to act in a particular way. For example, when you are confronted with a practice situation where you are unsure as to how to proceed you would ask yourself what you feel is the 'right' thing to do and reflect on what is motivating you to feel that way. Avery (2013) suggests that this approach offers flexibility but can lead to poor decision-making because while an individual may demonstrate all the required virtues, they may lack the required knowledge, education or information. He therefore advises that this approach is used in conjunction with others.

Relational ethics

A more recent ethical approach is referred to as *relational ethics*. Here it is proposed that ethical decisions are made in the context of relationships which should be based on mutual respect, responsibility for and engagement with others (Pollard, 2015). In the context of nursing, therefore, this means that when seeking to make ethical decisions we need to ensure that our focus is on caring *with* rather than *for* patients (Pollard, 2015). This reflects the values of person-centredness and working in partnership identified as underpinning learning disability nursing (Scottish Government et al, 2012). It is important to recognise that there may be situations where, as a practitioner, your assessment of what is the 'right' course of action can differ from those of the individuals you support. Nonetheless, a relational ethics approach provides us with a framework through which we can use our interpersonal skills in the context of the relationships we establish to explore options and either achieve an outcome that is acceptable to all or (where this is not possible) to achieve an understanding of why certain actions are required.

As can be seen from this brief overview of selected ethical theories, they all have differing strengths and weaknesses. However, understanding these varying standpoints and being able to consider how they might apply in any given situation enables us to consider differing courses of action and to assess their relative merits. They lead us to ask ourselves different questions such as what are the likely consequences of my actions (consequentialism)? What is my duty here (deontology)? How would a virtuous person act (virtue ethics)? How can I work with relevant others to ensure ethical decision-making (relational ethics)? In offering these different perspectives, they can help you to examine situations more fully and to consider wider perspectives.

Another tool you can use to assist your ethical decision-making is that offered by consideration of ethical principles. There are a number of such principles against which you can assess your thinking and your behaviour. Perhaps the most used framework in the context of healthcare, however, is that offered by Beauchamp and Childress (2019) who identify four such principles: autonomy, non-maleficence, beneficence and justice.

Autonomy

Autonomy is concerned with the capacity of individuals to be self-determining, and this is the key principle which underpins processes relating to consent and the capacity legislation referred to earlier in this chapter. Beauchamp and Childress (2019) argue that for autonomy to be achieved two conditions need to be in place, namely that an individual is free from external influences that may control their decision-making, and that they have the capacity to act in an intentional manner. People with learning disabilities, however, are often subject to the decisions of others, or their decision-making is unduly influenced by other people who are in positions of control. In addition, their autonomy may be limited by a lack of information in a format that is accessible to them. Some may lack the capacity to make an autonomous decision but even where they have capacity, they may be reliant upon other people to translate this decision into action. For example, an individual may decide that they wish to improve their diet to reduce their weight, but they are unable to achieve this as they live in a group setting where their daily diet is controlled by staff who do not feel there is a need for change.

Non-maleficence

Non-maleficence places a responsibility on us to act in a way that does not cause harm to other people and is commonly referred to in the context of healthcare as *'Above all do no harm'* (Beauchamp and Childress, 2019). While you are possibly thinking that this is self-explanatory for healthcare professionals such as nurses, it does require us to think critically about its implications both for practice and for research (which is explored more fully in Chapter 4).

Beauchamp and Childress (2019) argue that non-maleficence is linked to several moral rules such as do not kill, do not cause pain or suffering, do not incapacitate, do not cause offence and do not deprive others of the 'goods of life'. As learning disability nurses, these seem like good principles to guide practice but what about situations where we are required to cause pain by (for example) administering an injection? What about situations where an individual's capacity may be limited because they are not provided with information? There are, therefore, other things that we need to consider, namely whether in some situations a degree of harm may be justified. For example, an injection of insulin for someone who is diabetic may be both life-saving and (through achieving good glycaemic control) mean that long-term negative effects such as retinopathy or neuropathy may be avoided or reduced. The opportunity for longer term benefit may thus outweigh short-term pain. Furthermore, it is important to note that harm may be both active and passive. That is, it can arise from things that are done (eg administering the incorrect medication) but also from things that are not done (such as the failure to administer prescribed medication in a timely manner). Finally, by including the need to avoid causing offence we are reminded that harm may be both physical and psychological.

Beneficence

Beneficence is concerned with acting to promote the well-being (or benefiting) of others. It therefore moves beyond just seeking to avoid harm to actively seeking to promote well. In the context of learning disability nursing while it is important that we seek to avoid harm occurring this is not sufficient. If you think back to the values that underpin learning disability nursing (Scottish Government et al, 2012) if our practice is founded on being person-centred and strengths-based while ensuring promotion of human rights then a key element of our role relates to actively promoting health and well-being.

Justice

The ethical principle of *justice* is concerned with issues of fairness, equality and how various 'benefits' are distributed within society. As has already been noted in this chapter, legislation is in place to protect human rights and to promote equality. However, the evidence of health inequalities and premature avoidable deaths experienced by people with learning disabilities (Heslop et al, 2013) would appear to suggest that justice is not always achieved. It is also important to be alert to the potential for something that appears to be treating everyone equally (and therefore 'fairly') to have a different (negative) impact on people with learning disabilities. A recent example of this occurred at the beginning of the Covid-19 pandemic when the National Institute for Health and Care Excellence (NICE) Guidelines recommended that the Clinical Frailty Scale should be used to assess the suitability of individuals to receive treatment in intensive therapy units. However, when the tool was considered it was evident that it had not been validated for use for people with learning disabilities and that its use would be likely to lead to unfavourable decisions being made regarding their treatment. This was deemed to be unjust and therefore the policy was changed (NICE, 2020). However, there was damage done in terms of trust and implications for how valued people with learning disabilities and their families felt and the example serves as a reminder that there is a need to be constantly aware of the potential for people with learning disabilities to experience injustice.

While each of these principles has been considered separately here, they are interrelated and are often considered together when analysing a particular situation. For example, when determining an appropriate course of action, it may be important to weigh the various risks (non-maleficence) and potential benefits (beneficence) and to only progress if the latter is likely to outweigh the former. Similarly, you may encounter situations where seeking to promote the well-being of one individual you are supporting (beneficence) means that the autonomy of another may be restricted (autonomy) and you need to carefully consider what the most fair course of action would be (justice). However, as with the ethical theories previously discussed, ethical principles encourage us to consider a situation from differing perspectives and to explore alternative courses of action: they therefore form an important element of ethical decision-making.

Ethical decision-making

As has been seen in earlier sections of this chapter, applied ethics requires you both to make decisions and to provide a rationale for these based on reference to norms, values and principles that are commonly or widely accepted (Thompson et al, 2006). For this reason, it is important that as a nurse you develop the skill of ethical decision-making in practice.

If you look at different textbooks, you will see that several frameworks have been proposed to assist nurses with ethical decision-making. However, while they differ slightly, they also share many commonalities and therefore Figure 2.3 is offered as a framework to assist you.

Several things will be apparent from the framework offered above. First, you will see that it brings together each of the elements explored in this chapter (values, legislation and

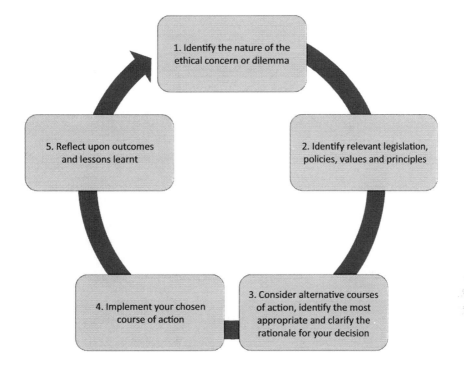

Figure 2.3 A framework for ethical decision-making

ethics) and shows who they are integral to the ethical decision-making process which in turn is integral to professional nursing practice. Second, you will note that it is presented as a cyclical (rather than linear) process and recognises the importance of learning from ethical decision-making, using this to inform our future practice and hence enhance our decision-making.

Each of the stages of this framework will now be explored. First, it is essential that we start by gathering as much information as we can regarding the situation and ask whether there is an ethical dilemma or concern and what is it about the decision that is needed that means it has an ethical dimension. Being clear about the nature of the issue then allows you to consider whether there are any standards or norms that you can use to inform your decision-making. For example, if we are confronted with a dilemma regarding whether someone you are supporting is able to provide consent for a particular treatment then we will need to refer to the relevant legislation concerning capacity and consent to determine what is the legally required course of action. You might wish to consider what your professional responsibilities are and therefore consult the NMC Code (2018b). You may also wish to reflect on which ethical theories or principles may be relevant. Returning to the example regarding consent to treatment it might be relevant to think about the extent to which an individual is able to exercise their autonomy, how maximum benefit can be achieved for them (beneficence), how harm can be avoided or minimised (non-maleficence) and therefore how justice can best be achieved. You might also reflect on what your duty is in this situation and what the consequences of acting (or not acting) might be.

Having considered all the above information, Stage 3 then requires you to use this information to consider the various courses of action available to you, to identify what is most appropriate and to understand your rationale for choosing this way forward. In some situations, having gathered this initial information there will be only one possible course of action. For example, if there is a legal requirement to act in a particular way then our professional code (NMC, 2018b) requires us to fulfil this requirement. However, even where this is the case it is important to remember that we may have options as to *how* we act. Sometimes fulfilling legal requirements can mean that there is the potential for distress, but effective communication and an empathic approach can minimise harm and hence offer a more ethically sound solution.

In other circumstances, it may be that there are alternative ways to address a particular issue or problem. Where this is the case then we need to carefully consider the options, what their likely outcomes are and weigh their various risks and benefits. By working through this process, we will then be able to provide the 'sound rationale' referred to earlier when defining applied ethics (Thompson et al, 2006).

Stage 4 requires that we then implement our course of action. However, while doing this it is important that we reflect in action and remain alert to the impact that our decisions and actions are having. It is also essential that we can adjust our approach if, and when, required. Stage 5 then involves us reflecting on our actions to identify what worked well and what might have been done differently so that we can use this learning to inform subsequent decision-making. Such reflection often takes place when we feel that things haven't gone to plan but perhaps less so when things go well, and important lessons may then be lost. When things do go well to, therefore, take time to reflect on why things went well and identify how you can generalise such practice to other areas and future challenges.

It is also important to remember that often decisions do not need to be made alone. As a learning disability nurse, you will have many opportunities to work in partnership with others. People with learning disabilities, their families, stakeholders and members of the MDT will have a perspective to bring related to ethical decision-making and its potential impact. It is important to capture their views, give space to thoughts and feelings, and make decisions in partnership wherever possible. There may also be situations where a higher level of scrutiny or thinking is required and, in such circumstances, it can be helpful if there is an ethics advisory panel within your practice area that can act as a space for thinking and testing ideas. Such panels are non-directional but bring other perspectives or challenges to your thinking for the benefit of the person with a learning disability, to ensure their rights are upheld and to reinforce values-based approaches.

Critical reflection 2.3

- Think about a situation in your recent practice where you felt you were confronted with an ethical situation, concern or dilemma and try to apply the above framework for ethical decision-making. Work through stages 1–3 of this framework, and then consider whether you would do things differently were you confronted with a similar situation in the future.

Chapter summary

This chapter has explored the importance of values, the law and ethics in relation to professional learning disability nursing practice. It has argued that these areas of knowledge provide an essential foundation for the development of ethical decision-making in all fields of nursing. However, there are specific challenges that arise when seeking to support people with learning disabilities as they are at increased risk of their rights not being upheld. As a learning disability nurse, therefore, it is essential that you both develop the required knowledge and skills in relation to values, the law and ethics and that you ensure that these are constantly updated and extended. Only by doing so will you be able to support people with learning disabilities to self-advocate or to advocate on their behalf. And hence ensure that their rights are not only recognised but also upheld.

FURTHER READING

Fisher, K, Robichaux, C, Sauerland, J and Stokes, F (2020) A Nurse's Ethical Commitment to People with Intellectual and Developmental Disabilities. *Nursing Ethics*, 27(4): 1066–76.

This paper explores the need for all nurses to ensure ethical practice in relation to people with learning disabilities and highlights the challenges that can arise.

Griffith, R and Dowie, I (2019) *Dimond's Legal Aspects of Nursing. A Definitive Guide to Law for Nurses,* 8th edition. Harrow: Pearson.

This book provides a comprehensive overview of legal aspects of nursing.

Hopes, P (2020) Joining up the Dots: Strategic Thinking Clinicians. [online] Available at: https://learningdisabilitynurseconsultant.home.blog/2020/05/17/joining-up-the-dots-strategic-thinking-clinicians/ (accessed 16 January 2022).

This blog discusses the important of values and strategic thinking.

McKenzie, K, Taylor, S, Murray, G and James, I (2020) The Use of Therapeutic Untruths by Learning Disability Nursing Students. *Nursing Ethics*, 27(8): 1607–17.

An interesting paper that explores the concept of 'therapeutic untruths' and the ways in which they are used in the context of learning disability nursing practice.

RESOURCES

What Are Human Rights?: www.equalityhumanrights.com/en/human-rights/what-are-human-rights (accessed 21 June 2022).

The Equality and Human Rights Commission website provides you with detailed information regarding equalities and human rights legislation.

Nursing Ethics Journal: https://journals.sagepub.com/home/nej (accessed 21 June 2022).

This SAGE journal provides a useful source of research and debate relating to ethical aspects of nursing education, research and practice.

3 Communication

Chapter aims

The aim of this chapter is to explore the importance of communication in learning disability nursing and to examine the essential skills needed to enhance opportunities to engage with people with learning disabilities and their families, carers and key stakeholders. Effective, person-centred and augmented communication is central to learning disability nursing, ensuring that people with learning disabilities are able to articulate their wants, needs and wishes when in receipt of care and treatment. This chapter explores key issues in communication with people with learning disabilities as well as with families and other professionals. Contemporary professional issues related to communication are also considered.

Professional standards and expectations

The Nursing and Midwifery Council's Code (NMC, 2018b) identifies that nurses should: *'use a range of verbal and non-verbal communication methods, and consider cultural sensitivities, to better understand and respond to people's personal and health needs'.*

The Nursing and Midwifery Council (NMC, 2018a) standards have a number of references to communication and relationship management skills, of which the following are examples.

- 1.11: communicate effectively using a range of skills and strategies with colleagues and people at all stages of life and with a range of mental, physical, cognitive and behavioural health challenges.

- 1.13: demonstrate the skills and abilities required to develop, manage and maintain appropriate relationships with people, their families, carers and colleagues.

- 4.3: demonstrate the knowledge, communication and relationship management skills required to provide people, families and carers with accurate information that meets their needs before, during and after a range of interventions.

The Equality Act (Gov.uk, 2010) is clear that we all have a duty to ensure that information is accessible, if you fail to make reasonable adjustments to your communication style then this increases the risk of vulnerability to the people in your care.

The five good communication standards (The Royal College of Speech and Language Therapists, 2013) highlight hidden speech and language issues for people with learning disabilities which can often be overlooked. In developing your professional practice, you must think about how people with learning disabilities can experience safe, compassionate and dignified care in environments that are not always augmented to their unique communication needs.

THE NATURE, PURPOSE AND IMPORTANCE OF COMMUNICATION

Communication is an essential skill in nursing. Making and maintaining connections with others is reliant on effective communication. In healthcare situations, communication is often thought about in a functional way, related to the management and organisation of care rather than to develop and enjoy a relationship. An understanding of communication and an ability to adapt or augment our communication style to work in partnership with people with learning disabilities and their families is fundamental. Within the learning disability nursing pre-registration programme, whole modules focus on the development of communication skills and standards.

Communication skills are essential to allow us to:

o   develop and maintain relationships with others;

o   understand messages being relayed by others;

o   express our own messages and relay information;

o   make sense of information from the environments we are in, supporting decisions about safety, etc;

o   interpret emotions such as anger, excitement, elation;

o   recognise underlying issues such as pain, distress, confusion.

Communication is a two-way process essential for the way we live our lives but also a fundamental right. There are many reasons that we need to communicate with each other based on much more than the use of speech and language. We often need to be able to communicate verbally, in writing and through other non-verbal methods. Non-verbal communication can be used to express many emotions, thoughts and feelings and can often be more powerful than the words being used (Ali, 2018). Supporting your communication with non-verbals can be very influential and positive within an interaction. It is also important to be aware of the unintended messages we may convey.

Critical reflection 3.1

- We are constantly communicating messages. Take a moment to write down the verbal and non-verbal styles you use when communicating.

BARRIERS TO EFFECTIVE COMMUNICATION

People with communication support needs may face barriers in their day-to-day lives. They may be excluded from activities or opportunities and can be discriminated against in environments and services that are not adapted to meet their needs. If language, jargon or terminology is used in communication with people with learning disabilities this can mean that there are challenges in decoding, understanding and acting on the messages. Healthcare communication is not always user-friendly; as a learning disability nurse there will be many times in your professional practice that you will need to interpret and modify language to enhance an individual's healthcare experience. Poor communication may lead to poor outcomes for a person and can lead to a breakdown in trust and relationships.

Stans et al (2016, p 2494) recognise the complexity in communication for healthcare professionals, highlighting that there can be challenges due to the matter being communicated but also *'due to time constraints, emotions, different expectations and factors in the social and physical environment'*. Exploring potential barriers in all means of communication – written, verbal, non-verbal, listening, presenting, multidisciplinary working and continuing professional development – is essential to the development of professional nursing skills.

Personal barriers

There might be things that impact on an individual's ability to communicate or receive a message. As a student nurse you will develop skills and confidence that allow you to grow professionally and improve the way that you connect with the people you serve and work with. Some of the personal barriers you need to be aware of are:

- skills;
- confidence;
- motivation;
- cognitive ability;
- auditory or visual impairments;
- physical health issues;
- cultural issues;
- language barriers;

○   lack of personal, financial or technological resources;

○   limited opportunities;

○   historical factors.

Environmental barriers

This can relate to the physical, social or attitudinal space that people live their lives in (Bornman and Murphy, 2006). Factors which might contribute to barriers from an environmental perspective you need to consider include:

○   lack of reasonable adjustments;

○   an environment that is heavily reliant on verbal communication;

○   poor culture;

○   lack of diversity or inclusivity;

○   limited opportunities for engagement;

○   lack of external exposure or scrutiny;

○   use of jargon or terminology;

○   time constraints;

○   the physical environment, screens, lighting, furniture position, noise;

○   lack of investment in technology, resource, opportunities, not seeing the need to adapt or evolve.

Completing the following critical reflection will support your understanding of personal and environmental communication challenges.

Critical reflection 3.2

Has there been a time when you have felt that you haven't been understood when communicating? Jot down the thoughts and feelings you link to that memory. Use the prompt questions below to develop your thinking.

•   What opportunity did you have to make your point?

•   Did you feel you had enough time and space to communicate your message?

•   What was happening in the environment that might have made it difficult to relay the message?

•   Was the person you were communicating with listening to you? Did you feel their barriers in their communication style that made it difficult for you to express yourself?

•   How might reflecting on this experience influence your nursing practice?

Reflecting on exercise 3.2 should highlight that both communication partners have a responsibility in the interaction to convey and receive a message. The partnership as communicators relies on specific skills and recognition of each other's needs. You need to be aware of the way you attend to your communication partners. If you work with people who may not have clear verbal communication, then you will need to work harder to listen, to demonstrate that you are listening and responding authentically and ensure that the person communicating a message is afforded the dignity, respect, time and space to assert their point. There are potential power imbalances in the relationships that you will have with people with learning disabilities and their families (Togher et al, 2010), so exploring alternative ways of communicating is important in affording dignity, respect and empowerment.

Recognising the potential for power imbalance

Where there is a power imbalance, you might see people with learning disabilities acquiesce, for example, by responding in a way that they think the person wants. Acquiescence may occur because of how a person has been socialised and due to expectations of compliance or conformity. Within your practice, be aware that using closed questions can cause problems for some people with learning disabilities. Our communication can be very complex; there is much that you will take for granted because of the way you have been socialised and the opportunities you have had. People may give what they perceive to be an expected answer or response where they have not understood the question or concept.

○   People with learning disabilities might be more likely to say what they think you want to hear.

○   The person may agree when asked, but may not have understood the question.

○   People may repeat a request but may not be able to retain or repeat at a later time.

○   A person with a learning disability might find it hard to say no to you, because they perceive you to be powerful and fear the ramifications.

This potential for acquiescence can be exacerbated in situations where the person is not well known or understood, for example, new appointments, unfamiliar settings or processes, and where there might be a requirement to use yes or no responses. The importance of supporting a person in line with their own needs and recognising their potential communication challenges needs to be fundamental to your practice. Find ways to build on the person's communication strengths: start by asking what is the best way to communicate with you? How do you need me to give you information? Making sure that the person who is supporting an individual with a learning disability is included in these conversations is important (where appropriate with consent) as they can support your understanding of an individual's needs. The use of a communication tool such as a health profile, communication passport or other personalised profile captures this information and gives the healthcare professional an insight into some of the more subtle intricacies of an individual's communication needs.

As a professional, it is beneficial to consciously look to develop your style of communication. If you become more aware of your communication skills, you will develop your approach and effectiveness as a communication partner. Increased self-awareness will be good for your confidence and ability to notice and respond to cues from those you support or care for. There is a responsibility to adapt, augment and articulate our messages in ways that people with learning disabilities, their families and fellow professionals understand. The way that we attempt to communicate with others can demonstrate the value we place on the individual, in other words there is no greater way to convey dignity and respect for an individual than to communicate with them in a way that they understand.

There can be times when professionals overestimate communication skills for some people, particularly within familiar routines or environments, in situations where there is a power imbalance or where communication occurs in a specific context. For example, when asking someone to get ready to go out, there are likely to be many other contextual cues that indicate this is the request. The person supporting might be putting their shoes and coat on, they may have picked up a handbag, shopping bag, car keys, shopping list, there might be other indicators such as closing internal doors, switching off the TV or radio.

Critical reflection 3.3

* Thinking about the scenario above, what are the implications for your nursing practice when communication skills may have been overestimated?

LANGUAGE DEVELOPMENT

There are complex requirements in using language which can be impacted on by level of cognitive ability. Understanding linguistic development and the context in which the person functions is essential to establishing meaningful communication, engagement and relationships. If you do not seek to understand this then as a professional, you can contribute to the further disabling of an individual, devaluing their voice, their potential and their opportunities for freedom in the way they live their lives.

As already explored, people with learning disabilities are not a homogeneous group, each person has a unique set of skills and abilities and you should never hold assumptions about the people you meet. Some people with a learning disability are able to communicate their wants, needs and wishes with little need for additional support. You may find that you meet some people who have learned to 'mask' their communication difficulties by a range of strategies, sometimes using 'cocktail party speech', this is where a person has learned some social rules that support them to get by in conversation without giving too much detail or technical information, for example, talking about the football, asking about your car or discussing the weather. The communication skills of people with Williams syndrome are sometimes referred to in this way, highlighting the social disinhibition and overly familiar, stylised way of engaging in conversation, there is a need to be hyper aware to the potential of overestimating a person with Williams syndrome ability due to their presentation. There are others who are likely to use language that would be developmentally appropriate but chronologically much lower than their actual age. Boardman et al (2014) highlight that there can be a tendency to rely on speech as the main communication method, although there might be evidence to indicate that this is not in line with an individual's needs.

Masking may be used due to the person being self-conscious about their learning disability, they may feel they could be stigmatised. You will need to be alert to the potential for the person taking a passive role in communication, using language that appears rote and repetitive, for example, saying something that is very colloquial, mechanical or jargon based. This can help a person fit in, saying something like, '*I don't know whether I'm at the park or the pictures*', to indicate they are confused, the person may have set, learned responses which help them to participate, get help or get out of more difficult communication. Awareness of non-verbal communication will help you to understand if the person is saying one thing when they mean another, does their body language match the tone, intonation, volume, speed and the story they are telling you?

Taking the time to get to know the person will help you to assess the level of skill and support the person needs. You may need to be more covert in your observation style and non-directional in your language to build up trust. Time to listen, speaking naturally and communicating with the person in a humanistic, age-appropriate, culturally normalised and in a way that does not demean or patronise the person is very important. Ask for feedback on your communication style, try to check the persons understanding and use the words and phrases that the person uses to make sure that you are on common ground and you are both talking about the same thing. One good example would be when asking about elimination and bowel habits as part of a nursing assessment, some people will use very specific terms and may not know that wee and urine are the same thing. Finding out the names and terms people use will help in building a relationship and trust. It is likely that there may be times that you are able to learn from the person and develop skills that will develop your professional practice by investing the time, being open and honest and reaching a common ground in the way you work with people.

Pre-symbolic, symbolic and verbal communication

Boardman et al (2014) identify three broad categories to understand the communication skills of people with learning disabilities: pre-symbolic, symbolic and verbal.

Those who use pre-symbolic communication are functioning at the earliest stages of communication, people who have a severe or profound level of learning disability. This might mean communicating using eye gaze, vocalisations or trying to position themselves closer to an item, the complexity and subtlety of the communication strategy can mean there is a strong reliance on those who know the person well to facilitate meaningful engagement. There are various skills that you can use in your practice to develop relationships, ascertain what's important to the person or anticipate wants, needs or wishes, these are explored later in this chapter.

Symbolic communication can encompass various modes, such as speech, symbols, signs or pictures. There are people who will be able to respond to simple instruction, engage in communication using basic, everyday phrases and language or be able to understand a sequence of event via a communication method such as a social story, sentence strip or other symbolic representation. When you support a person with a learning disability to use a resource to understand a message, you will find that although they may not have verbal language, they can convey emotion, feeling and behaviour that indicate meaning and response to the situation.

Although there will be people with a diagnosed learning disability who are able to demonstrate verbal communication, you must take on board the importance of ensuring that the level of receptive and expressive communication a person demonstrates is understood. As a clinician, it is important that you use language that is easy for a person to understand, avoid medical terminology, jargon or abstract concepts. Check the person's understanding as much as possible. You might ask the person to repeat what you have said and make sure that there is enough time for a person to process information, don't repeat the request or question too quickly as this might feel like an additional pressure or demand for the person. You can still supplement your communication with resources such as pictures, symbols, body maps or show me where tools, many of us benefit from visual prompts in our day-to-day life, for example, signage, calendars, diaries or visual instruction leaflets.

Another concept that it is important to be aware of as a learning disability nurse is echolalia, an automatic vocalisation that people make, where phrases or noises are repeated. This might be something that happens immediately, and may be a partial repetition: when asked a question, '*where shall we go today?*' the person may reply: '*go today*'. Echolalia is often a feature of language development in neurotypical functioning and Lovaas (1981) explored the concept that echolalia may be intrinsically rewarding for the person and that they get a sense of reinforcement from matching to what others say. An additional challenge for some people can be delays in processing time, meaning that you need to give extra time to receive and interpret information you have given. It is important to not repeat your instruction/request/question too quickly or the person might become overwhelmed.

LEARNING TO LISTEN

For some people listening is not something that comes naturally. As we have explored earlier in the chapter, communication is a two-way process and there are communication partners who will need to listen and be heard. In nursing and healthcare situations, there are often time pressures that impact on the space given to an individual. There are examples of nurses not responding well to identified needs, not recognising underlying issues which impact on an individual's ability to express their need. For a person with a learning disability, there is a need to observe and respond to subtle communication cues. The barriers explored earlier in the chapter highlight why it is important to make time and seek to improve the experience for the person as much as possible. Paying attention to details is likely to require you as a practitioner to say nothing for long periods of time, waiting and listening to understand rather than to respond. Listening well, for enough time, should support your understanding of the individual, identifying what is unique to them and their situation and improving the quality of the interaction.

The SAGE and THYME model (Conolly et al, 2010) (see Table 3.1) of communication is one tool that can support the development of effective listening skills, providing you with a structured approach to practising and implementing attending to a person in an interaction. It is key that you hold back from attempting to resolve an issue without completing the steps. This is an empowering, person-focused approach which seeks to appreciate underlying factors.

Table 3.1 The SAGE and THYME model

S	Setting	What's happening in the environment? Have there been incidents in the setting today that make it feel unsettled, are you expecting a new admission or referral.
		How private is the space? Are there distractions or tasks that you need to complete which might be a barrier to this communication, can you deal with them now so you can fully attend can you make the person aware you may be interrupted, for example, if you are required to respond to something and interrupt the discussion.
A	Ask	Find out what the person needs to communicate, for example, say 'you seem upset, can you tell me what has happened?' it is important to use the cures the person is giving you to start the conversation, their facial expression, body language, tone. It's not as simple as asking a closed question, for example, are you upset?
G	Gather	Reflect back to the person what they have told you, reflect their language and descriptions and gather as much information as you can about the issue or concern being discussed. Summarise the concern and check that you have all the information that the person wants you to know.
E	Empathy	Demonstrate that you have understood how the person is feeling, sensitively use a summary statement that starts with 'I can see that you feel ...' Showing compassion towards a person who is distressed or anxious is important. It is essential that you are not preoccupied with your own emotional responses during these interactions.
T	Talk	Find out if the person has shared their issue with anyone else, who do they have to talk to, do they feel people understand and are able to appropriately support them?
H	Help	Specifically check that the person has help, for example, you've told me you talk to your sister, how does she help you?
Y	You	Make sure that the person is empowered and prompted to think about what they can do to make a situation better, asking what they think can help is one way to do that.
M	Me	Find out what the person thinks/would like you to do to help. Confirm the steps you are taking, for example, 'you have told me that you think the medication you are taking makes you feel sleepy, I am going to help you with a recording chart so that we can find out what else might be making you sleepy'.
E	End	Ensure a clear ending to the interaction with clear actions agreed. Summarise the concerns, check that the person is happy to end the conversation for now and agree when action will take place.

(Conolly et al, 2010)

Emotional intelligence

The SAGE and THYME model indicates a need for a level of emotional intelligence during interactions, emphasising the need for sensitivity in addressing emotional concerns and using skills that hold and respect those concerns without applying solutions. Goleman (2020) describes emotional intelligence using five core characteristics: '*self-awareness, self-regulation, motivation, empathy and social skill*'. Familiarising yourself with the concept of emotional intelligence is important as there are implications for your practice and for the safety of those in your care. The core characteristics are essential for leadership and can be fundamental to the culture of an organisation. When in practice, it is important not to make judgements about the way things are done but to try and understand the values and drivers which influence attitude and behaviour.

As a learning disability nurse you will be faced with situations where you will need to manage your own and others emotions. The level of emotional intelligence you have will allow you to deal with stressful, difficult and challenging incidents. You may need to demonstrate empathy, calmness, clarity and respect in the face of those who are angry, upset, frightened or anxious. Being emotionally intelligent can allow you to cope with challenges in practice such as dealing with conflict, being able to reason, understand and manage the emotional aspects within yourself and your communication partner.

There are many specific examples where you need to focus on behaving in an emotionally intelligent way, understanding that what you say and how you say it influences others. Some examples highlighted are the potential for behaviour described as challenging and the use of humour. Communication issues can be a significant risk factor for behaviours described as challenging, '*as communication difficulties increase, behaviours that are considered challenging typically increase in frequency, intensity or duration*' (RCSLT, 2013). Mee (2012) advises caution when using humour. There are potential power imbalances which can change the context of the joke from being with the person to on the person. There are clearly some situations where humour can be valuable (and valuing); a shared joke can support bonding, relationship building and diffuse potential challenging situations. However, it is essential that the person with a learning disability can share and understand the joke in order to feature positively in the interaction.

Critical reflection 3.4

Think about a time in your nursing practice that you have needed to ask for help.

- How did emotional intelligence help you to know who to ask, how to ask and how to get the outcome you hoped for?

- What did you learn about asking for help?

MAKING INFORMATION EASY TO UNDERSTAND

While people who don't work in learning disability services might think that accessible information is only needed for those with literacy issues or learning disabilities, how many of us rely on signage, symbols and pictures to support our understanding or choice making? When travelling, there are some signs that are universally relatable, for example, bus stop or public conveniences. There are many professionals in the field who find it much clearer and less time-consuming to access easy read versions of lengthy reports and policies to support our ability to process and retain information. Accessible information can be of benefit to everyone, reinforcing the well-known adage, if you get it right for people with learning disabilities, you get it right for everyone.

People with learning disabilities are likely to need additional support to understand information. There may be complexities to take into account such as visual or hearing impairments as well as recognising that there are many people with learning disabilities who have not learned to read. Retaining information and remembering conversations can also be difficult for people.

You need to make sure, as a nurse, that you are able to communicate complex messages in a way that people with learning disabilities and their families can understand. There will be many situations where you need to support a person to make a choice or decision and there will be complexity in the message that needs to be broken down, adapted or presented in a different way so that it is accessible. Making something accessible is complex and requires a level of skill. It is much more than selecting images and putting them next to words. It is very important that you choose the right words and think about what the words mean that you select. Written information needs to flow and feel natural, there should be simple, easy to understand concepts which are consistent, for example, pick a word and stick to it such as 'jab' and not change to injection or vaccine within the document. Check with people with learning disabilities that they understand and use the words selected and give specific space to reduce confusion, for example, a clear definition of a new word where confusion might happen.

To empower people with learning disabilities, you have a duty to ensure that you have supported the person to receive information in a way that is meaningful to them. This is a legal requirement enshrined in the Equality Act (Gov.uk, 2010). For some people, this might mean providing information in a visual way, for example, using pictures, symbols, sentence strips or social stories. It is essential that in developing these resources as a learning disability nurse, you understand what the person's communication skills look like. Working together with a Speech and Language Therapist to understand receptive and expressive communication and to access specific guidelines on the best way to communicate with an individual will support your professional practice and development of skills.

The five good communication standards

The Royal College of Speech and Language Therapists (RCSLT, 2013) developed the five good communication standards (see Table 3.2), as part of the Department of Health (2012) Transforming Care report, which responded to the Winterbourne View scandal, an undercover investigation in 2011 by the BBC Panorama programme.

The emphasis in the standards is about the importance of making reasonable adjustments to communication as a way of improving experience, quality and safety. The standards are designed to be used proactively and practically, so that people with learning disabilities and their families as well as practitioners and organisations are able to know and respond to 'what good looks like'. Without good communication, there are implications for quality of life, partnerships, citizenship and that people may be dehumanised.

Table 3.2 The five good communication standards

Standard 1.	How best to communicate with somebody is clearly described, for example, in a communication profile, passport or care plan.
Standard 2.	There is clear demonstration in services of how they support people to be involved in decisions about the services they receive and how their care is delivered.
Standard 3.	The best approaches to support individual communication are valued and competently implemented.
Standard 4.	The opportunities, relationships and environments create conditions in which people with learning disabilities want to communicate.
Standard 5.	Opportunities are in place to support individuals to understand and express their needs related to health and well-being.

(Adapted from RCSLT, 2013)

For some individuals, written and spoken words may not be accessible even with reasonable adjustments; however, all people are able to communicate. For these individuals in unfamiliar situations the communication passport, hospital passport and the team around them as well as their family is essential in ensuring the best possible approach to facilitating effective care and intervention, supporting understanding, engagement and empowering the person.

Karas and Laud (2015) describe how a person with a profound and multiple learning disability may have communication options available to them that are less recognisable to those who do not work in the field. It may be that some people with profound and multiple learning disabilities have not developed intentional communication and they will be heavily reliant on those supporting them, their family, carers or support teams to interpret their presentation or recognise subtle changes which indicate a want, need or a change in their personal state. As is clear, there are multiple ways that people who have profound and multiple learning disabilities may communicate. They may not have verbal language but are likely to be able to communicate using other non-verbal strategies:

- ○ facial expressions;
- ○ vocalisations;
- ○ body language;
- ○ gestures;
- ○ behaviour;
- ○ responses to their environment;
- ○ use of objects or activities;
- ○ eye gaze.

Mencap (2015) has developed top tips for communicating with people who have profound and multiple learning disabilities. Emphasised in their guidance is the importance of talking to people who know the person well, asking what does this mean? Is this usual for this person? When would this person usually do this/show this? What does it mean if it increases/decreases? A useful resource which relates to this is the Disability Distress Assessment Tool (DisDat, Regnard et al, 2007) this can be used to document a wide range of signs and behaviours which may indicate distress or contentment. The DisDat tool allows for an understanding of an individual's personal distress indicators or vocabulary and helps to contextualise these behaviours related to potential experience of distress.

The skills of a partner who is able to interpret and respond to communication are essential and for a learning disability nurse, this will be a role that evolves as you become more experienced in your practice.

Resources to support communication

Beyond Words are books, leaflets or downloadable resources from an app, produced for people who do not read. These tools have been developed with groups of people with learning disabilities who advise on imagery and content to ensure that pictures in stories are fully accessible. There are stories to fit a broad range of scenarios including loss, grief, sexuality, love and safety. Some relate to specific health and social care issues such as having an injection, feeling down, being abused or living with dementia. In '*I can get through it*' (Hollins et al, 2009), a lady who seems happy going about everyday tasks is attacked by a man and pictures demonstrate how disturbed she is by the incident.

There is a level of professional judgement and skill needed to support engagement with Beyond Words because there may be some temptation to interpret the pictures and influence the individual's responses to the story. Some people will be able to use the resources without support, using their own storytelling skills. Most people with learning disabilities can follow the stories with support. It is essential that you familiarise yourself with the suggested storyline and the images within to ensure that you can support the individual as much as possible to get the best out of the experience. They might be useful to elicit information from a person, for example, 'do I feel safe?' or to prepare for an unknown situation.

Communication passports involve gathering, sharing and making explicit information about a person and their communication needs in order to help less familiar people recognise and make sense of the person's communicative behaviour: (CALL Scotland, nd). The communication passport can contain specific information about individuals' use of language, what augmented systems they may use, whether they have physical communication barriers such as visual or auditory impairments etc.

A communication passport may make individualised recommendations, such as:

○   use a person's specific tools, such as iPads, communication boards, sentence strips;

○   keep to concrete examples as much as you can;

o   think about how to ask questions – use simple either/or questions;

o   provide support in visual ways – pictures, drawing and signs or symbols;

o   reduce complexity, breakdown information into smaller chunks;

o   use a slower pace.

As a clinician or student nurse, you may be involved in informing the passport. Tools like this are only helpful to the individual if they are read and understood by those around them. Making sure that you understand the communication passport, give information where appropriate to keep it updated, and work in partnership with the person to reflect their preferred communication style and needs are essential.

Easy read information (sometimes called 'easier information') is an example of 'accessible information'. The process is a way of making information easier to read and understand for people with learning disabilities. It is much more than using sentences and pairing with pictures. Wherever possible it should be developed with people with learning disabilities who are able to scrutinise and inform the resource from their perspective. Easy read resources can be developed for a specific issue for an individual's use or to communicate resources or publications such as reports, policies and guidelines, and can cover topics related to health issues such as accessing services, what will happen at an appointment and so on. There are self-advocacy groups that develop easy read information and many resources are freely available online, for example, Easy Read Wales. During the pandemic in 2020/21, there were many calls from self-advocates with learning disabilities challenging the lack of accessible or easy read information and highlighting how people with learning disabilities and their families were being disadvantaged due to this.

Inclusive communication is an approach that seeks to reduce barriers to communication which can exclude members of communities and society. By reducing barriers, inclusive communication increases the likelihood that people will benefit from accessing the right service at the right time (Mooney et al, 2016). The Scottish Government (2011) explains the benefits of ensuring inclusive communication from a rights-based, legal, ethical, cost and individual perspective. By delivering inclusive communication, the service people receive will be more tailored to their needs, people will be more satisfied with the service they receive and rights will be upheld.

Intensive interaction: described by the Intensive Interaction Institute (online, accessed 28 March 2021) an approach designed to help people at early levels of development, working on early interaction ability (pre-verbal), supporting development of communication which is about enjoying being with others. Intensive interaction is an intervention used to support people with severe, profound, or complex learning difficulties and people with autism, to learn how to relate, interact, know, understand and practice communication routines. Hutchinson and Bodicoat (2015) explored the effectiveness of intensive interaction with some groups of people with learning disabilities and autism and considered the training and experience of practitioners. The review reflected on the potential perceived impact for people and their families, but recognised the challenge in quantifying the evidence of effectiveness. There are questions about the appropriateness and effectiveness of intensive interaction as a strategy. You may find in your practice that this can be a strategy that allows you to develop a connection or relationship with an individual.

Objects of reference: understanding real objects is the first stage of symbolic development and recognition of real objects is the most concrete way of representing a word. The systematic use of an item/object to represent an activity (wooden spoon for baking), place (goggles to represent the swimming pool), person (a piece of cloth to represent a person) or change in an environment (using a textured board to indicate transitions) can build predictability, reduce anxiety and support a person to understand what is happening at a moment in time. As a learning disability nurse, you will need to work closely with speech and language therapy colleagues to build the appropriate use of communication strategies into the care plans that you develop. Personalising the use of objects of reference to give meaning; for example, showing a washcloth to the person to indicate they are going to the bathroom or shoes to show they are going for a walk will be fundamental in supporting the individual in their day-to-day life.

Social Stories: Social stories are simple, accurate and concrete models which give individualised descriptions using life situations and people, the person writing the story must consider the perspective of the individual who will use the story. Gray and Garand (1993) recognised the value of the use of stories particularly for children with autism, highlighting that *'they have been used successfully to introduce changes and new routines at home and at school, to explain the reasons for others behaviours, or to teach new academic and social skills'*. They can help to prepare people with learning disabilities, work through life skills, including a planned way to respond in a situation. Social stories can be used to develop social skills, independence skills and what to do in an emergency or other difficult situation. A study by Samuels and Stansfield (2011) found short-term improvements in social interaction, people within the study and their support staff engaged positively in the use, however they also identified that there would be benefit from longer term intervention studies to strengthen the evidence base.

Talking Mats™ can provide a strategy for developing conversation with people of who require intervention to express thoughts or emotions about specific topics and is appropriate for all ages. Talking Mats™ use a visual framework which allows for the person to go into depth about a topic (Bornman and Murphy, 2006). You can engage people in the Talking Mats™ framework to allow for a topic to be explored fully with understanding and appropriate questioning. The use of a visual rating scale supports an individual to express their thoughts about a particular topic, for example, going shopping. Other pictures which make up the components of going shopping are placed by the individual in the area of the mat where the visual rating scale is. This allows for breaking down discussion about the things the person does and does not like about the topic and can support further exploration to try and find ways of overcoming issues that are challenging for the individual. For example, if the person likes all aspects of going shopping except packing the bags at the end, further work can be done to find out what the person does not like about this. As a practitioner, you would need to access specific training to support your ability to use Talking Mats™ with people you support. You may find in your areas that there are other professionals who are skilled in using them and can support your development of the intervention.

When considering new and innovative ways of communication, particularly through technology, apps and other digital means, we must be mindful of the potential for people with learning disabilities and their families to be disadvantaged by systems which rely on access to technology, for example, WiFi, social media and associated skills. It is inevitable that post-Covid-19 services which support people with learning disabilities may want to continue to deliver virtual services and capitalise on the resource and cost benefits of doing so. As learning disability nurses, we need to use local knowledge and person-centred practices to ensure that nobody with a learning disability is disadvantaged by these advancements. As the impact of technological advances is realised, learning disability nurses will need to advocate for the practices they want to take forward and further develop and be open about the need to let go of the things that are no longer effective.

Case study 3.1

Owen is 16 years old, funny, curious and fiercely independent. He is very keen to know when he might get a driving licence. Owen was born prematurely and spent several weeks in neonates. As he grew older he was delayed in meeting developmental milestones and assessment indicated that he had impaired vision and fluctuating hearing loss. Owen also had a diagnosis of cerebral palsy and moderate learning disability. As a teenager, sometimes Owen would lash out at others in tasks where he was being given direct instruction or where he was struggling to do something autonomously. If this happened his teachers or support staff would ask Owen, did that happen because they were too loud? Owen would repeat 'too loud'. One day Owen's community nurse was in the classroom when this happened, she approached him and asked him to sign 'too loud'. Owen was not able to sign this despite having a good level of Makaton signs. The community nurse concluded that Owen did not understand what 'too loud' meant and reviewed the recent behaviour recording charts to look at potential other antecedents to the behaviour. Owen had learned to use a phrase to stop staff from asking questions and making demands of him when an incident happened. The staff in his environment did not have a good level of Makaton and could not always effectively communicate with him. The community nurse could communicate in a way that Owen understood and this allowed for a deeper understanding of why Owen was using behaviour in these situations.

Case study discussion

In Owen's case study, we have touched on one method of communication, Makaton, that some people with learning disabilities learn which integrates speech, symbols and signing to teach communication. Often people will develop their own, idiosyncratic signing, which is personal to them and relies on people in their environment having the interpersonal skills to interpret meaning. Some of the key underlying issues which may present barriers to communication were also highlighted; Owen has little eyesight and a hearing impairment. When communicating with somebody it is very important to know what a person's visual status is, it would be important to ask when did the person last visit the optician or have their hearing assessed, not only as part of an initial assessment but also important in ongoing reviews. It is possible that Owen also uses echolalia and perhaps in the situation, repeating '*too loud*' is an example of this.

MAKING DECISIONS

The Mental Capacity Act (2005) is focused on ensuring an individual's right to make their own decisions and presumes capacity in the first instance (Principle 1). The second principle is clear that every effort must be made to encourage and support the person in making the decision for themselves.

As a learning disability nurse supporting a decision-making process, you have a duty to make sure the individual has the relevant information that they need to make the decision. Part of the process is finding out the persons preferred communication method and whether they have hearing or visual impairments, specific needs related to signing, use of symbols. It is essential that information to aid decision-making is presented in a way that is individualised to them and makes the situation easy for them to understand. Involvement of people who know the person well can be very important, but it is essential the uniqueness of the situation is taken into account, there are some situations where family members may feel it can be detrimental to their relationships to try to engage a person in a difficult conversation. An Independent Mental Health Advocate (IMHA) or Independent Mental Capacity Advocate (IMCA) might be better placed to support decision-making and advocating for the individual. For more information on using the Mental Capacity Act (Gov.uk, 2005) in practice read Mughal (2014).

Case study 3.2

Lisa is 47, she lives in a supported living service, she works in a café and is very popular in her local community. She had an older sister who died aged 45 after treatment for breast cancer and due to the family history Lisa is considered to be high risk. She has recently been referred to a consultant oncoplastic surgeon after attending her GP, she had reported to her support worker that her breasts looked funny and had experienced unusual discharge from her nipple. Lisa has previously attended '*check for change*' sessions from her local community learning disability team where the focus was on health facilitation and increasing awareness of potential body change which could be indicators of cancer. Lisa was diagnosed with suspected breast carcinoma and at the time of diagnosis a mental capacity assessment was carried out. Key individuals who are involved in Lisa's care were present for the assessment and were able to support Lisa to receive information and ask questions. At the appointment Lisa started to become angry when the topic of further investigations was raised. She appeared to not understand the severity of the situation and refused to engage in the conversation, she talked about her sister who died and seemed to be confused about what had caused her death. The professionals and family members who supported Lisa at the appointment felt that she did not have the capacity to make the decision about additional investigations and subsequent treatment options and they decided that there would need to be a best interest decision for Lisa.

Table 3.3 provides some communication strategies to support understanding of diagnosis and treatment options.

Table 3.3 Communication strategies to support understanding of diagnosis and treatment options

Education about risks of cancer	Visual aids/objects of reference
	Show me where tool
	Body maps
	Simulated body parts to touch and describe
	Group work exploring names for body parts and awareness of where and how changes might happen
	Individual sessions
	Support to supporters
Resources during assessment appointment	Support from somebody who knows Lisa well
	Pictures of the hospital, a map, an easy read guide to what might happen at the appointment
	Body maps
	Simulated body parts
	Show me where tool
Going for a scan	A personalised social story about what happens at the scan
	Watching a YouTube video or an environment-specific video from the hospital
	Time to plan in advance with a named person to reduce anxiety and think about what might happen
	Pictures of equipment
	Carrying out the procedure first on the person supporting so that Lisa can see what will happen
Overall reasonable adjustments	Partnership work with an acute liaison nurse
	Reducing distractions in the environment
	Minimising equipment which might cause anxiety
	Supporting Lisa in a chair instead of a trolley
	Allowing Lisa to keep her clothes on instead of wearing a hospital gown
	Try to minimise impact on routines and schedule appointments at the beginning or end of the day.

Critical reflection 3.5

- What are some examples of good practice within Lisa's case study?

- Who are the key people that should be involved for people with learning disabilities in planning care and treatment?

- What are the resources that learning disability nurses can employ to increase the confidence of people who do not routinely work with people with learning disabilities?

Lisa's scenario gives examples of many of the ways that communication can be adapted, supported and facilitated to support a person to understand important information relevant to their own health. It is clear that Lisa was not able to understand all of this information to facilitate her decision-making. In contrast Owenson (2018) describes a situation where no attempt to adapt communication or make reasonable adjustments were made to allow her daughter Rachel to access a minor clinical procedure.

o   An appointment letter arrives, not written in a way that Rachel can understand.

o   A blanket policy of all patients attending at 8am for procedures in the day unit meant that Rachel required anxiety-reducing medication for the appointment.

o   Medication was prescribed and dispensed without an explanation of how to use it.

o   A post-op patient information leaflet was written in an inaccessible way, Rachel could not understand or follow the advice.

Examples like Rachel's highlight the need for service improvement and a deep understanding of the service user and their family's experience. Finding ways to access feedback about the reality of the persons experience is essential to developing services that meet the needs of the people who use them.

PROFESSIONAL COMMUNICATION

Whenever there are investigations into scandals, poor practice and failures in care, there are reflections on communication. Poor communication is often cited as one of the most common causes of dissatisfaction with healthcare experiences. There are many potential opportunities for failures in communication in nursing practice.

The NMC (2018a) standards on communication and relationship management skills provide guidance on expectations about professional nursing communication, this includes:

1.11: Communicate effectively using a range of skills and strategies with colleagues and people at all stages of life and with a range of mental, physical, cognitive and behavioural health challenges

1.13: Demonstrate the skills and abilities required to develop, manage and maintain appropriate relationships with people, their families, carers and colleagues

4.3: Demonstrate the knowledge, communication and relationship management skills required to provide people, families and carers with accurate information that meets their needs before, during and after a range of interventions

4.2.5: De-escalation strategies and techniques when dealing with conflict

Critical reflection 3.6

- What are your expectations of professionalism when you are communicating with colleagues and people who you support?

- Write down some of the keywords that you relate to professional behaviour and conduct.

The importance of record keeping can never be underestimated, as student nurses you will have heard many times *'if it's not written down, it didn't happen'*. There are many registrants who have felt the devastating consequences of not ensuring that the records they complete are timely, accurate, and legible or linked to the individuals' care plan. It is essential, in the development of your professional practice, that you acknowledge your learning and development needs, exploring these with your clinical supervisor and line manager and take steps to address any deficit which you perceive related to your role, scope of practice and professional responsibilities.

We have more resources available to us than ever before, we can communicate virtually with colleagues across the world. There are technological solutions that allow for instant relay of information and communication. In 2020 during Covid-19 we saw the use of technology become embedded in our daily practice allowing nurses to connect with colleagues and service users in timely and responsive ways. Barriers to effective communication which may have existed due to inadequate technology, travel, cost or time allocation have come a long way to being resolved. However, with new ways of working there are potential additional barriers to be aware of. Many meetings are now held in virtual ways, requiring a structured approach, for example, hands up to speak or remain on mute unless speaking. There are some professionals who may not feel as confident in these forums, we are increasingly being exposed to meeting with people who we do not know well, do not have pre-formed relationships with and we may feel intimidated by these situations. Scott (2017) talks about the importance of looking out for the quiet ones in meetings, this can be particularly difficult in virtual platforms. In your practice, think about how you can be inclusive, how to draw out conversation and information from others and how to ease some of the challenges for teamwork. If you are in a position of chairing meetings, think about ways that you can encourage participation from all in a non-threatening way, some people do not respond well to being put on the spot. It is essential that there is good communication within teams, between teams and in the wider systems we work, this includes how we use social media platforms.

The NMC (2019c) gives specific guidance related to the use of social media. The NMC recognises the value in networking opportunities through social media as well as other benefits. While learning disability nurses continue to benefit from the use of social networking with specific Facebook groups, Instagram feeds and twitter chats which draw together colleagues with people with learning disabilities, their families and advocates to have open communication about the key issues relevant in contemporary practice, there are certainly potential challenges to professional practice which have to be acknowledged. There are generational challenges, media-savvy students and registrants can quickly manoeuvre through a myriad of apps, networks and sites which facilitate sharing, caring and networking. Others may not be so aware of the potential implications of sharing their views, recognising the possible implications of discussion in what feels like a private space, the potential for information to be taken out of context, shared more widely than intended or misused.

There are broad principles that learning disability nurses need to consider in order to uphold the expectations of the Code of Practice which reinforces the public and professional expectations.

o   The public have expectations of all Healthcare Professionals when on and off duty. This includes the use of social media.

o   You must be aware that your behaviour on social media should not bring your profession or the organisation that you work for into disrepute.

o   You can be implicated by liking or sharing materials; this can be perceived as reflecting an endorsement of others' views.

o   Screenshots can be taken and shared more widely than you may have intended. Do not think that because something is only on your wall, others will not potentially get to see it.

o   Social media is very powerful and therefore negative cultures can be reinforced; others may be intimidated or discouraged from sharing their true reflections because of the norms within the social media group.

o   Staff can face disciplinary processes potentially leading to dismissal and referral to their professional body if social media is used irresponsibly.

Appropriate, timely and accurate information is essential for effective work within teams and organisations. The SBAR is a tool which has traditionally been used in an acute, time sensitive situations to deliver information which is outcome focused and draws together a consistent approach to information sharing. SBAR (D) relates to Situation, Background, Assessment, Recommendation (Decision). The SBAR (D) can be very useful in drawing together a case presentation, a report or an issue which needs to be escalated to a senior decision-making forum. As learning disability nurses, thinking through the practice and professional issues you are faced with the SBAR can be a resource which assists in supporting the synthesis and dissemination of information. You can use the format to escalate issues, draw together ideas and raise awareness with your colleagues. For example, the SBAR below relates to a specific piece of work where lessons can be learned and good practice developed.

Table 3.4 SBAR to safeguarding committee to demonstrate good practice and information sharing

Prepared by: A.N. Other, Staff Nurse **Date:** 27.03.2021	
Situation	A safeguarding referral was made following a disclosure from an individual with a learning disability that they had been hit by a staff member. Accessible resources were used to ascertain views related to safeguarding process.
Background	There is a requirement to ascertain views of the individual when a safeguarding issue is raised. This does not always happen and sometimes referrals are made without consultation with the individual. On this occasion a decision was made to use a safeguarding DVD and accessible information leaflet to engage with the person who raised the allegation and gather their views about what they expected to happen in the process.
Assessment	The team who supported the individual reflected on their learning from the event. They were able to see the benefit of using augmented communication, resources and communication targeted at people with a learning disability to explore a challenging topic. They were able to evidence learning and increased awareness for the individual and develop a strategy to build good practice in safeguarding.
Recommendations	That a review of recent safeguarding referrals is undertaken. Data to be collected to understand percentage of referrals made where the person with a learning disability is not consulted and why. A scoping exercise for all use of safeguarding resources across the service to ensure accessibility and engagement with individuals throughout safeguarding processes.
Decision	Recommendations agreed, data collection to be undertaken and presentation back to safeguarding committee in three months.

Chapter summary

This chapter has explored the importance of communication, recognising barriers and potential challenges to good communication. Various concepts have been introduced to help you develop your practice in relation to how you communicate with people with learning disabilities, their families, professionals and organisations. As a learning disability nurse, it is essential that you develop the required knowledge and skills in relation to communication and reflect on ways in which you have communicated effectively and ineffectively in order to learn and grow from the experience. By doing so you ensure that you are able to uphold rights, recognise challenges and empower people to have the best possible outcomes. The importance of a person-centred approach, utilising evidence-based practice and working in partnership with key professionals who have specific skills and knowledge to support exemplary practice in communication has been a key feature of this chapter.

FURTHER READING

Nursing Times (2018) Communication Skills 3: Non-verbal Communication. 15 January. [online] Available at: www.nursingtimes.net/clinical-archive/assessment-skills/commun ication-skills-3-non-verbal-communication-15-01-2018/ (accessed 8 June 2022).

These are the NMC and guidance related to communication.

Fitzpatrick, L (2018) The importance of communication and professional values relating to nursing practice. *Links to Health and Social Care*, 3(1). [online] https://openjournals. ljmu.ac.uk/index.php/lhsc/article/view/193/204 (accessed 25 June 2022).

This article shows the importance of communication and professional nursing values.

RESOURCES

Person Communication Passports: www.communicationpassports.org.uk/home/ (accessed 21 June 2022).

This website contains resources to help create a personal communication passport, which helps people communicate information about themselves.

Talking Mats: www.talkingmats.com (accessed 21 June 2022).

Talking Mats is another resource to aid effective communication for those who find it difficult.

Royal College of Speech and Language Therapists: www.rcslt.org/ (accessed 21 June 2022).

This website contains important information about the role of speech and language therapists.

Communicating with People with a Learning Disability: www.mencap.org.uk/learning-disabi lity-explained/communicating-people-learning-disability (accessed 21 June 2022).

There are a range of materials available on the Mencap website related to communication and involvement of people with learning disabilities.

Beyond Words: https://booksbeyondwords.co.uk/ (accessed 21 June 2022).

This website has many examples of stories and resources that can be used to work with people with learning disabilities on issues affecting their lives; there are physical books and resources that can be downloaded onto apps.

4 Accessing, appraising, applying and developing the evidence base

---

Chapter aims

This chapter introduces you to evidence-based practice as a key foundation for learning disability nursing. It first explores the extent to which evidence-based practice has informed learning disability nursing and some of the challenges encountered. It then assists you with developing your skills in accessing and critically appraising evidence before examining some key areas that need to be considered when seeking to use evidence in practice. Finally, it explores the need to further develop the evidence base for learning disability nursing including the need to work in partnership with people with learning disabilities and their families and carers to make this happen.

Professional standards and expectations

The importance of evidence-based practice to the role of the registered nurse is identified in several of the platforms set out in the Standards (NMC, 2018a). For example, Platform 1 states:

> Registered nurses act in the best interests of people, putting them first and providing nursing care that is person-centred, safe and compassionate. They act professionally at all times and use their knowledge and experience to make evidence-based decisions about care.

It then goes on to specify that understanding of research methods, ethics and governance are needed so that registered nurses can critically analyse research evidence, safely use this evidence and apply research findings in practice to inform best nursing practice (1.7). It is also specified that evidence-based practice needs to be safely demonstrated when undertaking and delivering the skills and procedures outlined in Annexes A and B (1.20). Furthermore, evidence-based practice is also identified as required for the development of person-centred plans of nursing care (3.5), and the importance of being a role model for the provision of evidence-based person-centred care is explicitly stated. All these required areas of competence mean that developing an understanding of, and being able to promote evidence-based care, are integral elements of your role as a learning disability nurse.

EVIDENCE-BASED PRACTICE

As has been seen from the introduction to this chapter, evidence-based practice is a core feature of safe and effective nursing practice. Indeed, the NMC Code (2018b) states that as a nurse you must always practice in line with 'best available evidence' and ensure that any advice you provide is also based on such evidence. However, what does 'evidence-based practice' mean and what is the 'best' evidence?

Schalock et al (2017, p 115) state that evidence-based practices are those practices *'for which there is a demonstrated relation between specific practices and measured outcomes'*. This suggests that there is a focus on cause (interventions) and effects (outcomes achieved) and that ways of assessing the impact of the former on the latter are available. In turn, this requires that a systematic and scientific approach to assessment is adopted and hence that research is undertaken to explore the impact of interventions. However, it also raises the question as to whether all outcomes can be measured and has implications for the type(s) of research needed. This point will be returned to later in the chapter when considering the types of evidence needed.

Craig and Dowding (2020) argue that evidence-based practice *'aims to deliver appropriate care in an efficient manner to individual patients so that the optimum outcome can be achieved'*. Here the same link between care/interventions and the outcomes achieved is noted and this is concerned with the effectiveness of any interventions. In other words, 'does it work'? Indeed, all of us, when consenting to receive a particular treatment or intervention expect that it will work and achieve our desired outcomes whether that be cure or effective management. We would probably be reluctant to receive any treatment if a practitioner told us that there is no evidence that it works. However, in this definition another element is introduced – the need to provide care in an 'efficient' manner. Efficiency is concerned with making best use of available resources and avoiding waste. For example, if an intervention is not effective for an individual but it is continued then this would not be making best use of available resources.

The NICE plays a key role in assisting policymakers and clinicians to deliver evidence-based care through the critical appraisal of evidence and the development of evidence-based guidelines, care pathways and quality standards for a wide range of treatments and conditions. When considering effectiveness NICE also consider efficiency and the cost-benefits of interventions.

Critical reflection 4.1

- Visit the NICE website (www.nice.org.uk) and familiarise yourself with the resources available there.

Aveyard and Sharp (2017) suggest that evidence-based practice has three key integrated elements each of which has equal value:

1. best available evidence;

2. clinical judgement; and

3. patient/service user values and experiences.

Each of these elements are explored in turn.

'Best' evidence

As has been mentioned above, the NMC (2018b) states that as a nurse you should base your practice on the 'best available' evidence. However, what constitutes 'best' evidence and how do we recognise it?

If available, then research conducted to accepted scientific standards is usually considered to be the 'best' evidence since it is undertaken in a systematic manner and is less likely to be biased. Jolley (2020) therefore argues that where research is available then other sources of evidence can be viewed as '*less than adequate*' but that when relevant research is not available it may be appropriate to use other forms of evidence. Such alternatives may, for example, include opinion papers and policies. They also encompass clinical audit, benchmarking, established clinical expertise, tradition and experience (Jolley, 2020). Some of these sources of evidence might be viewed as anecdotal and it is important to exercise due caution when drawing upon them to inform your practice. However, Aveyard and Sharp (2017) suggest that they can make a helpful contribution to your clinical decision-making, can provide contextual information and can assist with identifying what is common practice.

Jolley (2020, p 4) defines research as '*any enquiry that is systematic in its approach and that seeks to ensure that the results of the enquiry cannot be criticised on the grounds of poor technique*'. From this definition, it is possible to see that when we are considering research it is important that we consider not only what has been researched but also how the research has been undertaken. For this reason, a later section of this chapter will introduce you to the concept of critically appraising research to ensure that when reviewing research to inform your practice you can be confident that it has been conducted according to accepted criteria of quality.

In terms of research, you are probably familiar with quantitative research (that which is associated with measurement and where results are presented numerically) and qualitative research (where data are gathered, analysed and presented as words and where the focus is on seeking to determine certain qualities). You may also have come across what is often referred to as 'mixed methods' research in which both quantitative and qualitative data are gathered.

In the context of evidence-based practice, it is common to refer to what is known as the 'hierarchy' of evidence in which randomised controlled trials (RCTs) and systematic reviews are viewed as the strongest forms of evidence at the top of the hierarchy. The rationale for this is that the design of RCTs means that they involve randomly assigning participants to two or more groups where one group receives a particular intervention or treatment (the intervention group) while the other group receives either no intervention or usual care (the control group). Randomly assigning participants means that each group should be similar in terms of (for example) age, gender, socio-economic status. This avoids any bias that might occur should the researcher decide who should go in which group. Given that each group should be similar in terms of characteristics any difference in terms of outcomes can then be attributed to the intervention or treatment since this is the factor that differs between two groups. To further strengthen the evidence in some studies there is what is known as 'blinding' which means that the participants and the researchers are not aware of which group an individual is in. This means that potential impact of thinking that an intervention will work (or not) is reduced. Of course, this is not possible in all situations since (for example) participants will know if they are attending an exercise class or not. However, in other situations it may be possible by (for example) providing placebo medication for the control group.

The RCT is therefore designed to be undertaken in a systematic manner, to reduce bias and to produce valid and reliable evidence. A systematic review will usually encompass several RCTs on a particular subject and therefore if similar results are found across such RCTs then this is viewed as even stronger evidence. However, while RCTs are the appropriate research design for determining whether an intervention is effective they cannot answer questions such as those that relate to issues such as how participants feel about the intervention or the perceptions of clinical staff. For this reason, many RCTs are also now encompassing a qualitative element to the study since (as discussed below) patient/service user perceptions of acceptability are a key element of evidence-based practice.

Rather than thinking solely in hierarchical terms of RCTs being 'strong' evidence and qualitative research being 'weak' evidence it is therefore better to consider whether a chosen research approach is appropriate to the research question it seeks to answer. If the question is focused on effectiveness, then an RCT is likely to be required. However, if the research question asks (for example) 'What do people with learning disabilities feel about ...?' then a qualitative research approach will be appropriate.

Clinical/professional judgement

Critical appraisal of the available evidence (see later section in this chapter) may demonstrate that a particular intervention is the most effective for a given condition. However, before this information can be used to inform practice then clinical judgement (the second element of evidence-based practice) needs to be applied. For example, a treatment may be 99.9 per cent effective but what if the individual you are supporting is one of the 0.1 per cent for whom it is not effective? Should you continue with that treatment because it has been identified as 'best practice' even where (in the context of a particular individual) it is ineffective, or should an alternative treatment be identified? Similarly, what if the most effective treatment for a particular infection is a form of penicillin and the individual you are supporting is allergic to penicillin?

As a learning disability nurse, therefore, it is important that not only are you aware of which interventions constitute best evidence but also that you have a good understanding of those you support and that you are able to make an informed clinical decision as to what is appropriate. Later sections of this chapter will assist you in developing the necessary knowledge and skills to access, appraise and apply evidence.

Individual/patient preference

The third key element of evidence-based practice relates to the preference of the individual who is the proposed recipient of an intervention. The reason for this is that even where a particular intervention has been assessed as being the most effective for a condition/problem, and professional judgement supports this view in relation to a specific individual, if it is not acceptable to that individual then it is unlikely to be effective. For example, a medication may be prescribed for an individual, but they feel that the side effects are not acceptable to them and hence they are not willing to take it. Alternatively, a particular behavioural support intervention may be recommended for an individual, but their family may feel that they do not have the resources to deliver it consistently.

Of course, it is essential that, where an individual has capacity to make a decision regarding their treatment, such decisions are respected even where others judge them to be unwise. However, if individuals are to make informed decisions regarding their care and support, they need to understand the nature of the intervention, any alternatives that may be available, and any associated risks and benefits (Dowding, 2020). In relation to supporting people with a learning disability, this means that it is important that information is provided in a way that is understandable to an individual, and this requires careful consideration of the format and content of the information as well as the pace at which the information is delivered. It is also important to check for understanding and to encourage questioning.

> ## *Critical reflection 4.2*
>
> Think of an individual with mild learning disabilities that you support and imagine that they have been prescribed a new medication for a long-standing health condition that has recently deteriorated.
>
> - How would you explain the new medication to the individual?
> - What methods would you use?
> - How would you check to see that they have understood and retained the information and were making an informed decision to take (or not take) the medication?

There will, however, be times when an individual who has capacity refuses to accept medication or another intervention and, as a learning disability nurse, it is important to try to understand why an individual is refusing. It might be that they do not fully understand what it will entail and that further clear explanation in a format they can understand with sufficient time being provided to process this information could address their concerns. Alternatively, it could be that they have a specific fear (for example of needles) or that they have previously had a bad experience. Here some desensitisation may be helpful. Listening to the concerns of the individual, providing information and exploring alternative approaches may thus enable an acceptable solution to be found.

Case study 4.1

Asif Aktar is 19 years old and lives with his parents and younger sisters. The family all attend the local Mosque, and their religion plays a central role in their lives. Asif enjoys attending the Mosque and is very proud to be Muslim. He has a mild learning disability and attends the local further education college where he is undertaking a life skills course for young people with learning disabilities.

Asif has experienced epileptic seizures since he was a young child. These are generally well controlled by medication and his parents have ensured that he regularly attends his neurology appointments, so he receives the most clinically effective treatment for his epilepsy. Recently, however, he started to have frequent seizures and his parents have become very concerned requesting that the community learning disability nurse visit to assess what is happening.

The community learning disability nurse spoke with Asif and he disclosed that although his parents had been giving him his regular medication he was not taking it. When asked why he said that someone at college had said they didn't think that people who are Muslim were allowed to take medication. This had concerned him as he then thought that he was doing wrong by taking his tablets but didn't want to upset his parents and so just stopped taking the medication. The community nurse arranged for the Iman from the Mosque to speak with Asif to reassure him that it was acceptable to take the medication, Asif recommended his medication and his seizures subsided.

EVIDENCE-BASED PRACTICE AND LEARNING DISABILITY NURSING

Kay (1995) stressed the importance of learning disability nursing, as part of the wider profession of nursing, having adequate research-based knowledge to inform professional practice. However, he also commented that learning disability nursing was some way from achieving this arguing that much of the knowledge base regarding learning disabilities at that time came from disciplines such as psychology, medicine and education.

Writing some five years later, Parahoo et al (2000) also concluded that *'For evidenced based practice to become a reality in learning disability nursing a great deal needs to be done'*. To effect change they argued that several actions were needed including greater access to research, training in the use of technology and a culture which is supportive of, and encourages use of, research in clinical practice. However, they also stated that there needs to be more research that is specific to the field of learning disability nursing.

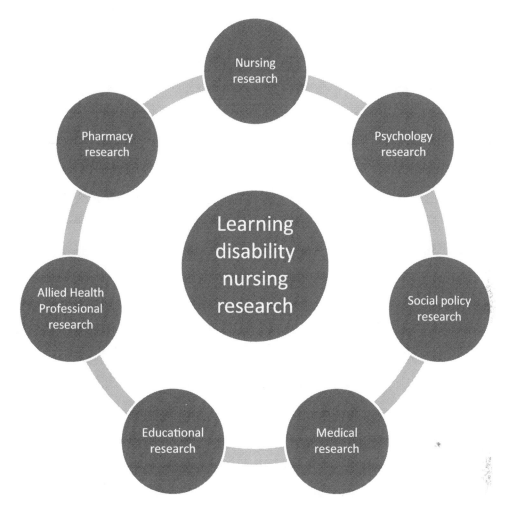

Figure 4.1 Locating learning disability nursing research in context

Gates and Atherton (2001) noted that much of the evidence that learning disability nurses draw upon in practice comes from different academic and professional backgrounds. Figure 4.1 identifies how learning disability nursing research is located in the context of other academic and professional disciplines and, to some extent, this is inevitable given that learning disability nurses work in an interdisciplinary context. For example, it is possible that, as a community learning disability nurse, you may be working alongside a psychiatrist, a psychologist and an occupational therapist to support an individual with complex behavioural support needs. In such a situation then the evidence used to inform a care plan is likely to be drawn from this range of disciplines to ensure the most effective care is delivered. In addition, when the effectiveness of interventions is being assessed then it is likely that the team delivering such interventions will be interdisciplinary. Finally, as a learning disability nurse you will also need to draw upon wider nursing research to inform your practice. For example, if you are supporting an individual who requires wound care then the wider nursing evidence relating to wound care will need to be accessed to ensure the most appropriate care.

This does raise the question: 'what is learning disability nursing research?' It might take many forms including:

o   research undertaken by learning disability nurses about any topic;

o   research which focuses specifically on the role of the learning disability nurse;

o   research that evaluates the outcomes of interventions delivered by learning disability nurses;

o   research undertaken by nurses (or others) that focuses on the nursing care of people with learning disabilities.

Griffiths et al (2009) undertook a systematic scoping review of learning disability nursing research. In the context of this study, learning disability nursing research was defined as that which focused on *the work of people in nursing roles (whether specialist trained or not) in any care setting (including the community or institutional settings) with people with learning disabilities, their carers and family members*'. It can thus be seen that a very broad definition was used and included not only those areas listed in the bullet points above but also research that focused on families and carers of those with learning disabilities.

One hundred and eighty relevant papers were identified and reviewed many of which involved small-scale convenience samples with few focused on the clinical outcomes of learning disability nursing or on care delivery by learning disability nurses. Griffiths et al (2009) concluded that, at that time,

> *the body of learning disability nursing research as a whole is not fully fit for purpose in terms of its extent, quality or quantity if a significant part of its purpose is to develop and evaluate interventions for practice and in practice.*

They therefore recommended the development of research focused on learning disability nursing interventions and services, and the experience of people with learning disabilities and their carers. To achieve this the development of high-quality programmes of research was advocated along with a collaborative approach (including international links).

In this context it is perhaps not surprising that the Strengthening the Commitment report (Scottish Government et al, 2012) recommended that there was a need to further develop the evidence base to develop the profession of learning disability nursing, to ensure that practice is evidence-based and to be able to demonstrate the impact of interventions. To achieve this, it was argued that learning disability nursing required support for:

o   research activity;

o   research training;

o   implementation of research findings in practice.

Subsequent sections of this chapter, therefore, focus on supporting you to develop the knowledge and skills required to access, appraise and apply research and other evidence in practice. It then returns to consideration of what needs to be done to further develop the evidence base for learning disability nursing.

ACCESSING EVIDENCE

The first step in evidence-based practice is identifying what evidence is currently available, and this requires that you possess the necessary knowledge and skills. In some instances, you may find that there are NICE guidelines which provide you with an overview of what constitutes best evidence-based practice for the condition or intervention that you are interested in. Accessing the NICE and SCIE (Social Care Institute of Excellence) webpages to see what work has already been undertaken in a particular area can, therefore, be a helpful starting point. Alternatively, you may identify a recent systematic review focused on your topic of interest.

However, in many cases you will not find that a current critical appraisal of evidence exists for a clinical issue or problem that you are interested in, and you will therefore need to undertake a literature search. When undertaking such a search it is essential that you approach the task in a systematic manner so that you (and others) can be confident that the search has been thorough and unbiased. One test of a good search is that someone else could take the search strategy that you have documented, follow it and obtain the same results. Documenting your decision-making and outcomes in relation to each of the following is therefore important.

o   What is the question you are seeking to answer by undertaking the literature search?

o   Which search terms did you use and how did you use them?

o   Which electronic databases did you use?

o   How many 'hits' did you get for each combination of search terms in each database?

o   Did you use any other strategies to identify possible items for inclusion in your search?

o   Which inclusion and exclusion criteria did you apply to your results?

o   How many papers/articles did you include in your review?

Each of these areas are discussed in turn.

Identifying a clear question

Identifying a clear question that you wish to answer when undertaking a literature search is important to ensure that the search is focused and so that you do not become swamped with information that is not relevant to you (Aveyard and Sharp, 2017). Your question is likely to start as an area of clinical interest – for example, you may be wondering how best to support a service user with diabetes. You might find it helpful to use one of the recognised frameworks such as PICO (Sackett et al, 1997) or SPICE (Booth, 2006) which support you to ensure that key elements are included in your question.

PICO (Sackett et al, 1997) stands for:

o Population – which population are you concerned with, for example, children or adults with learning disabilities. Are you concerned with all those with learning disabilities or just those with severe/profound learning disabilities or mild learning disabilities?

o Intervention – this might, for example, be a medication, behavioural intervention or psychological therapy.

o Comparison – it is not always possible to identify a comparison intervention, but you might, for example, wish to compare the evidence for the use of medication versus a psychological therapy or one medication versus another.

o Outcome – this might, for example, relate to effective glycaemic control (for diabetes) or a reduction in the number of seizures (for epilepsy).

SPICE (Booth, 2006) stands for:

o Setting – where an intervention or treatment occurs can have a bearing on how it is experienced, people's behaviours and beliefs.

o Perspective – whose perspective are you concerned with. In other words, who are the people who are the focus of the intervention.

o Interest – what is the phenomenon of interest? Is it a particular intervention or treatment?

o Comparison – what is the intervention being compared with (if anything)?

o Evaluation – how is the effectiveness or impact to be evaluated?

If the PICO framework is applied to the clinical question suggested above, you might end up with a research question such as 'How effective are adapted diabetes self-management programmes (intervention) in achieving glycaemic control (outcome) for people with mild learning disabilities (population) when compared with standard diabetes self-management programmes (comparison)?'. You can then see that by underlining the 'PICO' elements you have the basis for key search terms to include in your search.

Identifying your search terms

Having identified your key search terms from your question it is important to also identify synonyms for these keywords. So, for example, to continue the example above you might (in addition to 'diabetes self-management') also include 'diabetes management', 'DESMOND programme' (a recognised diabetes self-management programme) and 'diabetes education'.

Using alternative terms is especially relevant when undertaking a search in relation to learning disability since several terms have been used both across time and across the globe to refer to what we in the UK understand as 'learning disability'. Perhaps the most used alternative internationally is 'intellectual disability' and in Ireland this is the term that is used when referring to specialist nurses in this field of practice – they are Registered Nurses (Intellectual Disability). However, there are other terms that you may need to also consider using in a search such as 'developmental disability', 'cognitive disability' and (particularly if searching for historical material) 'mental retardation' and 'mental handicap'.

A couple of words of caution also need to be offered here regarding terminology. While the term 'developmental disability' is widely used in some parts of the world such as North America it is used to refer not only to those who, in the UK, would be considered to have a learning disability but also those with other developmental conditions such as autism and cerebral palsy (who may not have an associated learning disability). Second, while in the UK we use the term 'learning disability' in the US this term is used to refer to those with what we would term specific learning disabilities such as dyslexia and dyscalculia. This means that it is important to have clear inclusion and exclusion criteria (see below), that you carefully review papers to ensure that they meet your criteria, and to exercise caution when comparing studies undertaken in different countries as their inclusion criteria may differ.

When you have identified your key terms you need to then think about how you will use them in different combinations to ensure that you identify as many sources as possible. You need to carefully consider the term you use to link your individual search terms since they will give different results. These linking words are known as 'Boolean operators' and they include 'or', 'and' and 'not'. Examples of the different impact each word has are illustrated in Table 4.1.

Table 4.1 Use of Boolean operators in searches

Term 1	Boolean operator	Term 2	Results
Learning disability	or	Nursing	Papers that focus on learning disability and papers that focus on nursing but not necessarily on both. So, for example, you would be likely to retrieve many papers focused on other areas of nursing practice.
Learning disability	and	Nursing	Papers that focus on both nursing and learning disability
Learning disability	not	Nursing	Papers that focus on learning disability but which exclude any relating to nursing

Choosing your databases

There are several electronic databases which are available to assist you with searching for relevant papers to address your question. You should have access to these via your university or health board library. Different databases index different journals and so to ensure that you identify all available sources it is important that you search more than one database. Some useful databases for learning disability nursing are set out in Table 4.2.

Table 4.2 Some electronic databases relevant to learning disability nursing

Name of database	Key areas covered
CINAHL	Nursing, medicine and allied health professions
Medline	Medical and healthcare literature including nursing
PsychInfo	Primarily psychology literature but health, developmental and behavioural psychology are all pertinent to learning disability nursing
ASSIA	Health and social care disciplines including nursing, social work, psychology and allied health
ProQuest Central	Multidisciplinary database which includes nursing and medicine
NICE Database	Current evidence concerning treatments, interventions and technologies
SCIE Database	Evidence-based guidance and resources for social care
Cochrane Database	Database of systematic reviews

Each database will have slightly different functionalities – for example, CINAHL allows you to search using different categories such as whether your chosen keywords appear anywhere in the paper, in the title or in the abstract. It also allows you to search for 'intellectual disability or mental retardation or learning disability or developmental disability or learning disabilities' as one term rather than having to search separately using individual alternative terms for 'learning disability'.

It is worth familiarising yourself with various databases and their functionality. You may find that your university learning resources centre will either provide sessions on database searching or produce guidance. It can also be very helpful to enlist the support of a specialist librarian (located in your university or health trust library) when planning and undertaking a search.

Recording your 'hits'

It is important to keep a record of your search results and so you might find it helpful to construct yourself a table such as that below (Table 4.3) to enter all your results with each database.

Table 4.3 Example of table to record database 'hits'

Database			
Search term 1	Boolean operator	Search term 2	Number of hits

Using additional search strategies

In addition to undertaking database searches, it can also be helpful to use additional search strategies. One useful strategy here is to review the reference lists of papers you have found during your online searches to see if they cite any papers of potential relevance to your question that have not already been identified. Another strategy is to review the table of contents of key journals in the field to identify potential papers. If you use such approaches, make sure that you record the number of papers identified using this approach.

Identifying and applying inclusion and exclusion criteria

Having undertaken your searches, you will then need to review the results to identify the papers that are most relevant to address your question. You do this by clearly identifying your inclusion and exclusion criteria so that you can assess each 'hit' or result against these criteria to decide as to whether they are suitable for your review.

Examples of inclusion criteria might include:

o   papers published after a certain date (to make sure that you access the most current evidence);

o   only empirical research or systematic reviews (to access the strongest evidence);

o   only research using a particular study design (eg if you want to determine whether an intervention is effective you may need to limit your search to include only systematic reviews and experimental studies);

o   only papers focusing on a particular population (eg adults with learning disabilities);

o   only papers focusing on a particular location (eg community or hospital settings).

Examples of exclusion criteria might include:

o   papers published before a certain date;

o   opinion papers and editorials (depending on the focus of your search and the extent of literature available it may be appropriate to use these sources in certain circumstances);

o   papers focused on a particular population (eg if your area of interest is adults with a learning disability then studies that focus only on children with a learning disability might be excluded).

Finalising the papers included in your review

In your search results you will see some duplicate results (the same paper listed in more than one database). A first step is therefore to remove multiple copies and leave only one, making a note of how many 'hits' are excluded using this approach. Having done this you can then review the remaining hits against your inclusion and exclusion criteria retaining only those that meet all your inclusion criteria. In some instances, you will be able to do this by reviewing just the title of the paper and the abstract. However, in other instances it may be necessary to obtain the full text of a paper before being able to decide. For example, a title may suggest it is relevant, and the abstract supports this, but closer reading of the full paper indicates that perhaps either the study location is not appropriate or that the study population does not meet your inclusion criteria. Once again make a note of how many 'hits' are excluded having undertaken this review along with the reasons for excluding them (eg not meeting key inclusion criteria).

Having worked through this process, you should now be left with several papers that are relevant to your review and you are ready to proceed to the next stage of critically appraising them. Before doing so, however, remember to make a note of how many papers you are including.

Critical reflection 4.3

- Consider the following literature search question and identify synonyms for the words underlined: 'How effective are talking therapies when seeking to address mental health problems experienced by people with learning disabilities?'

CRITICAL APPRAISAL OF EVIDENCE

Not all research that is published is suitable for making decisions regarding care delivery and therefore it is important to develop the knowledge and skills required to critically appraise research (Lancaster and McCray, 2020). As Aveyard and Sharp (2017) observe, it is crucial you ensure that you have the best evidence available rather than just any evidence.

It is important not to confuse 'critical appraisal' with 'criticism' since while it is essential that any weaknesses in research are identified, appraisal needs to be broader than this. The aim is to take a systematic and balanced approach to identifying the strengths and weaknesses of a study and then to consider the implications of these in terms of the value that can be placed on the study, and its relevance to practice. Lancaster and McCray (2020) suggest that there are three elements to critical appraisal.

1. Is the quality of the research good enough to provide results/findings that can inform clinical decision-making?

2. Are the findings applicable in the setting you are working in?

3. What are the results and what do they mean for your patients/those you support?

There are many frameworks available to assist you with critically appraising a research paper. For example, many research textbooks will include a section or chapter which provides a series of questions to help you to determine the strengths and weaknesses of a study. Using such a framework can be very helpful as it will assist you with making a balanced judgement rather than trying to assess a paper in a random manner. This will strengthen the quality of your review.

There are also other frameworks available online to assist you with undertaking a critical appraisal. For example, the Critical Skills Appraisal Programme (CASP) provides a number of checklists that can be used to assess different types of research designs, such as RCTs, systematic reviews and qualitative studies (CASP, nda). It is important that you use the appropriate checklist to assess the type of study you are reviewing since using a quantitative checklist to assess a qualitative study is like using a ruler to try and assess the temperature of something: assessment using inappropriate criteria will not give you an accurate appraisal.

Other critical appraisal tools/checklists can be found on the Joanna Briggs Institute website (JBI, nd). In addition to the range of critical appraisal checklists, this site also provides a range of resources to support evidence-based practice.

When undertaking a critical appraisal of a research paper, it is possible that you will encounter research terms that you are not familiar with. If this occurs, then use one of the available research glossaries that can be found either in many research methods textbooks or on the CASP website (CASP, ndb) to provide you with a definition of that term. Doing this will not only extend your knowledge in relation to research terms and methods but it will also provide you with clear criteria against which to appraise the study.

For example, you may come across a study that describes itself as a RCT in which participants were allocated to either an experimental group (who receive an intervention) or a control group (who receive usual care). The CASP glossary says that in an RCT, participants should be randomly assigned to one of two or more groups but, in the paper you are reviewing, it is not clear how participants were assigned to a group. In this instance you might express concerns regarding the rigour of the study as it is not clear whether there was randomisation and, if this was not present, then this might impact on the reliability of the results.

You can also use research methods textbooks to assist you in identifying objective criteria against which to assess research papers. For example, a textbook might say that an acceptable response rate for a postal survey is X% but the study reported in the paper you are reviewing received a much lower response rate. You might then express concern about the reliability of the results and the potential to generalise from them due to this low response rate.

Critical reflection 4.4

Identify and download a research paper that you feel is relevant to your practice.

- Read through it and identify any terms that you are not familiar with and consult a glossary or research methods textbook to provide you with a definition.

- Having obtained the definition return to the research paper and assess whether you feel that the research described by the author(s) meets the criteria outlined in the definition.

- If it does not meet the criteria think about the implications of this in terms of how confident you would then be to consider using the research to inform your practice.

When critically appraising research studies in relation to a specific question, you might find it helpful to record key features of the studies in a table such as the example provided in Table 4.4. Additional columns can be added as required. This will assist you with being able to look across the various studies and to be able to identify similarities and differences in (for example) sample sizes, methods and key findings.

Table 4.4 Example of a table to record key features of papers reviewed

Author	Year	Reference	Sample/ participants	Methods	Key findings	Key strengths and weaknesses

Undertaking a systematic critical appraisal of research is an essential step in the development of evidence-based practice. However, once you have undertaken such an appraisal you also need to consider whether the evidence is appropriate to use in practice. To do this requires both consideration of its appropriateness to the patients/individuals you are supporting and consideration of the appropriateness to the context within this the intervention will be delivered. For example, you may be able to identify a good evidence base for self-management of diabetes in the wider population, but would it be appropriate to try and transfer it directly to supporting people with learning disabilities without considering the need to make adjustments? Similarly, there may be a strong evidence base for a particular intervention to be used in residential settings where there is 24-hour nursing support for people with learning disabilities, but could this be transferred to a community setting where only visiting nursing support is available?

If you have critically appraised the evidence and reviewed its appropriateness for the service user group you are supporting, and the context within the support will be delivered, and are confident that a change in practice is required (based on the evidence), you then need to think about how you will bring about that change in practice. This means that it is important to think about how to use evidence in practice and to understand how a culture of evidence-based practice can be developed and sustained (see also Chapter 10).

USING EVIDENCE IN PRACTICE

Thompson and Quinian (2020) argue that if organisational culture is not considered when seeking to implement research evidence then the change is likely to fail. An evidence-based culture, they suggest, is one that promotes decision-making in which appropriate weight is given to research evidence, patient preference, availability of resources and clinical expertise at all levels of an organisation. But this then raises the question of how such a culture can be promoted.

Recognising the need for strategic leadership at the highest level, the Chief Nursing Officer for England launched 'Making Research Matter', a strategic action plan for research in November 2021 (May, 2021). This document argues that a 'research-enabled' and 'research-active' nursing workforce is essential in promoting quality of care, protecting health and promoting public health. However, it also notes that support to use research in practice is essential if care is to be transformed. To achieve this, they argue that using evidence and contributing to research need to be made as accessible as possible for nurses so that the benefits of nurses engaging in such activities are realised. Actions are therefore set out in the document to translate the vision into practice, and it aims to provide guidance and direction to senior leaders within healthcare organisations.

If a culture of evidence-based practice is not in existence, then change is necessary and an important element of managing effective change is to be able to identify exactly what needs to be considered and addressed. Thompson and Quinian (2020) suggest that there are three key dimensions – the innovation, the individuals and groups involved and the system within which the innovation is to be introduced. However, they also add a fourth dimension which is the linkages between the other three dimensions since they are all interdependent. So, for example, if you were seeking to introduce a change in practice based on the best available evidence it would be important to clarify exactly what is the nature of change required (what is current practice, what is best practice and what needs to change). You would then need to consider who would need to be involved (eg their readiness for change, whether they possess the necessary knowledge and skills) and the system (eg what resources are available, what policies are in place, what support is there for change). Specifically, from the perspective of learning disability nursing it is also important to consider individuals with a learning disability themselves and their families/carers when thinking about who needs to be involved, to remember what was said earlier in this chapter about acceptability to patients/service users and ensure that they are provided with timely information in an accessible format.

Through consideration of each of the areas identified by Thompson and Quinian (2020), it is possible to identify any potential barriers to change and seek to eliminate these or to reduce their impact. A further consideration when implementing an evidence-based change in practice is the need to plan for evaluation from the beginning of the process. It is important to understand what impact any change in practice has and for this to happen it is important to compare before and after as well as to gather information regarding acceptability of the change to those involved.

This discussion about strategic plans and organisational culture might seem somewhat removed from your current role as a student nurse. However, there are things that you can do to help promote an evidence-based culture in clinical practice and to help others understand the value of research. For example, completion of your academic assignments (particularly a dissertation) requires that you search, analyse and synthesise the most current literature. Have you considered sharing your findings with colleagues in clinical practice? They might not have the time to research a topic and may not have the same access as you do to resources such as electronic databases. By sharing your findings, you will be assisting them in better understanding current evidence and discussion with them will help you (and them) to consider the implications for clinical practice.

Another strategy you might use is to set up a journal club. Here a specific paper is chosen, and everyone reads it prior to meeting. However, one person takes responsibility for introducing the paper and their impressions of its strengths and weaknesses before opening it up for wider discussion. Such an activity can help all involved to better under-stand research and enhance their skills in relation to critical appraisal in a safe setting.

DEVELOPING THE EVIDENCE BASE FOR LEARNING DISABILITY NURSING

As was noted earlier in this chapter, concerns have been raised concerning the limited evidence base within learning disability nursing (Griffiths et al, 2009) and the need to develop the evidence base has been noted (Scottish Government et al, 2012). Since 2012 there has been some development of the body of research relating to learning disability nursing both in the UK and internationally. This section of the chapter will, however, explore what is needed to further address this agenda and develop sustainable programmes of research.

Different roles

It is important to note that evidence-based practice is a professional responsibility of all nurses. Nonetheless, as Figure 4.2 shows, the nature of involvement with evidence and research will vary according to roles, responsibilities and chosen career path. At the left of the figure, it shows that all learning disability nurses have a responsibility to be able to access, critically appraise and use evidence to inform their practice. The earlier sections of this chapter have, therefore, sought to provide you with knowledge and skills to assist you in developing this element of your professional role. Some practitioners will progress to actively being involved in research studies and to undertaking their own research.

As the figure moves towards the right, the level of involvement in research increases and the number of practitioners involved reduces. Nonetheless, it is essential that the career of some learning disability nurses moves them into roles where they lead teams of researchers and have strategic responsibility for the development of research. This will ensure that learning disability nursing has a voice in strategic discussions regarding research and that there are individuals to provide leadership and mentorship for those wishing to develop the research elements of their role.

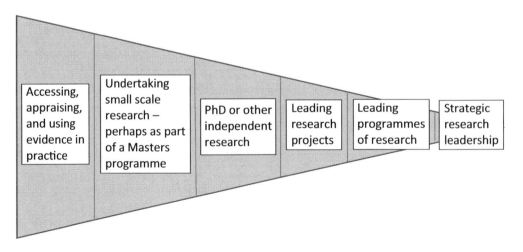

Figure 4.2 Levels of involvement in research

As a student learning disability nurse, the idea of leading research teams may seem a long way off or may be something that you have not considered at all. However, the foundations are being laid during your nurse education and this means that it is important to use this opportunity to develop your understanding of research and evidence-based practice. It is essential that the evidence base for learning disability nursing is extended and that programmes of research are developed in a sustainable manner. This requires the development of champions and leaders of research in both academic and clinical settings, and you are the future champions and leaders.

Research is very much a 'team sport' which requires on collaboration and on different individuals bringing different knowledge and skills to the process of planning, under-taking and disseminating research. For example, some bring experience and expertise in relation to research design while others bring strengths in relation to data analysis. Some nurses working in clinical settings may feel that they do not wish to be involved in undertaking research, but they can still play an essential and important role in the devel-opment of research through contribution of their clinical knowledge and skills. Research that is relevant to practice needs to be rooted in practice and clinical practitioners can play an essential role in identifying research questions, in advising regarding the practi-calities of undertaking research in their clinical setting and in analysing the implications of research findings for practice. They can thus be key members of a research team.

Critical reflection 4.5

Think about a clinical area that you have recently worked in and identify an aspect of practice where you think research might be useful.

- Identify a research question that would address this area of practice.

- When developing your question think carefully about whether it is a 'how', 'why', 'when' or 'who' question.

- How would you design research to answer the question?

Case study 4.2

Anna Smith is a registered learning disability nurse who qualified four years ago. Since qualifying she has undertaken a master's degree and as part of this she undertook a research module and submitted a literature review-based disserta-tion. She very much enjoyed the research module and her dissertation made her realise how little research there is in some areas of learning disability nursing. In her current role as a community learning disability nurse, she has recognised that a lot of her time and that of her colleagues is focused on promoting access to healthcare for people with learning disabilities but that they don't have any real evidence of the impact of their interventions. She would very much like to

→

undertake research in this area but doesn't feel confident as to where to start. Her line manager is supportive of the idea of this research as they feel that evidence of impact would assist the nursing team in securing senior management support to extend their staffing levels and to extend the range of services they can offer. They therefore suggest that Anna contacts the health trust's research and development department to discuss her ideas with them. Anna contacts them and they talk her through what would be involved, suggest other people she might wish to speak with and put her in contact with an experienced researcher in the trust who also has an interest in this area.

Promoting an inclusive approach to research

Working in partnership with people with learning disabilities and their families and carers is fundamental to learning disability nursing practice and this value base also needs to encompass our research practice. If we are to extend and expand the research base for learning disability nursing, this needs to be undertaken by working with people with learning disabilities as active partners in the research process, recognising the experience and expertise that they bring to the research team.

People with learning disabilities have often been excluded from active participation in research. There are two main reasons for this. First, historically people with learning disabilities (and other key groups) have sometimes been badly treated and harmed during research. For example, during the Second World War people with learning disabilities in Germany were subjected to unethical experiments which, in many instances, led to their death (Iacono and Carling-Jenkins, 2012). These practices were exposed during the Nuremberg Trials, which led to the Nuremberg Code and eventually to the Helsinki Declaration that sought to protect the rights of participants in biomedical research (Iacono and Carling-Jenkins, 2012).

Another example of harm being caused to individuals with learning disabilities in the context of research that is often cited is the case of Willowbrook Hospital in the US. Here, poor and overcrowded living conditions for children with learning disabilities within a state institution meant that viral hepatitis was widespread among those living there. In this context an experiment was established in which some children were deliberately infected with hepatitis with the aim of developing a vaccine. Those leading the study argued that, given the prevalence of hepatitis within Willowbrook the children would be at high risk of contracting it anyway and that those who were to be deliberately infected would be cared for in a special, well-staffed unit. They also argued that any additional harm that might be experienced by the children would be outweighed by the benefits of a vaccine. However, those opposing the research argue that it is never acceptable to knowingly infect individuals and that the standards for ensuring free and valid consent from parents for their children to participate were insufficient. Further information regarding Willowbrook can be found in the Resources section.

In both cases described above people with learning disabilities were experimented on with little or no regard for issues such as harm and valid consent. The Declaration of

Helsinki (World Medical Association, 2013) therefore states that '*some groups and individuals are particularly vulnerable and may have an increased likelihood of being wronged or of incurring additional harm*'. People with learning disabilities are one such group and hence it is essential that appropriate safeguards are in place to ensure that their rights are respected and upheld in the context of research. When critically reviewing research, therefore, you should always pay attention to how ethical issues within the research are identified and addressed. In addition, as a learning disability nurse you may be in the position of 'gatekeeper' where a researcher wishes to access those you support to participate in research. Being aware of the ethical issues that can arise and how they should be addressed is therefore an important element of your professional role.

While recognising the need to ensure that appropriate safeguards need to be in place, the fact that people with learning disabilities are viewed as a 'vulnerable' group in the context of research has sometimes made researchers and ethics committees reluctant to develop and approve research that supports their active participation. It is sometimes viewed as too difficult to do. However, it also needs to be understood that denying the right of people with learning disabilities to participate in research if they wish to do so has ethical consequences. If their views and experiences are not heard in the context of research that focuses on their lives, then questions need to be asked regarding the validity of that research. If people with learning disabilities are therefore not to be marginalised in the context of research we need to develop appropriate ways of working together – a point that will be returned to below.

The second reason that people with learning disabilities have often been excluded from participation in research is that they have often been viewed as being 'unable' to make a meaningful contribution and to possess the necessary skills to participate. Traditionally participating in research has involved being able to undertake tasks that require certain literacy skills. For example, being able to read and understand an information sheet, sign a consent form and complete a written questionnaire. Even where other methods have been used to gather data, such as interviews and focus groups, people with learning disabilities have often been perceived as not having the verbal skills required to participate in a meaningful way.

However, over recent years this perception has changed, and it is now widely accepted that people with learning disabilities are best placed to comment on their lives and that their views and experiences should be central to research that focuses on their lives. To facilitate this, attention has shifted to considering how the methods we use to undertake research can be adapted to support their inclusion. This has, for example, included the development of easy read materials to support the process of consent and using visual materials to support participation in interviews and focus groups. As a learning disability nurse you may, therefore, have a key role to play in supporting such participation using the knowledge and skills that you have in adapting communication to the needs of those you support.

The participation of people with learning disabilities in research has, however, moved beyond just supporting their participation in research undertaken by other people. They have been involved in setting the agenda for research (Northway et al, 2014a) thus promoting research that is relevant to their self-identified needs and priorities. They have also been involved in designing, undertaking and disseminating research being co-researchers within the context of both funded and unfunded research studies (see, for example, Tuffrey-Wijne and Butler, 2009; Tilly, 2015; Schwartz et al, 2020; Wake et al, 2020) and in securing ethical approval for research (Northway et al, 2014b).

While inclusive approach has, therefore, become much more common Frankena et al (2019) argue that it has tended to be used less frequently in the context of health research. They therefore developed consensus guidelines on how to undertake inclusive health research that identify the attributes, outcomes, reporting and publishing of inclusive research as well as future directions for research. They note, however, that since this is a developing area of research practice there is a need to continually reflect upon such practice and to further develop the guidelines as appropriate.

Support for developing research

As has been mentioned several times in this chapter the development of learning disability nursing research is an essential part of professional practice. Nonetheless, to take forward this agenda, support is required. This support may come in the form of academic support if you are undertaking an educational course such as master's course. You may also access such support if you decide that you wish to undertake a research degree such as an MPhil or PhD. However, even if you are currently not undertaking academic study support is available for those working in clinical practice.

All Health Boards and Trusts will have Research and Development Departments whose role is to support research and development within their service. They can provide advice and support with things such as research design, grant writing and securing the necessary ethical and research governance approvals. If you have an idea for research, or are interested in becoming more involved with research, they can be a good starting point for you to contact.

If you are considering pursuing a career in research then there are a range of National Institute for Health Research websites listed in the Resources section.

As has already been mentioned in this chapter, research is very much teamwork and therefore another helpful strategy if you are seeking to increase your involvement in research is to build and extend your networks. Your links with other people with similar interests and complementary knowledge and skills will be helpful when seeking to build a research team and may also give rise to invitations for you to participate in research lead by others. Further advice regarding networking is provided in Chapter 12.

> ### *Chapter summary*
>
> This chapter has argued that evidence-based practice is an essential element of learning disability nursing practice. As a learning disability nurse, it is important that you develop the knowledge and skills to access and critically appraise research and to use this to inform your practice with individuals you support and to develop effective services and supports. The material discussed in this chapter has aimed to assist you in the process as well as highlighting the need for further development of learning disability nursing research.

FURTHER READING

Craig, J and Dowding, D A (eds) *Evidence-based Practice in Nursing*, 4th edition. Edinburgh: Elsevier.

This book will assist you to further develop your understanding of evidence based care and its relevance to nursing.

World Health Organization Europe (2017) *Facilitating Evidence-based Practice in Nursing and Midwifery in the WHO European Region*. [online] Available at: www.euro.who.int/_ _data/assets/pdf_file/0017/348020/WH06_EBP_report_complete.pdf (accessed 18 January 2022).

This policy document provides a European perspective on the development of evidence based practice in nursing.

RESOURCES

Cochrane Collection: www.cochrane.org (accessed 21 June 2022).

This website contains information regarding the Cochrane Reviews and access the Cochrane Library

Evidence-based Nursing Journal: https://ebn.bmj.com (accessed 21 June 2022).

The website of this journal offers access to their podcasts, blogs as well as details of their articles which are commentaries relating to published research and 'research made simple' articles which provide helpful information regarding different aspects of evidence-based practice. The archive of the latter can be accessed via https://ebn.bmj. com/pages/collections/ebn_research_made_simple/.

Critical Skills Appraisal Project: https://casp-uk.net/casp-tools-checklists (accessed 21 June 2022).

This website hosts checklists to access different types of research design.

Joanna Briggs Institute: https://jbi.global (accessed 21 June 2022).

This website contains resources in relation to critical appraisal of research, systematic reviewing and evidence implementation.

Hepatitis Studies at the Willowbrook State School for Children: https://bioethics research.org/resources/case-studies/hepatitis-studies-at-the-willowbrook-state-school-for-children (accessed 21 June 2022).

This website from the Bioethics Research Center contains further information on the Willowbrook case.

National Institute for Health and Care Research: www.nihr.ac.uk/health-and-care-professionals/ (accessed 21 June 2022).

This website has a range of resources that provide a range of support (www.nihr.ac.uk/hea lth-and-care-professionals/career-development/) and educational resources (www.nihr. ac.uk/health-and-care-professionals/learning-and-support/) and a range of funding schemes (www.nihr.ac.uk/researchers/funding-opportunities/). Some NIHR schemes are only available to those based in England but similar support is available for those working in Wales (healthandcareresearchwales.org/), Scotland (www.nhsresearchscotland.org.uk/) and Northern Ireland (www.publichealth.hscni.net/directorates/public-health/hsc-research-and-development-wwwresearchhscninet).

Section 2

Dimensions of practice

5   Assessing need

Chapter aims

This chapter explores the importance of individualised, holistic assessment and the knowledge and skills that are required to undertake such assessments in partnership. Links to professional standards and expectations are made to support your professional development. There are opportunities for reflection on your practice and exploration of case studies. This supports practical application: working through examples develops skills for professional practice.

Professional standards and expectations

The Nursing and Midwifery Council's Code (NMC, 2018b) identifies that nurses should *'Make sure that people's physical, social and psychological needs are assessed and responded to'*. References to assessment are made throughout the following areas: prioritise people, practise effectively and preserve safety.

The Code of Practice is clear that nurses are required to assess, plan, implement and evaluate the care they provide in accordance with the nursing process first described by Henderson (1966).

WHAT IS A NEED?

Your perception of need may be different from that of the person you are assessing. The person's parents or carers might also have different views on need. Take a moment to reflect on why that might be. There are a number of ways of thinking about need. You will encounter within your practice variation across professions, services and society in how needs are defined and understood. There are also likely to be challenges in how services differentiate between social need and healthcare needs. Local authorities tend to have broader access criteria than health teams and so those who meet the threshold for eligibility for one service (social care) may not be able to access the services of the aligned health team.

Bradshaw's taxonomy of need (1972) reminds us that there are different perceptions of need and that these can change over time, often being subjective and dependent on a range of variables. Bradshaw's work on understanding social need is helpful for learning disability nurses due to the model of care in this field of nursing and the social history of people with learning disabilities. By understanding the taxonomy of needs, you will be more likely to deliver healthcare which addresses the social determinants of health. There are four areas used to describe need: normative, perceived (felt), expressed (demand) and comparative need.

- ○ The normative need is based on a standard which will be set by experts, professionals, administrators etc. There can be multiple factors at play where standards are set against a norm. Sometimes this norm can be class based or paternalistic. For example, the recommendations on how much fruit and vegetables should be eaten each day may not be attainable for some parts of the population, but will be based on a professional understanding of what makes a healthy, balanced diet. For some people where a standard is expected and that standard cannot be attained, this may lead to the decision of an unmet need.

- ○ The perceived (felt) need refers to the person's own assessment of their needs or requirement for care. This is about what the person wants. There are people who may think that they need help, but are not always deemed to really need it. There are others, who may not feel they require the support or service that professionals have assessed their need to be. Relationships are important in working together to identify and agree needs and manage the difference between want and need.

- ○ An expressed need (demand) refers to how the felt needs become an action. There is likely to be assistance sought and this relates to the way the individual expresses their feelings related to their perception of need.

- ○ Comparative need is based on understanding the characteristics of a population and using this to identify the needs of future service users. This predicts the needs of people and groups not currently receiving services.

The hierarchy of needs

Maslow's (1954) hierarchy of needs is presented as a pyramid (see Figure 5.1), where the needs lower down the hierarchy must be satisfied before the individual is able to achieve the needs higher up. Maslow identifies essential physiological needs, which all human beings have such as breathing, eating, sleeping, rest, having a safe place to stay, shelter etc. Only when those things are in place can a person then aspire and move onto achieve the quality of life factors such as work and play, sexual realisation and relational needs. After that, the person is able to progress to self-actualisation and achieving hopes, dreams and true potential.

Understanding the hierarchy is important in developing a therapeutic relationship and working in partnership. This is because being able to appreciate how needs are satisfied can help in the understanding of how to work with people who may have difficulties with the assessment and intervention processes. Ensuring that the person is safe and secure in the process and the relationship is the starting point for building a partnership as nurse and service user to understand and address need.

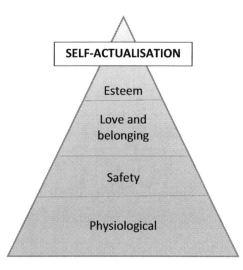

Figure 5.1 Hierarchy of needs
(Based on Maslow, 1954)

From a learning disability nursing perspective working through the hierarchy and recognising complexity is helpful for you in thinking about how to have the best inter- action and where barriers could be in place.

○   Physiological: make sure the person is physically comfortable, is able to concentrate because they are warm, nourished, hydrated and have access to any emergency medical equipment or sensory comforts etc they might need.

○   Safety: this can relate to physical and psychological safety. You will need to communicate with the person in a way that they understand, so that they feel safe and supported. Ensure that the person knows they can ask questions, take a break, say if they don't understand something and trust you to keep their information confidential. Consider the safety of the environment from the person's perspective. If they have sensory impairments then you will need to consider things such as noise, lighting, smells, visual distractions and so on.

○   Love and belonging: your assessment will need to consider relationships and loved ones. This can sometimes be difficult to explore and you will need to be sensitive to who the person is being supported by and how comfortable the individual is in discussing these things with others present. Find out if the person has caring responsibilities and if they have a carer. There may need to be a carer's assessment in place. It is important to know who is important in this person's life and if they could be experiencing loneliness or isolation, many people with learning disabilities report that they do. Do they have friends, a partner and are they safe in those relationships?

○   Esteem needs: does the person have a sense of purpose, do they feel valued, how do they contribute to society, are they confident, do they have self-worth. These are all things that might influence your ability to build a relationship. The person may not have had good experiences with professionals or those they see in positions of power. That might mean you have to work hard to ensure that the person is able to flourish, is heard and understands that they will be treated with dignity and respect.

○ Self-actualisation: When all other needs are achieved, people are able to realise their full potential. Within your assessment, you can support this attainment by thinking with the person about their goals (short and long term). A person might have aspirations of independent living but may be vulnerable due to their lack of confidence. In this example, until the esteem need can be addressed the self-actualisation need will not be realised.

Critical reflection 5.1

From a professional practice perspective, you might also find it helpful to think about your own needs in relation to Maslow's hierarchy.

- How are you able to function when you are hungry, tired or in pain?
- When you meet a new service user and their family/carers what steps do you need to take to ensure you are safe?
- Reflect on your lone working policy or mobile phone safety to consider how you take care of your well-being at work.
- Think about the needs you might have as a nurse in relation to:
  - love and belonging;
  - self-esteem;
  - self-actualisation.

Holism

Holism is a concept that encompasses an understanding of the whole person and their needs, rather than focusing on an individual part, which may present a problem for the person. Nursing a person holistically means understanding the person within a variety of contexts, for example, thinking about their physical, emotional, spiritual, cultural, religious and environmental needs. The holistic perspective is described by Byatt (2008) focusing on promotion of wellness as opposed to illness and using mutually agreed approaches to return to or facilitate optimum health. As with any other member of society people with learning disabilities have interrelated needs (social, psychological, spiritual and physical).

In learning disability nursing we often utilise the bio psychosocial model, seeking to understand the individual's needs in relation to the following.

○ Biological assessment takes into account the physical health information related to the person's needs and presentation. Considering history, diagnosis, health status, use of medication, impact of conditions and skills, strengths and resources. You will be able to gain insight into the person's perception of health and well-being and what they see as their skills and needs. This assessment may include your observation of the individual, how do they meet their needs within an environment, how do they communicate with others, how do they appear. A mental health assessment will include understanding of the person's presentation, their breathing, pallor, personal care, mood, interests pleasures etc.

○   Psychological information gives us insight into the person's ability to cope with demands, what resources they have, for example, communication, cognition and emotional well-being. Identifying psychological needs within the process supports understanding of how the person is best able to engage and communicate their needs.

○   Social assessment will help consider the person's personal experiences and history, their goals and achievements as well as the supports and networks they have. Understanding the education, employment and environmental experiences will help you to consider with them how they can achieve potential and focus on areas for development. Other things considered within the social element of the model would be:

–   family dynamics;

–   culture;

–   environment;

–   religion.

REFERRALS AND ASSESSMENT

Before the assessment begins, a referral will need to be accepted. It is not common for a person with learning disabilities to self-refer. More than likely the referral will come from another professional, such as the GP a social worker, health visitor or teacher. Sometimes the person's family or carers will make the referral. The trigger point for the referral to a specialist team or service might be because there is a challenge or need highlighted, perhaps due to behaviour, mental health or support needed to address a health issue.

In carrying out the assessment you will need to utilise a variety of skills, for example:

○   sensitivity;

○   communication;

○   observation;

○   listening;

○   history taking;

○   data collection;

○   analysis;

○   synthesis.

There will be initial discussions, which help you to consider the individual's needs and tailor the assessment. You will need to consider the most appropriate setting for an assessment to take place. This will depend on resources or equipment needed, how many people are going to be involved in the assessment, safety/risk elements etc. Health needs, mobility, mood, mental health, communication, activities and interests, likes and dislikes, self-care, awareness of risk/vulnerability, social and support needs, skills, education, finances and daily living skills are just some of the things that your nursing assessment might need to consider. If there are physical investigations that need to be conducted then you will need to consider privacy, dignity and the potential need for a chaperone. Understanding any history of contact with services will be helpful for you to prepare for the initial meeting, there may be things that can trigger anxiety, for example, notepads, medical looking equipment, lanyards or waiting rooms and knowing this reduces the chance of a negative first contact.

Starting your assessment will mean that you need to make contact, introduce yourself, explain your role and what a referral to your team means. The initial assessment will likely include a screening process, a risk assessment, consideration of the person's capacity to consent to assessment and their goals for your involvement. A referral to your service will have highlighted the referrer's perception of need. This should have captured the views of the person with a learning disability and their family but some-times this is not the case. Consent to the referral should be clear and if the person has been assessed as unable to consent due to capacity then this needs to be identified. It may be that a referral has been made in the person's best interests. Part of that initial discussion means capturing the individual's view on the assessment and referral. Are they in agreement, do they recognise there is a 'problem' or need? This is an opportunity for you to capture their views in their own words. Listen to what they say, note the kind of language do they use to describe themselves and their needs. Ensure that you accur-ately capture what the person says they hope to achieve from the assessment, what are the outcomes they are expecting. Ensure that their expectations are achievable and that the things they hope you and your service can do are realistic.

You will need to take some time to be clear about your role and what the service can do. You may need to make reasonable adjustments per the Equality Act (Gov.uk, 2010), this might mean thinking about augmented communication systems within this process. There will be people who you meet who have non-verbal means of communication (pre-viously explored in Chapter 3). Facilitating communication via pictures, symbols, signing or other means relies on understanding the person's preferred method of communica-tion and potentially working in partnership with others to prepare appropriate resources.

There can sometimes be conflict regarding eligibility and access, and as a learning dis-ability nursing professional you will need to engage within a range of forums and settings to think about the best way to meet individual need. For people with mild learning dis-abilities, complex histories and previous involvement with other services there may be a sense of falling between services. Sometimes when people have had limited educational opportunities or prolonged substance misuse this can impact on their presentation and can make it difficult to make an accurate assessment of need. Wherever possible there should be promotion of universal/mainstream services and the role of the learning dis-ability nurse or team should be about facilitating this and reducing the barriers to access.

Not all referrals will be appropriate and the initial assessment is the opportunity to work this through and consider more appropriate support, signposting if necessary. As a professional it is important that you are knowledgeable about aligned services and supports, community resources and groups and that you have a network you are able to draw on. Being connected in this way means that you can support smooth transitions to appropriate services, increasing access and reducing risk for the individual.

Take some time to think about how you would connect with different people and organisations in your role as a learning disability nurse. Jot down notes on how doing this will benefit you, the people you support and the service you work in?

Case study 5.1

Suzie has been referred to the community learning disability team. She is four years old, she has Dravet syndrome and cerebral palsy. Recently her nursery placement have told her mum that they are finding her behaviour difficult to manage, she is boisterous and finds it difficult to cope with the routines and expectations there. They have asked mum to think about reducing the placement to three days a week to try and build confidence and take some of the pressure off Suzie. Suzie's mum Sophie is worried about this, she has a small baby at home and another child at school. Sophie is a single mum with little support and was hoping that the nursery placement would provide respite as well as the structure she feels Suzie needs.

Critical reflection 5.2

- Thinking about the initial assessment, how will you consider Suzie's age, health, behaviour and developmental needs, the family support needs and the agencies you will need to work with to address these issues.

- How will you capture Suzie and her mum's understanding of who you are and what you will be doing in your assessment?

WHAT IS ASSESSMENT?

Assessment is a fundamental element of the nursing process, the first stage. The nursing assessment is likely to be one aspect of a wider multidisciplinary approach. Collecting information and data through assessment is recognised as vital in planning and promoting the delivery of personalised and meaningful care. Only once assessment has been undertaken can plans of care and subsequent evaluation be carried out. There are various ways of describing methods of assessment and it is essential that you think of it as an ongoing process. Assessment is not just the collection of information about immediate issues and circumstances. It is also about analysing the information to identify assessed need and make decisions on the most appropriate interventions.

Assessment may be used to describe the use of tools, for example, a pain assessment, an eating and drinking assessment or it may be used to gather an overarching understanding of the person. An assessment on admission to a ward or unit is likely to encompass a holistic understanding of the person. Gathering information about skills, concerns, wants, needs and wishes as well as physical and mental health status and essential information about how to communicate and motivate an individual as well as what to do if the person becomes distressed, angry or upset. The use of assessment can be likened to putting a puzzle together, gathering pieces of information to develop an understanding of how best to care for and support somebody, in line with their preferences and most importantly with them and their needs central to the process.

People with learning disabilities may require assessment from specialist learning disability services because they have needs relating to:

○ mental health, where specialist assessment, diagnosis and treatment are indicated;

○ well-being needs, promoting social inclusion, engagement in activities, co-production and self-advocacy;

○ specific therapy, for example, art psychotherapy, music therapy and specialist assessment;

○ autistic spectrum conditions/neurodevelopment disorders;

○ behaviours described as challenging;

○ epilepsy;

○ specialist assessment of skills, sensory needs and communication, dysphagia, nutrition and hydration;

○ acquisition of health, health promotion and health facilitation;

○ transitions, young people who enter services will require specific support and input in relation to continuing healthcare and complex placements.

When conducting an assessment the likelihood is that the nurse will gather and collate information from a range of sources, including the person, their family and other services. Sometimes assessments will be profession-specific, for example, a nursing assessment or speech and language assessment might be needed. Other times there are multidisciplinary approaches to assessment, particularly when a person is admitted to an inpatient setting such as an assessment and treatment unit or an acute admissions unit.

THE NURSING ASSESSMENT

Assessment is a key requirement in the nursing role and without an assessment of need it can be challenging to evidence the effectiveness or benefit of an intervention to the individual. When assessing the needs of people with learning disabilities it is not only important to select the right assessment tool but also to consider the method of assessment. How you assess an individual is as important as the tool you use. It is imperative that you keep the individual central to the process. There are other considerations for you as a nurse in understanding who to involve in the assessment and how and where to gather information from.

Assessing need can take a variety of formats, depending on the individual's presentation and the point at which the learning disability nurse becomes involved in their care and treatment. The depth and detail of the assessment must be proportionate to the person's needs and assessment should be supported by an appropriate evidence base. As you gather more information and the process builds you should be able to draw evidence-based conclusions about how best to address the individual's needs. Assessment may occur as a way of deciding on access to an appropriate service, a diagnosis, understanding an individual's support needs, physical or mental health needs or the presentation of behaviour.

Often families and people with learning disabilities can find assessments repetitive and sometimes difficult due to the need to continue telling their stories to each new professional they meet. Finding ways to record and report information that takes away the burden of the person having to repeatedly tell their story can be beneficial to relationship building, trust and improving the experience of care. One way that this might be captured can be in a health profile, or a health or communication passport (see the Once for Wales Health Profile from Public Health Wales in the Resources section at the end of the chapter for an example). This would also be considered a patient safety tool as this gives succinct and clear information about the person's immediate needs based on an informed assessment.

Practical considerations

Effective assessment relies on a number of professional nursing skills. The greatest being the ability to communicate effectively with an individual, using appropriate listening, questioning and engagement within the process. Social and interpersonal skills are essential to developing a relationship with the person, enabling trust and rapport to develop. It is important to be able to respond to verbal and non-verbal cues so that the assessment can be effective in gathering information in a way that does not challenge or distress an individual.

Gathering the information to make an assessment means asking questions, listening, recording, observing and engaging. There are specific skills required in formulating questions and eliciting further information to help inform an overall understanding. The assessment may be taking place in a busy environment (such as an outpatient clinic) or in an unfamiliar setting; there may be challenges for the individual in receiving and giving information or being asked questions which make them uncomfortable. You must always consider the influence of anybody who is accompanying the person and how they might be impacting on the person's presentation. Sometimes a chaperone will be required to support a physical assessment.

All care delivered must be provided in line with the evidence base; this means a detailed, comprehensive assessment is an essential tool in delivering quality care. As a learning disability nurse you will be skilled and able to:

○   undertake robust specialist assessment of need;

○   risk assess;

○   deliver therapeutic intervention;

- care coordinate and liaise;

- promote the rights of people with learning disabilities;

- educate and support others in the way that they make reasonable adjustments to meet the needs of people with learning disabilities.

There are things that you can do which will make the assessment process more engaging, relaxing and beneficial to the person being assessed.

- Find out the best way of communicating with the person.

- Ask the person if they want or need support.

- Recognise the contribution of carers and family members, where the person has given their consent.

- Think about dignity, respect, confidentiality and who else might be in the environment.

- Recognise that parents/carers may unknowingly influence the person's responses or behaviour within the assessment.

- Check the environment meets the person's needs, is it suitably accessible, would the person prefer a home visit?

- Offer choice within the assessment process, do what you can to promote self-determination and make the person's voice central throughout.

- Consider historical factors and the person's experience of professionals or assessments.

- Explain concepts in a way the person is able to understand, make sure the person does not feel like this is a pass/fail approach.

- Adapt information, use accessible resources, tools and leaflets.

- Schedule breaks and recognises when the person may be finding it difficult to maintain interest or attention to the process.

There may also be practical skills needed in assessment such as clinical observations, data collection, measurements and recordings. You will have achieved competence in the skills but there may be challenges within practice due to environment, use of equipment, the person's experience and potential anxieties within the process. Consider as much as possible how you can alleviate tensions and make reasonable adjustments to allow the person to participate within the process.

Some examples of where a learning disability nurse assessment might take place are as follows (each area will have pros and cons for you and the service user):

- an inpatient setting: assessment and treatment, secure services, specialist residential settings;

- a specialist community learning disability team;

- the person's own home;

o specialist roles, behaviour, autism, complex needs, forensic, consultant, advanced practice;

o continuing healthcare assessment;

o education or social care setting;

o a police station or prison.

Critical reflection 5.3

• Reflect on your experiences of assessment so far. Make a list of the nursing assessments you have been involved in, consider how they were impacted on by the setting, the identified need and any service or professional demands you have encountered.

THE NURSING PROCESS

Yura and Walsh (1967) described the nursing process and gave a clear model which helped nurses to put the patient (or service user) at the centre of decision-making. Using the process provides a clear framework for how care will be planned and delivered. As you develop confidence in your practice this standardised approach will underpin the way you use critical thinking and evidence-based practice in the assessment and treatment of people with learning disabilities.

Table 5.1 Working through the nursing process

The Nursing Process	
Assessment	Gathering information and data (subjective and objective) personal, family, medical, surgical medication, psychosocial history
Analysis or diagnosis	Using clinical judgement and interpretation of data to formulate an understanding of the person's need
Planning	Working in partnership with the person to develop a plan, incorporating goals and steps needed to achieve them
Implementation	Putting the intervention in place/delivering on a task
Evaluation	Used to understand how successful or unsuccessful the intervention was

There are a number of nursing models based on the principles of assess, plan, implement and evaluate. Yura and Walsh's model has the additional aspect '*analyse/diagnosis*' which relies on drawing together your clinical judgement, synthesising with the data and best evidence to make a decision about the person's needs.

Planning care needs to be based on assessment and assessment has to involve the person. Once needs are identified, you will need to agree how to best meet them. This is underpinned by a '*person-centred approach*'. Taking a person-centred approach means seeking to understand what is important to and for the person and working in partnership with them to achieve their goals. This relies on a flexibility within the service to be able to make positive risk-taking decisions and avoid paternalistic approaches. Individualised assessments and intervention plans are a key feature of a person-centred approach.

Models of care help to guide you in the way that you approach care delivery; however, they are based on the conceptualisation of human beings and predict outcomes which may not reflect diversity. For people with learning disabilities, models have often been adapted or implemented from a broader, generalist perspective, for example, Orem (1991) or Roper et al (1990). There has been criticism in the past that standardising approaches do not reflect the person-centeredness needed in nursing; Horan (2004) reflected this in identifying how many models in learning disability nursing have been '*borrowed*' from other fields. There are now more models specific to meeting the needs of people with learning disabilities.

Critical reflection 5.4

Take some time out to identify learning disability nursing models, compare to either Orem's (1991) self-care model or Roper et al's (1990) activities of daily living model.

- What do you notice about the theory underpinning the models?

- Why do you think it is necessary to have a learning disability nursing model?

- How do you think this will guide you in your practice and meet outcomes for your service users?

Working together to address needs

Sometimes the need will be patently obvious and will match the person, the referrer and the service understanding. A young person transitioning from children to Adult Services with a complex healthcare need and specialist input will likely to be known about in Adult Services and careful planning from a transition team or co-ordinator will ensure that a thorough understanding of needs is agreed. An older person who has lived semi-independently with family support and has started to lose skills and confidence may need some specialist input from a mental health or learning disability service to understand what the contributing factors are. A young man who is interested in making friends and developing an intimate relationship may need some joint work from members of the MDT dependent on what the barriers are and skills needed. This may include social and healthcare support.

Occasionally issues pertaining to health or social care can lead to professional conflict; it might be unclear where the responsibility for meeting this need lies and the professionals involved should do all they can to minimise the impact on the experience of the person with a learning disability. There are many excellent examples of nurses working in partnership with other agencies and increasingly being employed in social care or other non-traditional roles; however, in some areas there can be a distinction between health and social care which may become divisive.

There may be occasions where a person has been referred to a team or service and the referral is not clear about the person's need. Outcome measures help the nurse and service user work together to identify their needs, their goals for the episode of care and how they will know things have changed. There are a broad variety of outcome measures, some are profession-specific, therapeutic outcome measures. There are also symptom-specific outcome measures and intervention-specific measures. A tool such as the Health Equalities Framework (HEF) can be used to help an individual identify where their greatest area of concern is and target-specific pieces of work. There may be a mismatch between what the referrer has identified as the concern or need and what the individual highlights.

Outcome measures

Developing shared goals and measuring progress in achieving them contributes to the development of the therapeutic relationship. As a professional utilising an outcomes-based approach, you will experience the sense of achieving what really matters to the person. As a professional you want to be able to have impact, make a change and improve people's experiences. The use of outcome measures has to be embedded in your practice in order for you to evidence gains from a clinical and cost efficiency perspective. There are some tools specifically developed for use with people who have learning disabilities, while others have been adapted or adopted. Exploring tools and the benefits of use will help you to be clear on your role in improving health and well-being. This section introduces some tools, but there are many more and measuring improvement will be explored further in Chapter 10.

The care aims framework (Malcomess, 2015) focuses on outcomes for service users and recognises the challenge that practitioners can face in balancing the perceived need of the service user with the organisational and cultural practices of their team or service. There are suggestions that eligibility criteria and robust processes on access can create a sense of entitlement leading to inequity. Waterworth et al (2015) identified how using the care aims model could support a multi-professional team to improve outcomes for service users, improve professional working and encourage consistency in approaches. This was focused on a team who worked with older people and complexity and it is likely that the principles could also be applied to people with learning disabilities. An important aspect of the care aims model starts with language and the emphasis on considering requests for help (rather than referrals); this supports the partnership approach to meeting needs.

The Moulster and Griffiths model also presents an outcome-focused approach to the nursing process (Moulster and Atkinson, 2019). The need to identify, in partnership, the desired person-centred and health outcomes is fundamental as part of the assessment.

There is appreciation of the need to measure outcomes; this is emphasised at the start of the process. From a professional perspective it is expected that you will use outcome measurement in your day-to-day practice with service users. There are a range of outcome measures which can be incorporated into an assessment. There are a number of reasons for using outcome tools and gathering service user feedback.

○   People who use services, and their families and carers, want their views to be heard;

○   This helps to develop outcome-focused interventions.

○   Services and professionals can measure their effectiveness.

The Health of the Nation Outcome Scale for People with Learning Disabilities (HoNOS-LD) is a clinician-rated tool which detects changes over a four-week (or more) period; this provides a framework measuring risk and vulnerability (Roy et al, 2002). The ratings include 12 measures such as behaviour, level of impairment, presenting symptoms and social functioning. It has been promoted as an outcome measure by the Department of Health in England, recognising that measuring change in functioning due to mental health needs for people with learning disabilities required a specific tool. Other parts of the UK have not used the tool in a systematic way.

A measure such as the HEF can be helpful at the start of an assessment to help you focus on the actual needs of the individual, asking a range of questions which will give focus to the person's perception of the reason for referral and highlighting the area which causes the most challenge to the individual. The HEF enables nurses to demonstrate how nursing interventions can reduce the impact of social determinants of health (Atkinson et al, 2015).

Quality of life indicators are important for evaluating effectiveness of nursing intervention. Many people with learning disabilities experience loneliness, isolation, vulnerability and discrimination. Thinking about things such as mood, interests, pleasures, social activities and engagement can help to focus on areas for improvement.

There are challenges associated with the use of outcome measures, some clinicians may suspect ulterior motives for the data collection, or see the tools as routine and 'tick box' processes. From a clinical perspective there are potential limitations, for example, often it is not the person with a learning disability completing the tool or being interviewed, informant reliant tools may vulnerable to subjectivity, error or bias. There are also subtleties in symptom presentation, behaviour or communication that may not be detected in an outcome measure, particularly if this has been adapted from a general population tool.

There has been a growing importance placed on measuring outcomes and using these can help you to clearly identify need, set goals and evaluate the impact of your involvement. Demonstrating the effectiveness of learning disability nursing interventions is important in strengthening the evidence base of the profession. Outcome measures can also be used as evidence to support service development, evaluation and effectiveness of policy implementation (Delaffon et al, 2012).

Case study 5.2

Jordan is 25 years old and lives at home with his mum, dad and younger brother. Jordan's older brother got married and left home two years ago. Jordan is close to his older brother and aspires to living a similar life. Jordan would love to have a girlfriend and has been expressing this since his late teens. He is aware he has a learning disability and epilepsy; he is conscious about his seizures and describes a feeling he gets before having one which makes him anxious and upset. Jordan experienced some bullying at school and was the victim of mate crime as a young adult. Recently he has been articulating thoughts of low mood, low self-esteem and negative thoughts about his future. His parents can be very protective of him, his older brother supports his independence and encourages him to go out and about in the community, travelling independently etc however the family has recently requested additional support due to their concerns about Jordan's mental health. A referral has been made to the community learning disability team and you will be meeting Jordan for the first time.

Critical reflection 5.5

- Plan the assessment and think about what you want to ask Jordan about his goals.

- List the things that you will take into account from a nursing perspective.

- Research quality of life outcome measures which may be useful for you in understanding Jordan's experiences.

RIGHTS-BASED APPROACHES

Taking a rights-based approach to assessment means eliminating potential discrimination and removing barriers to access. It is imperative that you are aware of protected characteristics and your professional responsibility to reduce inequality within process and service delivery. Assessing needs with an understanding of diversity means that you will practice in a holistic and person-centred way. Building links with families, schools, advocacy and community groups and developing relationships across sectors will support your professional development in understanding diverse needs. This can take time, may be dependent on willingness and will likely develop from a shared understanding of goals.

Some people with learning disabilities may experience barriers and inequality at various points across the lifespan, employment opportunities are limited, access to higher education can be challenging, ageing can present barriers in accessing appropriate services. The role of the learning disability nurse focuses heavily on promoting independence and this may lead to conflict in some situations when assessing needs. There may be a potential for alienation if you do not build up appropriate relationships developing connectivity and trust before attempting to address issues such as gender roles, rites of passage, transition and adulthood. When working with people with learning disabilities and their families to understand wants, needs and wishes, there are likely to be some areas that can be contentious. If there are cultural sensitivities, you cannot impose your values and beliefs onto individuals, communities or groups. Exploring your own beliefs and potential bias will be an important step in allowing you to carry out careful assessment, extract hidden information and identify unmet needs.

There is evidence that people with learning disabilities from Black, Asian and Minority ethnic backgrounds can experience additional discrimination and inequality. This may be in combination with other types of discrimination (intersectionality), for example, gender, disability, age and can manifest in negative stereotypes, ignorance, attitude, professional ignorance, or service providers not taking into account associated needs and so on. These inequalities were further highlighted during the Covid-19 pandemic. Public Health England published figures in 2020 identifying that deaths of people with learning disabilities from all causes were 1.9 times higher than in 2018 and 2019 for those in White groups (PHE, 2020). For people who are in Asian and Asian-British groups it was 4.5 times higher and in Black and Black-British groups deaths from all causes were 4.4 times higher. NHS England (2020) highlighted that there could be additional challenges for people with learning disabilities living through the pandemic and reinforced the importance of people accessing medical care and attention where needed (Covid-related or not).

Listening to what people and their families say they want and need will help you to remain person-centred and demonstrate your value base. This supports skills in partnership working and gives opportunities for learning and your ongoing development.

Do with me, not to me

Critical reflection 5.6

- Think about the assessments you have used in practice, how do you ensure that you involve the person in their assessment?

- Can you reflect on a time when you have experienced barriers in engaging a person in the assessment process?

- What steps did you take to address those barriers?

As a healthcare professional, you will have power that you may not recognise. You will have acquired a level of competence and knowledge through professional training and practice. You have become skilled in gathering and providing information to support and develop a clinical assessment and understanding of need. This can result in an allocation of resource, equipment, time and provision of a service (or not). In times of working in prudent ways and managing budgets, responding to scrutiny and upholding Professional Standards, it is essential to always remember that there are people at the heart of what we do.

The importance of people with learning disabilities being involved and collaborating in their care is recognised by NHS England (2017) highlighting how a partnership approach supports people being able to make sure their care addresses what matters to them. This is supported by NICE (2019), who say that people with a learning disability should be able to lead an assessment. It is important to recognise that being able to lead relies on having enough information and time to prepare for the process. This includes deciding where and when they would like to meet with the professional, ideally a person they feel comfortable with.

The accessible version of Strengthening the Commitment (2012, p 6) made a powerful statement demonstrating the views of people with lived experience:

> *Learning disability nurses need to believe in people's rights. They should work in a person-centred way. They should see what people are good at, not just what they cannot do. They should support people to do the things they want to do in their lives.*

This message reinforces the rights-based, holistic understanding of an individual, considering the physical, emotional, social, economic and spiritual needs of the person which is embedded in learning disability nursing practice.

Services often identify their goals of recognising the service user's voice, listening to the views of the family and involving, collaborating or coproducing with them. In reality there continue to be large steps to take that make this the norm. The person with a learning disability should be able to identify who else should be involved in the assessment. Someone in the person's support network might be able to reduce anxiety, assist in communication and describing symptoms/presentation and can ensure that the person is able to truly express their needs, wants and wishes. There may be times when this presents additional challenge, partnerships between professionals and parents (or other family members) can depend on a culture of trust and respect. This means taking time to understand each other, appreciate perspectives, experience and opinions and sometimes building confidence in the relationship. Developing these relationships and investing time in understanding what families what and need will help you to develop your approach to assessment.

Some professionals have the power to decide whether somebody accesses a service or not, this may be through the labels applied to them: challenging, disabled, complex and due to eligibility criteria that means they do, or do not receive 'input'. This can be very distressing and confusing for people with learning disabilities and their families who sometimes experience unnecessary delays, complexities in process and barriers to access. Often people with learning disabilities and their families identify a need and can struggle to find the right service to meet it. There are many advocates for needs-led services.

Learning disability nurses seek to develop a partnership with the person with a learning disability. Working together to identify needs and address issues to improve access, promote rights and choice and independence and facilitate quality of life. People with learning disabilities want to be respected and valued and have equality in all aspects of life, as a learning disability nurse you can ensure this by the way that you demonstrate value and respect to the person within your delivery of the nursing process.

Making decisions and using tools

Decision-making tools are available to help nurses and other professionals rationalise their decision-making processes, supporting logical and evidence-based decisions. Often people with learning disabilities have not been given opportunity to problem solve, make choices or decisions for themselves.

Working together with other professionals, the person and their family brings benefits to the assessment process and supports person-centred care as an outcome. Finding opportunities to provide flexible and appropriate care irrespective of administrative boundaries between health and social care services can be challenging, and it is essential that the person and their needs remain central to the assessment. When professionals work together in the best interests of the person being assessed and the person's (and carers') views and wishes are central to the assessment process then the assessment can build a rounded picture of the need and context.

It is important that as a nurse you recognise your consciousness in the process of decision-making. This relates to when deciding which evidence to use and what decisions are relevant for the individual. Clarity and transparency of decision-making is essential, between not only nurses but also when nurses are involved in multi-agency and multi-professional working. Clarity is also important for service users, relatives and carers.

Critical reflection 5.7

Thinking about the last person with a learning disability you assessed, reflect on their family situation.

- How old were their parents and family members who contributed to the assessment?

- What generational and cultural issues did you need to consider?

- Write down what benefits and challenges you heard the family talk about as a result of their relative's learning disability.

CARE MANAGEMENT

Assessment is not a one-off piece of work. There should be a rolling programme with clear identified stages where assessment and reassessment is indicated. As a learning disability nurse you may have a role in co-ordinating this; however, there may also be other best placed professionals who are able to take on this role. Dependent on where you are in the UK and what type of service you work in this role may have a variety of titles: care manager, care co-ordinator, key worker etc. Regardless of whether the assessment is focused on a specific need or is part of a broader more comprehensive assessment there should be transparency, timescales and a clear process.

A group of registered learning disability nurses with various levels of experience were asked to reflect on key areas of primary nurse responsibility. Almost all identified care-coordination in terms of taking the lead in assessment planning and designing complete plans of care. Nurses do sometimes take on responsibility as 'key-worker' and this can bring an element of co-ordination and management. Understanding risk, minimising like-lihood of harm and working in partnership were the focus of the descriptions. There were challenges highlighted: time, administration, reliance on others doing their part and the conflict between clinical and co-ordination duties.

There can be added benefit for people with learning disabilities where a nurse takes on the role of care management. However, there are sometimes challenges relating to the role and how professionals work together to address this. In the evolving role of the learning disability nurse there can be requirements to undertake thorough and com-prehensive assessment to make decisions related to health and social care access, funding streams and continuing healthcare provision. This can mean that there feels like a process-driven, rather than needs-driven assessment and this may feel problem-atic for the healthcare professional. We have a duty to understand the needs of the indi-vidual through person-centred, needs-led assessment; however, many learning disability nurses express their frustration at the 'case co-ordination approach' or 'case manage-ment'. This can mean administrative co-ordination, drawing together professionals and resources and needing to organise meetings, reviews, completion of specific documen-tation and being a point of contact. There are also likely to be elements of managing resource and budget. There can be challenges for the professional in maintaining the focus on the health needs of the individual when drawn into the role of care manage-ment. Working together with others, maintaining relationships with the local authority and other partners is essential to allow nurses in care management roles to deliver on health outcomes.

As a learning disability nurse you will support people with learning disability to reach their goals, utilising person-centred approaches and co-producing plans to live their lives as fully and independently as possible. The role and contribution of the learning dis-ability nurse is explored by Moulster et al (2019) clarifying that all people are entitled to the same standards of care and that the learning disability nurse has expertise in key areas: 'assessment, communication, health promotion, education and empowerment'. The role of care co-ordinator is explored by Ruiz et al (2020), recognising that this can be a key role for people with learning disabilities in having their needs recognised and met. Many learning disability nurses perform care co-ordination and are responsible for drawing together the elements which make up a package of care, monitoring and evaluating the effectiveness. However, care co-ordination can be a challenging and contentious aspect of the nursing role; there are views that the management and organisation of care can take away from and challenge clinical practice, therapeutic relationships and the ability to address the nursing aspects of care for an individual.

Case study 5.3

Sioned has been living in a single person service since she left college; she was assessed on transition and was identified as needing the support of three nurses day and night to maintain safety, support community participation and ensure health and well-being across a 24-hour period. For the last six months Sioned has been telling her staff she is sad, lonely and wants to live with other people. Her only relationships are with the people paid to care for her and she has been increasingly upset this year as her requests for a change in her living situation have not progressed. There have been three occasions in the last month where she has displayed behaviours described as challenging, hurting herself and others, damaging property, screaming and crying and saying how unhappy she is. Twice the police have been called and on one occasion she has attended A&E. Sioned needs to have her views heard and listened to and the team around her need support to continue to keep her safe. A suggestion that she may need an inpatient assessment has been challenged and the decision is that a joint assessment from psychiatry and nursing should take place.

Critical reflection 5.8

Reflect on the things that the nurse will need to take into account and what the differences might be with a psychiatry assessment.

- How will you work together with the doctor to understand Sioned's needs?

UNMET NEEDS

All needs identified in assessment must be recorded and reflected in the subsequent plan of care; there will sometimes be needs identified as unmet. Where needs are identified as unmet it is essential that there is discussion and agreements made as to why these are unmet needs. This may be due to the person's aspirations or service limitations and attempts to draw the two together have to be made. This means developing actions that you will support the person to work towards.

Chapter summary

Throughout this book, we have explored the needs of people with learning disabilities, across the lifespan. The role of the learning disability nurse in assessing and understanding these needs is unique within health and social care. The objective of enabling people with learning disabilities to access services designed around their needs can be achieved by providing the support of learning disability nurses at key times.

Each individual you meet with a learning disability will have unique skills, strengths and abilities. People with learning disabilities sometimes need extra help to stay healthy, safe and have the best life they can. The level of support needed will look different for each person. While some people will live independently needing little or no involvement from specialist services, there are others who may be very vulnerable in society and may experience barriers, leading to health inequalities. Some people with learning disabilities can have difficulty with everyday activities, self-care, eating and drinking, performing household tasks, socialising or managing money. With the right support many people with learning disabilities are able to lead independent lives and aspire to do so. Knowing what an individual's needs look like means conducting a thorough and focused assessment.

This chapter has explored the role of the learning disability nurse in assessing need. It is clear that this is an essential element of learning disability nursing practice. Assessment has been highlighted as both a one-off and ongoing process. There must be focus on identifying actual and potential issues for a person, working together with them to find solutions, resources and supports to address unmet need.

Key relevance to your professional practice relates to holistic, person-centred, needs-based assessment, encompassing culture and values and promoting rights, choice, self-advocacy and empowerment. You will become skilled in delivering values-based assessment of individuals regarding their current needs and how they can be met. Integral to this is developing an understanding of people's aspirations and desires for the future, including how they might like to be assisted to live a more independent life. The role of the nurse in improving health outcomes for people with learning disabilities relies on assessing and understanding need.

FURTHER READING

Gov.uk (2018) Reasonable adjustments for people with a learning disability. [online] Available at: www.gov.uk/government/publications/reasonable-adjustments-a-legal-duty/reasonable-adjustments-a-legal-duty (accessed 21 April 2022).

Moulster, G (2020) Identifying Pain in People Who Have Complex Communication Needs. *Nursing Times*, 116(2): 19–22. [online] Available at: www.nursingtimes.net/roles/learning-disability-nurses/identifying-pain-in-people-who-have-complex-communication-needs-20-01-2020/?msclkid=cee81f94c32311eca0b834e55ea0f598 (accessed 23 April 2022).

NHS England and NHS Improvement (2019) People with a Learning Disability, Autism or both Liaison and Diversion Managers and Practitioner resources. [online] Available at: www.england.nhs.uk/wp-content/uploads/2020/01/Learning-disability-and-autism. pdf?msclkid=55853dbdc32311ec8fd34bf52e03950c

NICE QS187 (2019) Learning Disability: Care and Support of People Growing Older. [online] Available at: www.nice.org.uk/guidance/QS187 (accessed 30 November 2021).

Royal College of Speech and Language Therapists (2021) Eating and Drinking with Acknowledged Risks: Multidisciplinary Team Guidance for the Shared Decision-making Process (Adults). [online] Available at: https://gala.gre.ac.uk/id/eprint/34689/?mscl kid=9328c895c32211ecb2657e55c94a521f (accessed 21 April 2022).

RESOURCES

Disability Distress Assessment Tool: https://prc.coh.org/PainNOA/Dis%20DAT_Tool.pdf?mscl kid=ed73df03c32111ec89655f12379792b6 (accessed 22 July 2022).

The Disability Distress Assessment Tool was specifically developed to capture a baseline understanding of an individual communication and how this might manifest when communicating 'pain'.

Learning Disabilities Goals and Outcome Measures: https://cks.nice.org.uk/topics/learning-disabilities/goals-outcome-measures/ (accessed 21 April 2022).

Setting goals and outcomes are important in assessing impact of the role of the learning disability nurse. Use this resource to understand more.

NHS: Annual Health Checks: www.nhs.uk/conditions/learning-disabilities/annual-health-checks/?msclkid=3f1f4daac32111ec8fe37ab30242547f (accessed 23 April 2022).

Annual health checks are essential in reducing health inequality and understanding the health needs of people with learning disabilities. This link gives further information on the resources to support annual health checks taking place.

Nursing Notes: A–Z Guide of Clinical Assessment Tools for Nurses: https://nursingnotes. co.uk/resources/guide-nursing-assessments/?msclkid=9fe8cad1c32111ecb5ed3cfc3 289b5d1 (accessed 21 April 2022).

This link provides a toolbox of relevant nursing assessment material, you can easily dip in and out of this resource at key times as you progress in your development.

The Once For Wales Health Profile: //phw.nhs.wales/services-and-teams/improvement-cymru/our-work/learning-disability-health-improvement-programme/health-profile/health-profile-for-professionals/ (accessed 21 April 2022).

Planning and delivering care in partnership

Chapter aims

Within this chapter you will develop understanding of care planning at an individual and service level. You will further explore your understanding of the concepts and principles of service user involvement, shared decision-making, promoting independence and self-care, co-production and person-centred delivery of care.

Professional standards and expectations

The NMC (2018a) is clear that care planning is a fundamental role of the nurse and identify the nursing process as the most desirable way to achieve this.

The Equality Act (Gov.uk, 2010) reminds us of our obligations to ensure information is provided in an accessible format. The NHS England (2016a) accessible information standard also sets out these expectations.

NICE guideline NG197 (2021) shared decision-making reinforces the need to incorporate this into everyday care and treatment in health and social care.

Critical reflection 6.1

- Take some time to think about the following areas in relation to care planning:

    - communication;
    - consent and capacity;
    - dignity, respect, values-based approaches;
    - equality and accessibility;
    - person-centeredness;
    - self-advocacy;
    - safety and safeguarding;
    - co-production.

- Why do you think these factors are important?

- Are there other areas you think of as essential for learning disability nurses?

What is care planning in nursing?

A care plan is a document that outlines an individual's needs. It should be evidence based and developed following assessment. The care plan is essential as a communication tool between the person, their carer, family or supporters, as well as professionals and other services. The nursing care plan guides how a nurse will deliver care to an individual. As a nurse in practice, you should read through a person's care plan and get a sense of who they are as an individual.

In learning disability nursing, the importance of promoting independence, teaching skills and enhancing opportunities reinforces that the care plan needs to be formulated together with the individual. This makes the plan user focused and enables the individual's ownership in maximising potential health outcomes. Effective care planning is dependent on a process of communication, negotiation and decision-making. The nurse and the individual need to be able to appreciate and understand each other's views. It is important to co-produce plans of care that bring together the wants, needs and wishes of the individual and meet their assessed need from a health and social care perspective.

It is important to be clear that a care plan cannot be a 'wish list' and there may be a challenge to you as a professional if you are unable to agree something that the person or their family want incorporated within it. You must work within the frameworks of your role, service and profession. This can mean managing resources, working within budgets and rationalising the decision-making. Another challenge can be the co-ordination needed to ensure that care plans work together. Creating an overarching plan of care avoids any confusion from conflicting guidance in separate care plans. You may need to influence professions and providers on the way they deliver their services. Professional relationships, dealing with conflict and challenge and being able to present evidence in a meaningful way are some of the factors which you need to explore within your practice.

Others involved in the development of the care plan might include families, carers, other health professionals and partner organisations. Those involved are making a commitment to deliver actions identified within the care plan and the named leads are accountable for the review and evaluation of them. If the person does not give their consent to share their care plan with carers/family members then in some situations general information in relation to support, safety and well-being may still be provided. There will need to be a robust, well-documented decision-making process around this and it will need to be a MDT, case-by-case decision. At the same time, you should make every effort to gain consent from the person by explaining the benefits of sharing this information, while respecting the person's right to confidentiality. There may be times when the care plan is utilised as evidence, this might be in legal proceedings, internal investigations, disciplinary process or involving the regulatory bodies. Nurses must always be mindful of the quality and content of the care plans they produce and ensure they are accurate, truthful and transparent. Would you be comfortable if the care plans you have recently developed were reviewed as part of an audit or in legal proceedings?

Safety and risk management need to be considered within the care plan as well as crisis or relapse indicators. This can often present challenge; there will be different perceptions of risk and often consideration of historical behaviour and presentation can influence how a person is understood. In your professional practice you will face the dilemma of supporting choice making and risk-taking, balanced with your duty of care and Code of Practice. There may appear to be simple solutions, which reduce risk for the individual; however, this may not be what is in the person's best interests. You will be mindful of the need to reduce restrictive practice within your practice and there may be others who are more risk-averse or naturally go to restrictive approaches as solutions.

The plan of care must:

o   be based on a thorough assessment and present the identified needs;

o   record the individual's views, wants, needs and wishes; including goals;

o   outline treatment, interventions and expected outcomes;

o   clarify psychological and other therapeutic support to promote recovery and prevent deterioration;

o   detail all prescribed medications and specific needs related;

o   be clear regarding any risks to self or others, including carers, family and anyone providing support;

o   clearly stipulate action needed to address physical health problems or reduce the likelihood of deterioration in health;

o   identify who will carry out the actions needed to address needs;

o   be shared with appropriate others (those who are implicated and involved in the development);

o   be written in an accessible way;

o   provide information for the person, their carer/family or identified supporter about what to do in the event of deterioration;

o   include contact details for the named Care Co-ordinator or Lead Professional and all named parties involved in providing support;

o   stipulate plans for future discharge, or other transfer/transition;

o   include the next planned review date.

o   A detailed, evidence-based and up-to-date care plan shows that the person's needs are being assessed and addressed on an ongoing basis. There are many ways of writing plans of care. This might be structured specifically dependent on the health need being addressed or the type of service the person is in receipt of. In developing the plan, however, you will use the same skills and techniques to formulate it.

Writing SMART care plans

SMART is a well-known acronym for Specific, Measurable, Attainable/Achievable, Relevant/Realistic and Time-bound/Timely/Time-limited. Using these headings supports systematic approaches to producing clear, easily implemented and evaluated plans of care. They are well described, including the origins, in Tempest (2012).

Specific

Be clear on the goals for the service user. This needs to be well defined within the care plan, everybody, especially the individual, needs to understand what you are trying to achieve (other professionals, family members, your team members).

Measurable

Identify the criteria for measuring progress. Be clear on the metrics that will be used. If the goal is not measurable it will be difficult to evidence achievement.

Attainable/achievable

Be realistic. The plan should not be setting out to achieve things that are unattainable; however, an attainable goal might still be difficult to achieve.

Relevant/realistic

Make sure that the goal is realistic, it can be very demoralising if objectives are not achieved. If you are setting out to teach a skill, how much will this improve the person's circumstances? An achievement that aligns with the individual's overall goal such as reducing anxiety to increase social activity may need many defined in steps that work towards the eventual goal. From a nursing perspective you will need to be honest with a person who has unrealistic expectations. Working together on finding a realistic goal is essential.

Time-bound/timely/time-limited

Committing to a time scale within the plan will help to keep the person and the care team focused. It is important to be realistic and recognise additional pressures or barriers which may interfere with initial goal setting. Although there will need to be a clear start and end point you may also need this to be flexible.

CARE PLANNING FRAMEWORKS

There are various care planning processes you will be responsible for in your role as a learning disability nurse. Some examples are explored within this chapter; however, there will be different frameworks guiding your practice depending on whether you work with children or adults. There can be the legal expectations, for example, Section 117 aftercare, Court of Protection or Care and Treatment Planning under the Mental Health Measure in Wales, as well as organisational and Professional Standards.

Person-centred planning

A person-centred plan (PCP) is co-produced with the person. There are specific skills in developing PCPs and all aspects of the individual's life are considered within the plan. This may result in a pictorial representation of the agreed plan dependent on the person's communication skills and needs. Using a person's own words is very important. Mee (2012) asks if a service can be truly person-centred if the words used in a plan are not the person's own. The person's circle of support (those people important in their life) will be fundamental. There are also clear aspects related to personal strengths, aspirations and support needs (Smull et al, 2004). You will need to take time to make sure views and aspirations are captured, adapting your communication style to ensure the person is fully included and think about how the person can share their plans with others.

The Health Action Plan

The Health Action Plan (HAP) is developed from the annual health check (AHC). The HAP should establish clear goals for the individual following the AHC and there may be many professionals who have a role in supporting achievement of the plan. The plan should be coordinated by the health facilitator (this can be anyone who supports the person's acquisition of health). The plan will describe the person's health needs, the professionals who support these and any appointments they have to address. It is likely that you will be fundamental within the HAP as a learning disability nurse because you have the knowledge and skills to support reasonable adjustments and ongoing acquisition of health for people with learning disabilities. You are able to work co-productively with key providers, people with learning disabilities and their families to support rights-based healthcare.

Case study 6.1

Joey's HAP draws together some concerns about his physical health including his weight and diet. The last AHC identified that he is pre-diabetic and Joey has been advised by his GP to monitor his diet and try to lose weight. Joey's support worker will support him in a walking group twice a week, his mum will join slimming world with him and the supported living service he is in has set up an activities list looking for interest in a five-a-side team. Joey knows that he wants to lose weight to be healthier and happier; he needs social support and accessible information to help him stick to his plan.

Critical reflection 6.2

- What can you do as a learning disability nurse to develop a care plan that promotes choice, inclusion and goal setting for Joey?

Activities of daily living care plans

You will sometimes have responsibility for developing plans of care related to their activities of daily living, eating and drinking, personal care, breathing, elimination, sexuality, relationships, occupation etc. Sometimes you will need to develop care plans that outline individual's routines, for example, morning or bedtime routine, this might be to specify an individual's needs to a staff team.

Often these kind of care plans can be structured visually and supported with accessible resources such as pictures or symbols. There may be skills teaching elements incorporated within and an MDT approach to supporting activities of daily living might be considered. Utilising a communication assessment to pitch the plans at the right level as well as an occupational therapy assessment to ensure that the goals are achievable and meaningful can be appropriate for some people. You may need to negotiate and support input from other professionals, supporting reasonable adjustments and partnership working. Sometimes there may be access barriers dependent on an individual's primary need, staff skills and confidence and how service delivery is structured.

Acute admission care plan

Table 6.1 Basic care plan format for specific need

Identified Need	Desired outcome	Action	Person responsible	Date for evaluation

Some care plans may be developed with very little information, for example, shortly after admission. This should specifically set out the plan for the initial assessment and will need to be quickly reviewed in order that a more detailed, informed and evidence-based plan is in place. Where somebody has transferred at short notice from another area existing care plans may be utilised, it is the nurse's responsibility to review and update these as quickly as possible with the most up-to-date evidence about the person's needs.

Case study 6.2

Karl is an acute liaison nurse in a large district general hospital. A referral has been made for a 55-year-old lady who needs investigations for a stomach complaint. June has been withdrawn for the last 4–6 weeks, losing weight, hitting her tummy and has seemed distressed on multiple occasions; her GP has referred her for investigations. June has been described as challenging and the team planning her care has decided that it might be an appropriate reasonable adjustment for June to be sedated in a vehicle before bringing her into the hospital. Karl has some concerns about this suggestion.

Critical reflection 6.3

- What should Karl do to raise his concerns?

- What professional skills will he need to utilise in this situation, where might he get some additional support?

- What legal and professional frameworks will need to be considered in developing the care plan?

Critical reflection 6.4

- Read the following article: 'Woman with learning disability can have teeth removed, court rules' (BBC, 2020), and think about the development of a care plan to support this person's needs.

- What might be the role of the nurse prior to the decision for a dental clearance and afterwards?

Case study 6.3

Now consider Rachel Johnstone's sad and avoidable death, a 49-year-old lady who died in November 2018 after having all of her teeth removed. Rachel was described by her family as a lovely girl who loved her life, music and dancing. She lived in a residential service, staffed by nurses and had been experiencing pain in her mouth preventing her from eating. Her mum was anxious about Rachel having so many teeth removed in one go and the decision was made to do so while she was under general anaesthetic. Post-procedure there is some contra-diction and little evidence as to the information provided to her carers. The carers say they were given some paperwork and no advice on how to care for Rachel after having 19 teeth (and fragments removed) under a general anaesthetic. At the inquest it was recognised that registered nurses where Rachel lived failed to carry out appropriate physiological observations post-surgery and did not escalate concerns about her presentation to get the emergency response she needed. She died of cerebral hypoxia and aspirational pneumonia as a result of neglect.

Critical reflection 6.5

- What should a care plan have looked like for Rachel post-operatively?

- Imagine you were the nurse in charge after a person had just undergone a major procedure such as this. What would you want and need to be in place?

Behaviour focused

There are a range of ways of writing care plans for those whose behaviour is described as challenging. Some of this is explored in Chapter 9. It might be that the person has a comprehensive positive behaviour support plan or a specific, discreet plan related to one aspect of their behavioural needs. The plans may be pro-active or reactive. There might be specific plans on teaching coping mechanisms or skills for the individual as well as reinforcement programmes, engagement styles or functional communication systems.

A very simple way of helping others to support a person who might have behaviour described as challenging is the use of a know this/do this plan – see Table 6.2 (Smull et al, 2004). The structure is very accessible and can be something that you work on together with the person or their supporters to bring their voice and perspective into their plan of care.

Table 6.2 Sample: when this is happening plan

When this is happening	And X does this	We think it means	And we should

A worked example might state very simply:

o When this is happening ... *Joe hears his staff talking about their plans for the day or working out what the other service users in the setting will be doing that day*

o And this happens ... *Joe repeatedly says, and Joe will? And Joe will?*

o We think it means ... *Joe wants staff attention and for staff to remind him of the nice things he has to look forward to*

o And we should say ... *and today Joe will be ... seeing mum/do a jigsaw/go swimming (see the list of preferred activities)*

Section 117 aftercare

A plan is produced for an individual entitled to aftercare under Section 117 of the Mental Health Act 1983. This is specific to meeting assessed care needs after a person has been detained on certain sections of the Mental Health Act (1983) (Section 3, Section 37, Section 47, Section 48 and Section 45A). Services are planned with the person before they are discharged from hospital. The person must have an allocated lead professional (historically a CPA co-ordinator); this may be a learning disability nurse. In this role you will need to organise a yearly review and focus must be on maintaining the person in the community, recognising the potential factors which contribute to deterioration and contingency planning. ADASS (2018) set out the importance of reviewing individual needs and making decisions together about when it might be appropriate to discharge from 117 aftercare. A clear example of when discharge from 117 might occur would be if a person's mental health improves to the point that they no longer need services to meet their needs arising from or related to their mental disorder. However, this is not the case for all, some people may still need aftercare to prevent relapse or deterioration.

Case study 6.4

Tina will shortly be discharged from hospital under Section 117. She has had an assessment by the local authority. Those involved in the assessment feel that Tina's needs will be best met within a supported living service. She will need to have support from the local community learning disability team to maintain her mental health and well-being. Support will be provided to prompt her to take her medication on time, help her with budgeting, cope with her anxiety disorder and make connections in her local community.

Critical reflection 6.6

- How will you review Tina's needs and determine the ongoing level of input she will require from your service?

Care and Treatment Planning

The Mental Health (Wales) Measure (2010) introduced Care and Treatment Plans (CTP) for people with mental health problems in Wales. Part 1 is focused on improving access in primary care for people with mental health needs. Part 2 ensures everyone in secondary care has a care co-ordinator and holistic CTP. Part 3 enables adults to self-refer to secondary care services following discharge. Part 4 focuses on the importance of advocacy and the rights of those subject to the Act to have support from an IMHA (Welsh Government, 2020b).

When involved in CTPs and possibly acting as a care co-ordinator the learning disability nurse is responsible for ensuring best practice, compliance and inclusion of the views of people with learning disabilities and their families. It is important that the CTP has specific goals, identified outcomes and is reviewed within the indicated timescales (to a maximum of 12 months). There is a need to coordinate the review with the risk assessment and ensure if there is a change in status, for example, admission to secondary care, that the plan reflects accurately the individual's needs and situation. You will need to work closely with the person and the MDT to agree outcomes and achieve effective care and support.

Court of Protection

Increasingly learning disability nurses are involved in complex care management and co-ordination. This may involve preparing or presenting information to the Court of Protection. Sometimes the services that you work in will need to make checks on whether the provisions they have in place are infringing on people's human rights, and independent reviews of this may lead to Court of Protection referrals.

The Court of Protection (England and Wales) is able to make decisions on behalf of those who lack capacity to make their own; they may give the decision-making power to another person (a deputy). This Court mainly deals with issues of welfare, property or medical treatment (Young and McKinney, 2016). They are in place to act in the best interests of an individual, this is not the same as deciding what a person would want, should they have had capacity.

In R(J) v Caerphilly County Borough Council (2005), legal expectations of care planning are clearly set out:

> *A care plan is more than a statement of strategic objectives – though all too often even these are expressed in the most vacuous terms. A care plan is – or ought to be – a detailed operational plan. Just how detailed will depend upon the circumstances of the particular case. Sometimes a very high level of detail will be essential. But whatever the level of detail which the individual case may call for, any care plan worth its name ought to set out the operational objectives with sufficient detail – including detail of the 'how, who, what and when' – to enable the care plan itself to be used as a means of checking whether or not those objectives are being met.*
>
> (46)

There are occasions when care plans do not meet these expectations, this brings into question the quality of care and service being provided. The person in receipt of the care needs to be considered at all stages, if the care plan is of poor quality how do they know and trust that they will get the care and intervention they have been assessed as needing.

The Court of Protection has worked very privately to protect identity and maintain confidentiality of individuals, there have been challenges to this, the court can allow publication or public hearing where there is 'good reason' to do so (MCA, 2005). The Court of Protection involvement can be challenging for families and nurses. The practice issues of dealing with legal process and teams, the language used and how clinical information is expected to be presented can be daunting and unfamiliar. In addition to this, nurses need to know what to expect in court hearings and what the requirements of them from a professional element will be. This may not be something you feel prepared for at a pre-registration level; however, increasingly new registrants are entering community teams, holding caseloads and expected to work within these frameworks. Seek out policy and practice guidance, ensure you access training and supervision. It is important to be clear about the process and expectations and to access appropriate support in preparing materials and gathering information. However, ultimately professional nursing practice does prepare you for the evidence-based approaches needed.

Some of the situations where you might need to be involved in the Court of Protection processes include:

o   issues related to residence, where should the person live, where are their needs best met, decisions on whether the current place is meeting their needs;

○ safeguarding issues, possibly related to property decisions or safe contact with family members;

○ decisions related to finances and who supports the individual to manage them;

○ decisions related to Deprivation of Liberty Safeguards (DoLS), for example, where restrictions are in place in a person's home and the health board or local authority have responsibility for the package of care;

○ other aspects of DoLS challenge.

Risk and care plans

NHSE/NHSI (2021) describes how a personalised approach to managing risk is fundamental within the process of care and support planning. The risk assessment and subsequent care plan will take into account current and past presenting problems. You can seek to understand how an issue has been addressed in the past by gathering history. Using your communication skills to elicit this information requires sensitivity, dignity and respect. Some people will have had traumatic histories; interventions and approaches to management of behaviour and risk have evolved over time; however, some people will have experience of approaches, which they find difficult to share. There might be some element of shame related to discussing past events and sometimes people will want to distance themselves from their past presentation and behaviour. It is essential, as always that you maintain professionalism, do not judge and demonstrate value towards the person in this process.

Making choices in real terms can still be difficult for people with learning disabilities, while services and providers may appear to support choice there can be significant barriers. Skills of those supporting, the values of the service, financial aspects, availability of options and understanding the consequences of the choice are just some of the challenges that you will need to take into account when promoting choice. This is important in thinking about positive risk-taking. Learning disability nurses can support positive risk-taking to enable independence; however, this may not be strongly embedded within the services you support people in (Seale et al, 2012).

Case study 6.5

Brad is 44, he has often expressed that he likes to wear women's clothing, he does this in private at home. Brad identifies as male and presents as male, he has short hair and a goatee beard. He has recently been asked to leave a number of clothing shops in his local community after attempting to access the female changing area to try on women's clothes. Brad has become angry when challenged about this and feels he is being treated unfairly. He has limited support when accessing the community and the supported living service are finding it difficult to address this with Brad. Brad and his sister are very close but she has been quite embarrassed to approach this with him.

Critical reflection 6.7

- What do you think the risks might be to Brad in this situation?

- What are some of the things that will help you in developing a risk care plan? Think about the tools you will use, the people you will engage with and the process you might follow to develop this.

Sometimes people will make choices that increase the risk that they become a target for bullying or abuse, for example, they may choose to wear their hair, make up or clothing in particular ways that draw attention to them. As a nurse you may feel that you want to protect people from this and support them to be successful in the community. We have to ensure that the person's ability to experiment and learn is not cloyed by over protection in services or families. Equally finding opportunities to help the person to deal with the potential negative experiences can be built into the care plan.

Case study 6.6

Jack lives with his grandparents, he is 15 and is keen to exert his independence. Jack helps his grandad on his allotment and he loves his gran's home-cooked dinners. The family live close to a local shop, approximately ten minutes' walk and every day (more than once when given the opportunity) Jack will walk to the shop, he loves to talk to the shopkeeper and buys fizzy drinks and chocolate bars.

His grandparents are not concerned about risk to Jack in terms of road safety or community presence. He is well known and appears to be well liked in the community. Jack can make his needs known, he has verbal communication, he knows how to ask for help. He also has a mobile phone.

When Jack returned to school after the summer holidays his uniform was very tight and the school nurse has contacted his grandparents to say she is concerned about his weight gain. An MDT has been called and you will need to think about your role in understanding what Jack and his grandparents need, what they, the school nurse and school want and what the perceived and actual risks to Jack are.

When balancing the risks to Jack it is essential to consider the pleasure he gets from this activity. A care plan might consider his overall health, teeth, potential for diabetes or other weight-related issues. It would also need to consider the need for independence, for growth and for generalising these skills into other areas of Jack's life. The evidence related to Jack's height, weight and BMI will be important as well as thinking about his oral hygiene and visits to the dentist.

Positive risk-taking should always be built into a care plan; however, there will be some risks that also need to have a robust level of support. Sexual offending is one of these risks. There may be some people who are safely supported and cared for in an environment that reduces the likelihood of them being able to carry out such offences. However, without robust multidisciplinary input, care planning, risk assessment and environmental management this risk is unlikely to reduce. Griffiths et al (2013) identify some of the factors that might lead to sexual offending, poor social and interpersonal skills, combined with limited opportunities for appropriate sexual relationships as well as a degree of sexual naivety and limited education about sex and relationships.

Capacity and care planning

We should always presume capacity and work under the principles of the Mental Capacity Act (Gov.uk, 2005). This means recognising that all adults have the right to make their own decisions.

In situations where you have a question about the person's capacity to be involved in the care planning process you should explore the following.

- Has the appropriate level of information been provided to the person (and those supporting them) to enable them to make the decision?

- Has information been shared and communicated in a way they can understand?

- Are there other reasonable adjustments that might support the person to make the decision, for example, a more helpful environment, a particular person or activity that supports the person to fully engage.

- Where there may be options, has the person been given information on what the choices entail?

- If the person is not in the best place to make a decision, can it wait?

- Does the person have an advocate or anybody else who might be able to help them with making their needs known?

Covid-19 and access to the vaccine for people with learning disabilities has raised some questions about capacity and consent. From a practice perspective this should be considered in the same way as any other situation where there is a person who does not have capacity to consent to a procedure/intervention or piece of work. Sometimes there is a challenge due to family wishes being expressed rather than the views of the person.

Scorer (in Thomas, 2022) makes the issue very clear:

The decision to have the vaccine or not is an individual one. The Mental Capacity Act starts from the principle that people with a learning disability are assumed to have capacity to make their own decisions and should be supported to do so in a way that is suitable for their individual needs.

From a nursing perspective, the principles of the MCA (2005) need to be applied and efforts made to involve the person and their family where possible, trying as much as possible to work with them on making a decision in the person's best interests. This is for the clinical team on a case-by-case basis. If the family is not supportive then it may be that legal advice is needed.

The team will need to:

o   evidence the engagement with the family and actions to explain the risks
    and benefits;

o   identify what actions the family is taking to keep their family member safe and
    assess the impact that this may have on the person's well-being if they aren't
    going out etc;

o   document MDT best interests assessment and if necessary apply to the Court
    of Protection.

Some family members may present reasons to object to the vaccine for their relative but
if the vaccine is considered to be in the person's best interests, an application should
be made to the Court of Protection. Obviously, you would want to work together to try to
come to an agreement before it comes to that stage.

Promoting independence and self-care

Supporting people to manage their own care plan can be achieved in many ways, there
may be elements that the individual takes responsibility for such as administering their
own medication, recognising when they need to make an appointment for review or
engaging in interventions such as dialectical behaviour therapy (DBT). There may be
other elements of the plan that the person is not interested in taking responsibility for,
for example, paying bills, preparing their own food.

If the person is not in agreement or aware of their needs, but the care team feel there
are things that have to be considered essential in their care and support, there needs to
be some thought about how you will record this.

It may be useful to have a 'how best to support me' section in their care plan.

o   Joe will need you to provide reminders to take medication with food.

o   Sam doesn't like it if they feel nagged, give them a loose timeframe to complete
    the task, for example, this morning Sam, we need to write a shopping list. Sam
    will take this on board and will approach you at some point with a pen and paper.

o   It is really important that you say what you mean when you talk to Delyth, she
    takes things very literally and it is really hard for her to understand if someone is
    sarcastic or joking.

Crisis or contingency care plan

There will be times where contingencies are necessary, and although you must make
every effort, it may not be possible for the individual to be fully included in the development of the plan. This might be due to the level of crisis presented and the person's
own level of need at that time. A crisis plan is really an agreement of how the individual
can be best supported when they are having a deterioration in their mental health and
well-being. If the person has only recently become known to services, then there may be
limited knowledge on what they want and need at times of crisis. You will still attempt to
gather this information; however, there can be limitations in detail.

An advanced directive might be one way that you are able to support a person to make their needs known should there be a crisis. This might be difficult to raise and explore as you will be asking the individual to tell you what they want the care team to do at the time when they feel most out of control or vulnerable. The importance of having the conversation with the person cannot be underestimated, there may be reactive care plans that describe how restraint, PRN or other restrictive practice might be used and they should be very clear about what should be said and done. The person may describe a 'most to least' preferred option and as the nurse documenting the discussion you will have to agree with the individual what the trigger points will be for progressing through the levels.

What do you think are the key components of a crisis plan? Take a moment to jot down the supports and communications that someone experiencing a deterioration in their mental health and well-being might need? Think about the skills you will need to utilise to involve the person and capture their true views, particularly where the person is non-verbal or has communication challenges.

Options appraisals

Following assessment, you will need to consider the clinical information and make an analysis of how to achieve the desired outcome. It is important that you are able to demonstrate why you have considered or discounted approaches and one way of doing this is through an options appraisal or a 'balance sheet'.

By doing this you can work in partnership with the person and their family, carers or others involved to identify that you have considered risks and benefits of intervention. For example, one decision might be to do nothing, this should be described and the benefits and costs of doing nothing should be made clear.

Table 6.3 demonstrates one way of working through options to support development of a care plan. The list is not exhaustive, there may be many other things suggested, it is important that each one is noted and explored. Views of the person and family members need to be clear within. You will also need to include things that have been suggested by others even though as a professional you do not think this is in a person's best interests.

Table 6.3 working through an options appraisal

Presenting problem	When anxious John can self-injure, this has led to A&E intervention in the past due to severe head banging, causing pain, bleeding and damage to the environment.
	John has had four episodes of severe self-injury in the last two weeks, each requiring hospital treatment.
Identified need	An assessment has identified a range of factors which increase John's anxiety.
	• John needs support to manage his anxiety.
	• The team need to consider the environmental management and John's safety needs.

→

Desired outcome	Environmental management and skills teaching to reduce John's anxiety under specific conditions.
	Staff will have skills to reduce antecedents to anxiety and to respond when John shows symptoms of anxiety.
	John will not self-injure to the extent that he causes damage to himself or the environment.

Options appraisal		
Proposed intervention	**Benefits**	**Disbenefit**
Do nothing	Not possible to identify a benefit for this option.	Potential for serious harm or even death.
		Negligence on the part of the staff team and service.
		Morally challenging.
		Ethically inappropriate.
		John does not learn new skills.
		The team do not learn how to support him during episodes of anxiety.
GP appointment	Potential to rule out physical health issues.	Difficult to support John to a GP appointment × 3 staff needed and waiting is challenging.
		He may not engage.
		He may become anxious.
		He has recently had four hospital admissions and so physical health factors should have already been ruled out.
Ask for a medical review	John can be seen by a psychiatrist.	Does not consider environmental factors which influence anxiety.
	Detailed knowledge of anxiety and influences.	Can take 4–6 weeks to have treatment effect.
	Potentially medication can be prescribed to reduce anxiety.	John may not take the medication.
	Reducing anxiety in the short term can allow other assessment to be carried out.	If the medication has a good effect then there might be less desire to seek to change other influencing factors.
	Medication has been successful in the past.	

Conduct in house behavioural assessment	The staff team prefer this option. They have been gathering data since the behaviour escalated. This will allow them to develop their relationship with John and his family and their understanding of his needs. They can seek external supervision and support on the tools and plans.	The team are not as skilled as the specialist team. Could be time-consuming there would still need to be referrals for broader members of the MDT input.
Refer for communication assessment	John's communication will be assessed. The staff team will be able to better understand and meet his needs. John could be taught more appropriate ways of communicating anxiety and distress.	Could be time-consuming, there is a waiting list for speech and language therapy. John may not engage with unfamiliar staff. While waiting for the assessment there could be further occurrences putting John and the team at risk. May not reduce some of the environmental factors which influence anxiety.
Refer for specialist behavioural assessment	The staff team will be able to better understand and meet his needs. Behavioural assessments lead to comprehensive support plans. John could be taught more appropriate ways of communicating anxiety and distress. An overall positive behaviour support plan will be useful throughout John's life and transitions.	Is time-consuming. John may not engage with unfamiliar staff. The staff team in the environment may feel disempowered by an external lead on the behavioural assessment. John's family has had experience of behavioural work in the past and does not feel this helped them or John.
Use a restrictive device, for example, headwear	John's mum's preferred option. They had a padded helmet for him in childhood and would use this at the earliest indication of increased anxiety. This can prevent serious injury.	This is disabling and John does not like wearing the helmet. It does not address the underlying issues of anxiety. It does not teach skills. There is a risk of injury to John and staff when the helmet is only used in response to escalating behaviour.

→

| Restrain John when he starts to self-injure | Potentially the behaviour can be quickly stopped, preventing serious self-injury.

This is the least preferred option for all. | It does not address the underlying issues of anxiety.

It does not teach skills.

There is a risk of injury to John and staff when attempting restraint. This has happened on occasions in the past.

John's relationships with others could be damaged by this intervention. He has experienced abusive practice in the past and this could be re-triggering as an approach. |

Critical reflection 6.8

Consider the options set out above. There are attempts to bring in views of others, recognising the practical and relational issues, for example, the fact that the sub-stantive team may not work effectively with a specialist team. John and his family's past experiences and views are incorporated in a number of areas. Where there is a risk, this has been quantified, for example, John's history of trauma related to restraint and potential risk to staff and John.

- What other options might there be to support John and the team at this time?

- Do you think any of the above solutions in isolation could address this issue?

- As John's named nurse, how would you make sure his views are included?

- If you were to draw a conclusion, which option do you think is in John's best interest and why?

EXPERTS BY EXPERIENCE

Historically, people may have been encouraged to be passive recipients in the receipt of care, the very word patient makes us think of people who are able to wait, tolerate, remain calm and may even be long-suffering. There has been more recent recognition of the need for power to be shared, views to be heard and changes to be made based on the experiences of service users. Involving the person is essential, however is not always prioritised. Nurses can play a key role in ensuring that the person is involved and informed their care plan. Do you provide care plans to service users in an accessible format?

How are the needs of carers considered when you plan care? People with learning disabilities and their families can be considered Experts by Experience due to their personal experience of using services. The importance of listening to and working together with Experts by Experience is increasingly recognised by services and organisations. Experts by Experience have been recruited into education, review teams and inspectorates such as the CQC and Regional Partnership Boards.

Books beyond words ™ have been referred to throughout this book as one way of utilising accessible communication and engaging people. In terms of involving people in their care, there are some specific titles, which you can access for care planning. Hollins and Banks (2015) draw together short stories using pictures which can help people describe their needs for care and treatment, understanding how good someone thinks their care is and what they would like in terms of outcomes. Using resources, which allow the person to share thoughts, process images and respond to questions, is one way of demonstrating dignity and respect for the individual.

Critical reflection 6.9

People need to be involved in their care as much as possible. It is important that they are able to question aspects of their care and raise concerns they might have about the way that care is delivered.

Take a moment to think about the last person you planned care with.

- Did you encounter any challenges in capturing their views?
- What were the enablers in their life that allowed their perspective as an expert by experience to be recognised and valued?

Now reflect on the following questions.

- Can you do more to support the development of knowledge, skills and confidence to support a person to manage their own health and well-being?
- Do you feel you are able to offer meaningful choice to service users when it comes to the provision of care or support services?

Co-producing care plans

There are various levels of service user involvement that you will need to be actively aware of in your professional practice.

For the purpose of this chapter, in relation to service user involvement in care planning, this means the individual actively participating in shaping their individualised plan, based on their experience with services, personal awareness and knowledge of what works best for them. There is an expectation that the individual will sign and keep a copy of their plan; however, what is more important is that the person has been involved in the actual development of it.

As a nurse you must make every effort to maximise involvement. There may sometimes be reasons for not sharing a care plan with an individual, it is essential that this decision is clearly recorded. You will also need to prepare for the possibility that somebody does not want to be involved in planning their care. What are the potential reasons that somebody may not want to be involved?

Being familiar with your organisations engagement or at risk of disengagement policy is important in these situations. You might need to get additional support where a person is unwilling to engage in their care plan. Working with the MDT, the carers and other professionals who know the person can help you in approaching the challenge. You may want to develop an engagement plan, which has specific timescales and review points. There may be challenges for the person in terms of their experience, confidence, level of communication and insight into their needs. Also, people have the right to make a choice. The Mental Welfare Commission for Scotland (MWCS, 2019) describes situations where people have identified the best time for them to be involved in planning care and working in partnership. It is acknowledged that this might not be the best time for an individual early into an admission.

There are key principles of co-production and sometimes this term can be misapplied. It is important to understand the principles and ensure efficacy to them to avoid tokenistic representation. Co-production means producing or making something together, based on the idea that people who have used services are experts in designing and developing them. In nursing it is essential that you seek to achieve genuine and meaningful engagement. Co-production is fundamental to achieving this. From a care planning perspective, this means that you must collaborate with the individual to plan their care.

Your care plan discussion will need to bring clarity to the following questions.

○   What is important to them?

○   What are their hopes, and what are the barriers in achieving them?

○   What they think works well, who supports them?

○   What might they like to change?

○   How would they like to be supported?

○   What are their long-term goals?

Recording responses to these questions will ensure that you incorporate the person's voice into their plan. Developing the care plan using peoples' own descriptions, their words and phrases will make sure that you avoid jargon or complicated professional language which the person may be uncomfortable or unfamiliar with.

Personalised care plans reflect the principles in statements that describe what the person will do, in a language they understand, for example:

- My care team will help me to do my deep breathing exercise if I have an anxiety attack;

- I will work with my psychiatrist to review the medication I take for depression at my next appointment in January;

- I will attend the 1:1 sessions with my psychologist for support with my anxiety every week;

- I will talk to someone in my care team when I start to think sad thoughts, they will help me to use mindfulness in that moment;

- At the end of the sessions I have for anxiety I will talk to my care co-ordinator about a discharge plan from the community learning disability team.

Ham and Davies (2017) describe the full involvement of a service user in the development of their positive behaviour support plan and the subsequent training of the new staff team who would support him going forward.

Case study 6.7

You are a learning disability nurse in the youth offending team. This team supports young people (aged 10 to 18) in identifying their abilities and needs when there is potential for involvement with the criminal justice system. This team is essential in accessing the right services and ensuring that any implemented Court Order takes account of the person's unique needs and skills. James is 14 and has recently been accused of stalking his former teacher, Mr Brown. James has struggled since being excluded from school and has made frequent direct and indirect contact with him. There has been a referral to your team and James has told you that he wants to feel better heard and understood. He has clearly articulated that he wants to be supported to make decisions about what matters to him. He is keen to return to school and feels that people around him need support to understand his diagnosis of learning disability and autism. There are times he feels vulnerable in school and has been experiencing bullying.

Following detailed assessment and sessions to help James agree appropriate strategies and supports you agree that James will support you in providing training to teaching staff to support a smooth transition back to school. James' support needs will be clearly identified in the plan and will be shared with the teaching team in a way that helps them respond to James' needs to prevent outbursts. James describes how he needs the staff to approach him directly, get down to his level and support him to take deep breaths when he displays initial indicators of anxiety and distress. They also agree that he will have access to fidgets on his desk which he will distract himself with, if he perceives that other young people are making fun or attempting to 'trigger' him.

Case study 6.8

Reflective practice in nursing care plans

Suzy is 6, she is adopted and has lived with her mum and dad since she was 11 months old, before that she was with a foster family. Suzy's parents have been married for 18 years and have experienced a number of failed pregnancies and losses; they have longed to be parents. Suzy has increasingly displayed behaviour described as challenging since starting school, her family has been more concerned over recent months as she has damaged things in their home and other family members' homes. She hits out at her mum, spits, throws food, refuses to dress or get ready for school. Her mum has had to give up work due to the challenges of being called away due to Suzy's behaviour in school. You visit the home regularly during the assessment and feel that there are some family dynamics that make the behaviours more likely to happen. You are worried that you may be judging the family, you find her mum very emotional and loud, she struggles to remain calm and appears scared of Suzy sometimes. You access support during clinical supervision and decide to call a professional meeting to think about the support needs of Suzy and the family. You manage to arrange a respite provision which will allow the parents to have some space and the respite service will provide an assessment in a new environment. While Suzy is out of the home you plan to develop your relationship with her mum to try and set some terms of reference to your input and agree some goals with her.

Iorizzo and Ames (2019) describe the importance of reflective practice in care planning. Spending time reflecting on aspects of interaction and assessment can support the development of person-centred, meaningful care plans. The investment in reflective practice is emphasised throughout nurse education and contributes to the ongoing professional development needed to revalidate and maintain registration. Without reflective practice you may find that you become stuck in your thinking and development. It is important to take time to work through decisions you have made, the things you did or didn't do and what might have been different if you had tried something else. Reflecting allows you to learn from your actions and inactions and consider how you will behave differently and anticipate a different outcome. Bringing this into care planning is one way of supporting an informal approach to evaluation and developing additional approaches to meeting needs.

Imagine you are supporting a person at a dental appointment. You have been asked to develop a care plan for Millie, aged 12, because she needs four fillings. She recently had an appointment for a check-up and her parents were distressed that they had to hold her legs and arms throughout. The dentist feels that there are additional reasonable adjustments that can be made but also feels that Millie's mum and dad are too emotionally close to allow them to let Millie engage in a less restrictive way. You speak to Millie, her parents, the dentist and the dental nurse. They help you to develop a plan and realise that you will need to spend some time developing your relationship with Millie so she can be comfortable in your presence at the dentist. You go to the house three times and do a checklist of reinforcers, you find out lots of things that Millie likes (and doesn't). She tells you how much she loves glitter and you see lots of evidence of this in the home. You agree with the dental receptionist that the appointment letter will be accessible and have glitter inside the envelope, the dentist and you decide that you will both wear sparkly t-shirts during the appointments. You also purchase some glittery card and make a certificate for Millie to show her parents when she gets home from the appointment. The appointment goes really well.

Critical reflection 6.10

- What will you need to think about for future appointments?
- As Millie gets older what might you want to work on with her and her family?

Reviewing care plans

Every time a nurse delivers an intervention in line with a care plan, they will make a record of how this took place. In this there will be a level of review. The nurse who designed the care plan will read the records and assess how effective the plan is, making changes within a formal review; however, there should also be clear indicators that a review of care is needed.

There will be timescales set for reviews when plans align to specific processes such as Continuing Health Care (CHC), Care and Treatment Planning (Wales) Ministry of Justice (MoJ) or the Mental Health Act (MHA, 1983).

Critical reflection 6.11

Reflect on how you have reviewed care plans.

- Was the person involved?
- Who did you consult with?
- How do you feel this influenced the outcomes for the person?

All care plans need a clear review date. This is a planned opportunity to identify and celebrate any progress made. It is essential that individuals are also involved in reviewing their care. If people are to be truly involved this means a level of creativity and adapting to an individual's specific needs. You may use audio or visual tools that relate to the individual's need and preferences. Mood charts, behaviour monitoring tools, weekly evaluations or daily reflections can all be modified for people with different levels of ability and incorporated into an evaluation of a care plan. Perhaps you could spend time with the individual before the review meeting if they find the professional structure difficult, or you might suggest they stay for the beginning, share their views and then come back at the end to be involved in the decision-making. What is important is that the attempts to include a person in a meaningful way are made and their voice is heard.

This might mean developing an accessible format for capturing views. An approach to being inclusive could be to use simple questions and utilise this in the review.

Table 6.4 A basic tool for collecting feedback

	What is working well?	**What could be better?**
I think …		
My family think …		
My carers think …		
My health professionals think …		

Chapter summary

Care plans are essential in ensuring that people receive evidence-based, person-centred approaches to meeting their needs; within this chapter a variety of care plans have been explored. The importance of including people and their families in the development of care plans cannot be underestimated. The people who are responsible for delivering the care plans may not be nurses and so you must develop and maintain effective working relationships with others who will implement and evaluate the care. In your practice care plans will allow you to improve the lives of others, this might be through management of risk, safety, behaviour, developing skills, independence and relationships. Within your professional practice you will utilise a variety of skills in care planning, reflective practice has been emphasised in this chapter and is a tool that will allow you to continuously improve, work with others and demonstrate how you value the individuals you support.

FURTHER READING

Royal College of Nursing Wales (2022) Learning Disability Nursing. [online] Available at: www.rcn.org.uk/wales/-/media/Royal-College-Of-Nursing/Documents/Countries-and-regions/Wales/2022/Learning-Disability-Nursing-report-Apr-22.pdf (accessed 23 April 2022).

Smull, M, Sanderson, H and Allen, B (2001) *Essential Lifestyle Planning Manchester.* North West Training Development Team.

RESOURCES

Woman with Learning Disability Can Have Teeth Removed, Court Rules: www.bbc.co.uk/news/uk-england-lincolnshire-52774498 (accessed 6 May 2022).

This article provides a media perspective on a distressing situation where a lady with learning disabilities had teeth removed.

Webinar: Developing Innovative Ordinary Housing Solutions for People with Complex Needs and Behaviours that Challenge: www.bild.org.uk/resource/webinar-developing-innovative-ordinary-housing-solutions-for-people-with-complex-needs-behaviours-that-challenge/ (accessed 23 April 2022).

This webinar gives great insight into the developments in housing solutions and person-centred developments for people with learning disabilities.

7 Working across the lifespan

Chapter aims

This chapter explores the contribution that learning disability nurses make to promoting health and well-being across the lifespan. It details some of the issues for people with learning disabilities and their families within screening, diagnosis, child development, transition, relationships, growing older and end of life care. The context of understanding and working in partnership with the family of the person with learning disabilities is emphasised. The way that learning disability nurses can provide the right support, intervention and treatments to facilitate access to services and resources for people with learning disabilities throughout their lives is explored with opportunities for personal reflection and suggested activities.

Professional standards and expectations

The NMC (2018b) have clear standards related to how nurses meet needs across the lifespan examples can be found in standards 1.11, 1.12, 2.6 and 3.14.

NICE guideline (NG93, 2018a) for learning disabilities and behaviour that challenges recognise lifespan approaches for improving outcomes.

NICE (NG96, 2018b) guidelines on care and support of people growing older with learning disabilities make recommendations for identifying changing needs, planning for the future and delivering services including health, social care and housing.

THE ROLE OF THE LEARNING DISABILITY NURSE

As people with learning disabilities live longer with increasingly complex conditions, learning disability nurses are well placed to work in partnership to understand and respond to changing needs. The breadth of the learning disability nursing role means that there are a range of specialisms underpinned by academic, professional and practice-based approaches to improving life and health outcomes for people with learning disabilities at all stages of the lifespan.

A learning disability is a lifelong condition. People with learning disabilities will experience life events and health issues as all humans do and helping them understand and process these events is fundamental to the learning disability nurse role. The understanding of human growth and development across the lifespan is essential as the learning disability nurse may have many encounters with service users and their families during each stage of development.

Learning disability nursing is often referred to as the purist form of nursing (Gates et al, 2015) and you will see this in your practice experiences: you will care for people when they are well and unwell, at all stages in their life. This is not just a cradle to grave approach: due to the way that learning disability nurses work and the broad range of roles undertaken there will also be opportunities to work in the field of learning disability nursing pre-birth and post-death. There are examples at either end of the lifespan, which demonstrate this such as genetic screening and the genome project or working with parents who have learning disabilities, siblings and extended families, in preparation for the birth of a child. Post-death, you may contribute to the review of deaths, learning lessons from events, supporting families, carers and teams in filling the void left when a person with a learning disability has died, helping people through the grieving process and managing their memories and bereavement needs.

A rights-based approach

The role of the learning disability nurse is essential in upholding rights-based approaches. Learning disability nurses have a key role in making sure that the individual is seen as having the same rights and needs as those who do not have a learning disability. As people with learning disabilities grow older their life course will be influenced by personal, socio-economic, environmental and political factors at micro and macro levels. Everyday experiences, identity, interpersonal relationships, housing, education, access to health and jobs are all influenced by how people with learning disabilities are seen and supported in society.

Legislation and policy influences how people with learning disabilities are viewed and treated; the agendas can shape the way that you deliver care. Learning disability is often described as a social construct – something that is socially defined. Dependent on the political, social, academic, medical or economic influences at the time, those who are more powerful are in a position to define others who are less powerful, with implications for how people with learning disabilities are labelled, perceived, valued and treated.

The social constructionist theory highlights the multiple barriers and exclusions people with learning disabilities can face, hypothesising that with the right support, and a more inclusive society, people with learning disabilities can overcome these restrictions.

Historically, life expectancy has been lower for people with learning disabilities and a significant gap still exists today; on average people with learning disabilities die 25 years younger than the rest of the population (LeDeR, 2019). There is more detailed discussion related to these issues in Chapter 8. Covid-19 brought many challenges in 2020 for people with learning disabilities including moral and ethical issues for nurses. There was a need to reinforce the unique needs of individuals in order to increase the opportunities for fair and equal treatment, for example, vaccine planning or escalation of care. Many people with learning disabilities described how they felt left behind and not considered in some of the planning and preparation for Covid-19 responses. Examples include the rapidly developed NICE guidelines and use of a frailty score (NICE, 2020), shielding, access to testing, blanket restrictions and potentially inappropriate application of DNA CPR (CQC, 2021). Services had to think about how to deliver learning disability nursing through and post-Covid-19. The locked-out report (Welsh Government, 2021a) highlighted many of these experiences and evidenced the exacerbation of pre-existing socio-economic inequalities in our society and the impact on health outcomes.

We know that there will be more people with learning disabilities in the future due to advances in healthcare technology meaning increased survival rates and treatment interventions. As people grow older with learning disabilities we continue to learn about potential multi-morbidities and the impact of conditions associated with ageing. This has implications for the role of the learning disability nurse. You will encounter changing needs across the lifespan and will continue to work in new and emerging roles as the unique needs of people with learning disabilities are further understood. There will undoubtedly continue to be a need for advocacy and education of others who are not directly working with people with learning disabilities day to day.

CHILDREN AND YOUNG PEOPLE

As explored in Chapter 1 learning disabilities may be identified prenatally, at birth or as a child moves through developmental milestones. For some, a learning disability may be acquired, for example, due to the impact of injury or trauma (this must have taken place before the age of 18 to be considered a learning disability).

Global developmental delay is used when a child is delayed in meeting two or more developmental milestones, for example, motor, language or social-adaptive skills at the expected timescales (Foster et al, 2015), the description is usually used before the age of five. The term 'delay' might cause confusion for families, they may feel their child will 'catch up'. There needs to be careful discussion with a family about what the issues for their child are and what they might mean in the longer term. Some children will go on to have a formal diagnosis as their needs and presentation are better understood. Adlington et al (2018, p 1) describe how *recent advances in clinical genetic techniques and pathways have meant genetic testing now offers more diagnostic information than ever before* and highlight the complexity of having discussions about genetic testing due to issues such as consent, capacity, communication and ethical factors.

It is essential that you understand child development. If you have knowledge of developmental milestones, this will help you to recognise the potential areas where children with learning disabilities might need additional support. You will also be able to help others with their knowledge and ability to meet the needs of children and young people. The learning disability nurse will hold knowledge related to other agencies who can support, as well as strategies and practically implementable interventions. As well as the need to understand child development from a bio-psycho-social perspective it is also important to be aware of developmental theories. Nunkoosing (2011) describes how theories have application to practice and by working through them, we are enabled to think about what we do (as learning disability nurses) and what this can mean for people with learning disabilities. There are various developmental theories, which explore processes of socialisation, growth and learning in relation to others, taking into account environmental, cultural and interpersonal factors. One theory related to psychological safety and relationships is Bowlby's (1988) theory of attachment.

Attachment theory

Attachment describes the emotional bonds and patterns in relationship with parents or caregivers. The way the parent and child interact with each other will form patterns for how future relationships will develop and how a person feels about themselves and others.

Attachment difficulties can cause significant issues for children and families and there are factors which may increase the likelihood of developing poor attachment (from a parenting and child perspective). Most parents seek to satisfy their children's physical and emotional needs, there can be barriers which impact on the ability to do this which may influence the relationship before the child is born. The parents' own childhood experiences may impact on their thoughts and feelings towards their baby, mental health and well-being, physical health, socio-economic factors, educational attainment, job security and family dynamics are just some of the possible issues influencing attachment. Bowlby's attachment theory suggests that attachment is an evolutionary process which allows the child to survive by forming attachments to others. Babies are very vulnerable and dependent on others for meeting all of their needs; Bowlby (ibid) suggested that behaviour such as crying, screaming, being clingy are instinctive responses that served to avoid separation from a parent or caregiver. The attachment theory recognises the need for a holistic understanding of children, thinking about their environment, relationships, family and personal experiences and understanding the overall influences on our development

Critical reflection 7.1

- Carry out a literature search on one of the following developmental theories to learn more and consider its relevance to learning disability nursing.

Theory of development	Outline
Bowlby (1988) Attachment theory	Attachments develop in stages and continue to develop impacting on future relationships and feelings about self.
Piaget and Cook (1952) Cognitive theory	Explores new knowledge learned at each stage of development and how this builds cognitive skill progression.

→

Theory of development	Outline
Bandura (1977) Social learning theory	Considers that behaviours may be learned vicariously, from watching others and the importance of role models emerges in the work.
Vygotsky (Cole et al, 1978) Sociocultural theory	Describes how fundamental the role social interaction is in the development of cognition.
Erikson's (Orenstein and Lewis, 2020) Eight phases of development	The theory identifies stages of development which are mastered or unachieved and each stage builds on the one before. There is a belief that there are conflicts at each stage of development where a person develops a positive aspect, for example, in adolescence the young person will emerge with established identity or role confusion.

There will be opportunities for shared learning within pre-registration theory and practice placement. Learning disability nurses will sometimes learn alongside children's nurses and health visitors or midwives and access placements in schools, nurseries and other areas where children and young people are. A range of roles for learning disability nurses with children and young people are captured in the recent RCN (2021) report connecting for change: for the future of learning disability nursing. Examples are provided of nurses working in respite, community, schools, pupil referral units, hospices and transitions. There are many circumstances where the understanding origins of behaviour and presentation are needed in supporting a child or young person with a learning disability and their family. Learning disability nurses can often work with children from a very young age, many community teams accept referrals from the age of two. These will be children who have a specialist need, above the universal service offer. Learning disability nurses may be involved in supporting parents and carers to understand a range of needs including those related to sleep, sensory issues, anxiety, behaviour, continence and skills development.

There can be challenges in accessing, understanding and adapting to a diagnosis. Some families will never have a specific name for their child's presentation, many children will not demonstrate specific identifiable markers or characteristics that can help with identity and understanding. Learning disability nurses can be in a position to support parents in understanding their child's diagnosis, behaviour or developmental needs. Often educational programs focused on understanding diagnosis and parenting groups rely on partnership working between learning disability nurses, specialist health visitors, teachers, social workers and other key professionals to create space for learning, reflection, growth and development.

As with all parenting there can be challenges adapting to roles and responsibilities and there are likely to be additional challenges for some families at different stages. Beighton and Wills (2017) describe how parents may describe stress in relation to raising a child with a learning disability; there is also acknowledgement of many positive aspects.

Seven key aspects related to positive parenting experiences are identified and some of these focus on the strengths and achievements of the child, while others relate to the resilience and capability of the parents (Table 7.1)

Table 7.1 Positive aspects to parenting a child with a learning disability

Key theme	Examples
Increased sense of personal strength and confidence	Advocating for their child. Handling 'the situation' and prepared for handling other issues because they parent a child with learning disabilities.
Changed priorities	Identifying as less materialistic. Undertaking opportunities and new challenges such as career changes.
Greater appreciation of life	More appreciative of 'simple things in life' and less concerned with societal expectations.
Pleasure in the child's accomplishments	Celebrating small things, seeing the child accomplish something they were told they wouldn't be able to do, for example, walking.
Increased faith and spirituality	Taking a philosophical approach and a 'what's meant to be attitude'.
More meaningful relationships	Finding out who their true friends were and strengthened relationships with partners and family members etc.
Positive impact of the child on the wider community	Engagement from their child helping people to see beyond disability and increasing awareness of learning disabilities in society.

(Beighton and Wills, 2017, reproduced with permission)

In reflecting on these seven themes, learning disability nurses can gain awareness of the potential issues for parents of children with learning disabilities. The insight into how families can feel like they need to fight or battle to have their child's needs met and rights upheld is an important message for your professional practice. This is described in Blair et al (2016):

> in the early days I fought against the system, I fought against the fact that suddenly your life was not your own, that even 18 year-old student nurses could sit and read notes about your child that you were not allowed to look at. Lives on view for all to see, every emotion, every outburst.

Sometimes it can be difficult to access supports families want and need for their child and themselves. Understanding well-being and the interventions that can support parents and children's resilience, mental health and coping strategies is important. When working with children it is essential to understand their needs in the context of the family situation and the role that the parents take as advocates for their child's rights and needs. As a learning disability nurse you will need to undertake assessments of specialist need and work in partnership with the child and their family at key stages leading up to adulthood and transition.

Critical reflection 7.2

Think about developmental milestones.

- What are some of the 'firsts' that you think about in typical child development.

- What might your role be as a learning disability nurse in supporting children and families through these stages?

Safeguarding recognising Adverse Childhood Experiences

Some childhood experiences can have long-lasting impact and need to be considered within your practice. Remembering your potential role in safeguarding and recognising the risk factors for children with learning disabilities is important for your professional development and practice.

The Children Act (Gov.uk, 1989) is clear that children must be seen as children first and their rights must be upheld under that key principle. Understanding the Act is relevant to all learning disability nurses because inevitably you will meet children in your practice regardless of whether you have a direct role with children and young people. The 1989 Act sets out the current framework and the 2004 amendments give guidance related to the importance of inter-agency working and communication, changes in relation to safeguarding were made following the death of Victoria Climbie and Lord Laming's (2003) damning review. There may be safeguarding issues for the children and young people you support in your practice. The importance of accessing robust supervision, maintaining your CPD and mandatory training plays an important role in your ability to safeguard.

Critical reflection 7.3

- There are factors for people with learning disabilities that might increase their vulnerability to abuse and barriers for professionals to identify concerns. Make notes on why it might be difficult to identify safeguarding issues for children and young people with learning disabilities. Compare your ideas with those in Table 7.2.

Table 7.2 Barriers in identifying safeguarding issues

For the person	For the family	For learning disability nurses
Communication issues, having the words and capability to describe the situation or experience.	Not being able to get information from the child or other carers.	Explanations from family or carers, not able to have the child describe the situation.
Ability to understand what is happening and respond to risk.	May have their own history of abuse or vulnerability.	May not have the necessary skills or supports to recognise safeguarding issues.
A familiarity with being cared for by multiple adults.	Explanations given by staff or carers which seem plausible.	Seeing marks or bruising that could have been caused by accident or in daily living tasks.
Dependency on others for personal care.	A dependence on others to care for their child.	Reluctant to identify or suspect abuse and may take explanations at face value.
Physical dexterity and mobility may be used to explain cause of injury.	Parent may not see their child as vulnerable.	It may be difficult to help parents understand their child can be vulnerable. A careful balance is needed in the conversations.
Being labelled as making allegations or history of not being believed when speaking up.	A fear of raising a concern in case they are blamed or seen as struggling.	Challenges communicating with family members or staff teams who may be sensitive to allegations.

Adverse Childhood Experiences (ACEs)

There is developing understanding in safeguarding of the potential impact of ACEs. These are described as '*highly stressful, and potentially traumatic, events or situations that occur during childhood and/or adolescence. They can be a single event, or prolonged threats to, and breaches of, the young person's safety, security, trust or bodily integrity*' (Young Minds, 2018). Learning disability nurses may be in a position to support early intervention and take steps to minimise the potential for long-term trauma. There can be opportunities to work in partnership with families and provide support, structures, education and safe spaces to explore ACEs and ways that changes can be made. Some examples of ACEs include:

o   exposure to domestic violence;

o   emotional abuse;

o   sexual abuse;

○ physical abuse,

○ living in a family where there is addiction;

○ a family member who has gone to prison or who has a serious mental illness.

The more ACEs a person experiences, the higher the risk of negative physical and mental health outcomes. Learning disability nurses will have skills in supporting conversations about the impact of ACEs on children and working together with families to be aware of risk factors and protective measures. The child may benefit from having their own therapeutic work if they have been exposed to ACEs and need support in processing and understanding the impact. A trauma-informed approach (see Table 7.3) is necessary to recognise and respond to the potential difficulties a child or young person may present with. The Learning Disability Senate (2020) has produced an accessible version of ten tips for trauma-informed approaches (bild.org).

Table 7.3 Understanding a trauma-informed approach

What is a trauma-informed approach?
Being trauma informed means seeking to understand the impact of traumatic experiences that people have had and how that shapes their presentation and experiences going forward. Rather than asking 'what is wrong with you? we ask what happened to you?' (Perry and Winfrey, 2021)
What can learning disability nurses do to provide a trauma-informed approach?
Create positive, safe environments with therapeutic, sensory-based activities for discussion and exploration of issues.
Educate children, young people and families, educators, carers etc about the importance of understanding trauma.
Avoid the use of labelling (Johnson, 2017) suggests talking about 'bad things' or 'worse times' as a way of minimising this.
Develop trust, keep things predictable, use structured and consistent approaches.

There is evidence to suggest that exposure to ACEs can have an impact on the development of mental health challenges in later life (Scheffler et al, 2020). Mental health is everyone's business and all nurses should be in a position to offer general advice and intervention for lower-level mental health issues, contributing to conversations on good mental health and well-being and mental health promotion. The RCN (2014) identifies some of the core themes that can influence the presentation of mental health problems, including long-term conditions, bullying, experience of abuse and the use of restrictive practices. These may be experiences that are relevant to children and young people with learning disabilities. Maguire et al (2018) identify that pupils with learning disabilities are one of the most bullied groups in schools and communities. The learning disability nurse is likely to be able to advocate for the child, liaising with other key professionals in the child or young person's life. Some learning disability nurses work in paediatric and specialist health visiting teams or child and adolescent services (CAMHS) and bring specialist knowledge and understanding to the assessment and understanding of needs.

Rites of passage

There are significant events in all of our lives that indicate a growth and development, change in status, social movement and transition. Recognising these events within a family and community may involve historical ritual or embrace more modern values and concepts. In societies milestones such as birth, maturity, marriage, reproduction and death are recognised and celebrated in diverse ways recognising cultural values and beliefs. In some cultures there may be specific ceremonies or rituals related to the transition or passage, often associated with religious beliefs and tradition. These rites and traditions have broadened out over time and in contemporary society many 'firsts' are given status and recognition, often captured on social media. A contemporary example is the first day at school, where children pose in front of the fireplace or by the front door in their school uniform, ready to make those first steps to the classroom.

There are likely to be rites of passage that many young people and their families take for granted. These occasions can sometimes be problematic for people with learning disabilities, there are many examples of parents who did not have positive experiences associated with birth and celebration because of the responses of those around them. Binger (2020) emphasises this describing being told 'sorry' when pre-natal screening indicated her unborn son had Down syndrome. It is important for learning disability nurses to promote a positive image of the people they work with and challenge outdated ideas, stereotypes or misconceptions. This might be achieved by contributing to interprofessional learning, sharing good practice examples and educating non-learning disability clinicians. There are a number of campaigns (Don't screen us out, Wouldn't change a thing, Down side up) raising awareness of the impact of screening programmes and the messages given to families as well as people with learning disabilities especially those with Down syndrome about the perceptions of having a child with a disability. There are advocates who feel learning disability nurses should be involved in the delivery of the diagnosis of learning disability due to the rounded perspective and reality-based information they have about supporting children and families (Blair et al, 2016).

Saltmarsh et al (2016) describe challenges for children and young people with complex needs in being heard and having opportunities to speak up. Increasing opportunities for independence is a key feature of growing up and may also become a source of conflict as children seek to be more independent, developing their confidence and skills, parents may feel they need to restrict activities and exert authority in the adult, child relationship. It may also be that because others find it difficult to capture views and responses from some children and young people with learning disabilities, they do not take adequate steps to include and listen to them.

As children with learning disabilities grow up, their parents can find that they need to continue to advocate for them and boundaries may not be well established or maintained. Some children and young people will be dependent on others for aspects of personal care and daily living, and this may mean parents continue to address these needs for as long as the child remains at home. Parents will have an awareness of their child's physical development in a much more intimate way than parents of children who are typically developing. There is a need to broach these sensitive topics and work together with a family, the child and other services. Some examples of issues related to dignity and respect can be challenging to address but have implications for wider access and quality of life etc.

> ## *Critical reflection 7.4*
>
> Take some time to think about your experience of growing up and the opportunities you had to develop confidence and competence as a teenager and young adult.
>
> - What were the key rites of passage that shaped your growth and development?
>
> - What mistakes did you make and how aware were your parents of them?

Once you have considered your own experiences, think about the lives of young adults or teenagers with learning disabilities. The likelihood is that the parents or carers of individuals will have been involved in many of the big decisions; they may have been informed of mistakes their child has made, by teachers, respite care workers or other professionals in the young person's life. The experiences, opportunities and practical application of independence may not be well supported for a young adult with a learning disability; the family may be heavily involved in some of the personal care needs of the young person and may be more aware than other parents of how their child is developing physically and emotionally. The rites of passage that teenagers experience such as independent travel, handling money, attending parties and social events, going to the cinema or playing sports are precious opportunities to learn and develop, make friendships and experiment, test boundaries and learn safety skills. For those with learning disabilities it is more likely that these experiences are shared and supported by adults. Promoting the child or young person's potential relies on the individual being supported to access opportunities, being asked about their wants, needs and wishes and being able to aspire to them. Supporting choice and increasing awareness related to body image, dress sense, hairstyle etc may need careful and thoughtful interactions with parents and carers to help the individual assert their own ideas.

Life events such as leaving school, living independently or starting relationships may not occur at expected times with the usual excitement, because there can be a need for rigorous planning and engagement with a broad range of professionals who are integral to the process. Support during these times may need to focus on practical issues such as access, transport, financial support and how physical health needs will be addressed. These transitions do not always bring the celebration and recognition of the event that we anticipate and embrace in wider society. McGrath and Yeowart (2009) capture case studies which focus on transition and recognise the way that supports can be put in place to facilitate young adults achieving their aspirations. There are also examples of transition planning which has not met needs and has a negative impact on the young person's well-being, reducing their quality of life and impacting on the family dynamic and relationships. For these reasons it is vital that transition is perceived as a journey and young people are allowed to gradually make the changes and learn the skills required for adulthood.

Transition

Transitions happen often in our lives; we grow, learn, develop and are exposed to new challenges, opportunities and situations. From a learning disabilities perspective, we often think about transitions in an educational context. Leaving school is a major step for all young people, for those with a learning disability it can be even more daunting. The process can trigger a whole range of concerns: what choices may exist in the future, will future services promote a fulfilled life and the fear that important sources of support may fade away.

Achieving the best for young people with learning disabilities in relation to transition is a key ask of the Children's Commissioner for Wales (2018). Exploration of families, children and young people's experiences highlighted the challenge many families face and fear; however, it also demonstrated good practice examples (Children's Commissioner for Wales, 2020).

A number of things are highlighted within the report in terms of wants and needs for a successful transition including the following.

o   Involvement: young people want to be heard and want the opportunity to participate in planning.

o   Family life: services need to recognise the broader issues related to parenting a child with a learning disability.

o   Support: a variety of aspects are recommended, some very practical (transport, respite, finance), some of a social nature (friendships, life skills, independence) and reference to choice, flexibility and quality information.

o   Getting services: this element highlights the particular challenge when children have been placed out of area and families and services start to plan for their return. The financial (budgetary) issues are also recognised and a perception that services can be inflexible.

o   Quality of service: poor communication is highlighted as a barrier to effective transition and access to good, joined-up working to provide a quality service.

o   Good practice within services: where professionals work with the person, coordinate with each other and liaise with other professionals in a needs-based rather than diagnosis-based way transition can be smoother and a more positive experience.

o   Friends, social life and transport: services that support socialising are incredibly important to children and young people who want to access friends and develop relationships. Transport and access can greatly improve the opportunities but is often a barrier.

o   Hopes for the future: many young people with learning disabilities want employment opportunities and recognise the need for responsibility, routine, structures and purpose.

Learning disability nurses can involve people with learning disabilities in their transition planning, engaging in person-centred planning, making information accessible, supporting development of skills in relation to health, risk, safety and socialising. There need to be excellent links with education and local authority to create opportunities, and the role of an advocate can ensure that young people are heard and that their contributions are listened to. Bridging the potential gap between children and Adult Services is something that learning disability nurses are able to lead on, bringing people and services together and sharing appropriate information to smooth the process.

Critical reflection 7.5

Most people live in one space, work in another, exercise, access recreation and socialise elsewhere. You will engage with a range of different people in different settings, some of your choosing and some not, for example, you may choose where to work but not necessarily who you work with, you may choose an exercise class but have no control over who else will be in the space. When you choose a mentor, a friend to go to lunch with or who you will sit next to in class there are likely to be many influences.

* How do you live your life?

* Now think about the life of a person with a learning disability: who do they live with, what other environments do they access, what does their day look like, who do they get to choose to be around?

ADULTHOOD

Many adults with learning disabilities will live independently with little need for specialist support; however, for those that do, there are various reasons why an adult may benefit from the input of a learning disability nurse. Meeting specialist health needs and offering assessment and intervention is a key role. There are some people who will have regular support from learning disability teams, this might be for health facilitation and health promotion, specialist assessment related to mental health, challenging behaviour or help in adapting to a new need such as the diagnosis of diabetes or epilepsy. Sometimes assessment will happen in the community, the person remains in their home, accessing their usual support with short-term input from a learning disability nurse who works in partnership with the individual to meet that recognised need. For others, a short-term admission to a specialist unit might be needed; this might be a learning disability or mental health assessment and treatment unit where a multi-professional team work to address the health issues and support transition back home or onward, to a new home. Learning disability nurses can conduct thorough and informed assessment of mental health. The ability to recognise changes in a person's behaviour and understand what is typical for that person is fundamental to making the correct decisions about intervention. For people with learning disabilities it is especially important that a mental illness is not misdiagnosed, there are significant risks of overprescribing or inappropriate use of antipsychotics and associated side effects can be debilitating or deadly for some people (STOMP, antipsychotics).

There is potential for a mental health issue to be overshadowed by the presence of learning disability. In the past people with learning disabilities may not have been treated appropriately, in line with the general population, when experiencing mental distress. In overcoming this, as services have evolved there are learning disability nurses who work in mental health liaison and identify the specific supported needed at that time. Prisons are also areas where learning disability nurses can have specialist roles and work using skills to support the needs of inmates with learning disabilities, learning disability nurses can be involved in assessment, healthcare delivery and supporting understanding information for those in contact with the criminal justice system. Marshall-Tate et al (2019) describe the role of the learning disability nurse in recognising potential indication of learning disability in the criminal justice system and the importance of meeting potential unmet need for those who may be vulnerable and find it difficult to process the experience.

Due to the level of complexity and potential multimorbidity of health conditions, some adults are likely to frequently access multiple aspects of care, including health (Kalseth and Halvorsen, 2020). Some people may need specific input from a liaison nurse who facilitates access to health appointments in primary or secondary care; this might be on a planned or unplanned basis. Lynne (2020) describes the role of a learning disability nurse working in an emergency department (ED); the role is specific to supporting reasonable adjustments, providing information in accessible ways, reducing anxiety and improving the hospital experience. There are also training elements to the role, ensuring that nurses and staff in the ED are able to identify people with learning disabilities and respond to their unique needs.

Learning disability nurses may work in roles with adults outside of nursing, such as advocacy, therapy, education or in non-clinical roles: care management, commissioning, service management or social care settings. Learning disability nurses increasingly support people to live well with a learning disability using transferable skills and influencing developments in service delivery.

The AHC is one part of this and while in some parts of the UK this is accessed from the age of 14, in others the AHC begins in adulthood. Primary care is responsible for the completion of the AHC and there are many learning disability nurses who work in partnership with practice nurses and GPs to facilitate access for people with learning disabilities. The intention of the AHC is to provide a proactive approach with health protection and promotion as the main goals. AHCs and HAPs are considered a vital component in addressing the hidden inequality in healthcare for people with learning disabilities. Where the AHC is comprehensive and conducted appropriately then individuals would have a HAP with steps to take for health promotion and achieving optimal health in between their AHC. Unfortunately, however people with learning disabilities and carers say that they experience difficulties with accessing a health check. Appropriate reasonable adjustments are often not made and the health check does not always meet expectations.

There are some parts of the health check that may not be completed for various reasons; one of the more challenging and difficult areas for people with learning disabilities may be related to the questions about sexuality and sexual behaviour. This might be because they are asked private questions in front of their carers or family members. Sexual identity and behaviour is one area that can be neglected or overlooked for people with learning disabilities. This will be explored in some detail within this chapter. Seeing people with learning disabilities as sexual beings with rights and needs is still a challenge for some, and the learning disability nurse can have an impact on enabling individuals and environments to achieve their wants, needs and wishes in relation to this.

Enabling sexuality

Rights, independence, choice and inclusion may have impacted on attitudes towards people with learning disabilities but sex and sexuality can often remain an overlooked area of need. As a professional working with a person with a learning disability you may need to consider sexual identity and behaviour within an assessment and care plan. This is likely to be something that will need sensitive and careful consideration. Often people with learning disabilities have not had access to good sex education; they may have limited experience of relationships and may have been protected or prevented from developing a sexual identity (Schmidt et al, 2021). There may be challenges within people's support networks on having conversations about sexuality and sexual behaviour and there are many ethical considerations for you as a professional in trying to support the development of confidence and competence in exploring these issues appropriately with people with learning disabilities at all ages.

Critical reflection 7.6

- Think about the steps that you might take as a learning disability nurse to provide understanding and awareness of the sexuality support a person with a learning disability might need throughout the lifespan.

- Who will you need to work in partnership with?

- How and where might you need to deliver education and support with resources?

- What might the challenges or barriers be?

- Compare your ideas to the role of the learning disability nurse identified in Table 7.4.

Trueland (2021) explores the challenge for people with learning disabilities in dating and suggests there may be a role for learning disability nurses in facilitating relationships. The Love project (University of Kent) carried out research into dating agencies and the experience of people with learning disabilities, highlighting that there are far more men joining agencies than women and recognising the friendship needs of people as much as the romance needs. As a learning disability nurse you may be able to refer people with a learning disability to a dating agency. Encouraging referrals from professionals may act as safety and security measure from the agencies' perspective, however, can be challenging as professionals are sometimes reluctant to provide them. Could this be related to the taboos of relationships and historic, paternalistic attitudes and beliefs? Ndadzungira (2016) reflects that although attitudes are changing:

> *people with learning disabilities, like everyone else, have a need for affectionate and intimate relationships. Yet many people with learning disabilities don't get to have this type of relationship because of a lack of social and practical support, and society's negative and stereotypical attitudes.*

Table 7.4 Understanding sexuality in lifespan milestones

Stage of development	Behaviours and features in typical development	Examples of learning disability nursing activities
Birth to early childhood	Exploring own body Sexually stimulated by own touch/ rocking or rubbing onto objects Become aware of language to describe genitalia Inquisitive about body parts Emerging ideas about sexuality	Educate parents and carers Advise on developmentally appropriate behaviours Work in partnership with health visitors, paediatricians and other healthcare professionals Provide resources
Pre-adolescence (ages 8–12)	Changes in the body, onset of puberty More self-aware and self-conscious Self-exploration with intent, may start to masturbate	Educate the child, parents, carers Advise on developmentally appropriate behaviours Work in partnership with teachers, local authority and other health care professionals Provide personalised, accessible information
Teenage years	Bodies mature and the primary and secondary development of sexual characteristics takes place Hormonal changes, mood, interest and behavioural differences may emerge Regular masturbation more common and may be discussed with peers Interest in forming relationships (sexual and romantic) May have their first sexual encounter with another person More confident in own sexuality and identity May need access to contraception	Promote access to information and resources Undertake specific pieces of work with the young person Liaise with primary care, family planning services on needs of children and young people with learning disabilities Support relationship and developmental work around intimacy and boundaries

→

Stage of development	Behaviours and features in typical development	Examples of learning disability nursing activities
Adulthood	Experience of relationships, commitment and heartbreak More confident in understanding own wants and needs in a sexual relationship May explore ideas and desires with a partner (or multiple) May want to commit and think about having children May experience pregnancy Access to screening programmes starts	Support meaningful understanding of appropriate behaviour and social situations advise and signpost to appropriate services. Liaise regarding support needs, promote reasonable adjustments and accessible information Work in partnership with the person and appropriate services
Older adults	Menopause, changes in the body Hormonal impact and may see change in behaviour, mood, interest and pleasure May be less interested in sex and desires may change Men may start to experience erectile dysfunction and other challenges	Education on changes in the body. Nurses need to be aware of the physiological changes in older age Facilitate and advocate for access to appropriate support and treatments Work in partnership with other services to ensure reasonable adjustments and reduce inequality

It is important to recognise that people with learning disabilities have a right to a sexual identity and to be recognised as sexual beings. The World Health Organization (WHO, 2015) is clear that sexuality includes: 'sex, gender identities and roles, sexual orientation, eroticism, pleasure, intimacy and reproduction'. It is also important to recognise that for people with learning disabilities, their awareness of their bodies, their desire and needs may not develop in line with the typical stages identified above and there can be a range of factors which impact on the outward expression.

Critical reflection 7.7

- Are you aware of any policy in your practice that supports people with learning disabilities to develop their sexual identity and address their sexual needs?

- How do you see this as relevant to your professional practice?

Promoting healthy sexuality: identifying and addressing barriers

There may be multiple barriers for people with learning disabilities in exploring and understanding their own sexuality. Taking a rights-based approach means seeking to understand these issues in your professional practice and considering ways in which people with learning disabilities can be supported in a holistic way. Your role in increasing autonomy and awareness as well of achieving quality of life means understating the issues related to sexuality. There are many implications for health equality if people with learning disabilities are educated to understand their own bodies and supported to meet their sexual needs and desires. Sinclair et al (2015) draw together evidence related to the sexual education needs of people with learning disabilities and highlight that people can be empowered through education, not only in being able to meet their needs but also to protect themselves from abuse, avoid sexually transmitted disease and unplanned pregnancy. This is also supported by McDaniels and Fleming (2016) highlighting the paucity of evidence in relation to sex education and people with learning disabilities and that there is a need for specific educational approaches. Enabling people to recognise and protect themselves from unwanted sexual interactions is essential, without educational approaches people may not have the awareness, language and skills to highlight their experiences to others. Willott et al (2020) recognise the implications of under-reporting sexual assault for people with learning disabilities.

People with learning disabilities may lack knowledge about the mechanics of sex and the physiological factors, it may be part of your role to educate people with learning disabilities, to know their body parts and understand their function. If a man with a learning disability does not know that he has testicles, because he has never explored his body, asked questions about it or been encouraged to understand how it works, then how would you approach awareness of testicular cancer or 'checking for change?'. You will need to think about how you find common language so that the individual is clear about the issue being discussed.

Women of child-bearing potential who have epilepsy need to be informed of specific risks dependent on the type of medication they use. Sodium valproate (Epilim) is known to be particularly harmful and the PREVENT (pregnancy prevent) program stipulates guidance which must be adhered to when prescribing Epilim to women who could potentially become pregnant. Your role may be in providing support, education and accessible information on medication, appropriate contraception and monitoring of regimes. This is likely to be done in partnership with the consultant psychiatrist, specialist epilepsy nurse or neurologist who oversees the individual's management of epilepsy. There are many other medications where there needs to be awareness of potential complications and harm during pregnancy. It is important you understand the specific issues for the people you support and potentially administer medication to.

Clawson et al (2020) describe the demographic of forced marriage for people with learning disabilities in the UK. Access to the UK Governments Forced Marriage Unit data evidenced that people with learning disabilities are at five times greater risk of forced marriage than people without learning disabilities. In the general population, women are more likely to be forced to marry than men, for people with learning disabilities it is equally likely that both men and women may be forced to marry. Clawson acknowledges that many cases go unreported and there is a role for all healthcare professionals to understand the issue of forced marriage as a safeguarding issue. Learning disability nurses can work in partnership with social care, education and criminal justice to raise awareness, minimise risk of harm and educate people with learning disabilities, their families and the services who support related to these potential issues.

Parents with learning disabilities

Critical reflection 7.8

- Read the blog 'Caring for Women with Learning Disabilities' from Maushe (2020) (see Resources section for more details).

- How do you think the VALUE ME tool could improve the experience of those with a learning disability who are in contact with maternity services?

- Are there other areas of practice where you think this approach could be taken?

- To what extent do you feel learning disability nurses are prepared to advocate with people with learning disabilities who are or wish to be parents?

Historically there have been active attempts to prevent procreation for people with learning disabilities, forced sterilisation and the eugenics movement perpetuated false beliefs about moral corruption and societal damage from people with learning disabilities becoming parents. Women with learning disabilities can feel devalued as parents or expectant mothers; they may feel stereotyped or excluded from the typical experiences, and they may feel judged or unsupported in their decisions. Gould and Dodd (2013) researched experiences of mothers with mild learning disabilities where their children had been removed, mothers interviewed reflected feeling there was scrutiny of their parenting style, that they were presumed to be incapable of parenting and that there were issues related to power imbalances, understanding rights and knowing how to have them upheld.

Case law from 2015 (Medway Council v A and Ors) highlights a situation where a parent with a learning disability had not been treated fairly by the local authority. The case highlights the importance of recognising a parent's needs related to their learning disability and that assessments that professionals carry out must consider the implications of the learning disability and potential impact on children. The emphasis is placed on not prejudging and assuming that because somebody has a learning disability this means they cannot learn new skills. The point is made that although a person with a learning disability may require long-term support that does not automatically mean they are not able to take care of their family.

Working together to safeguard children (Children's Act, 1989) emphasises the roles of professionals working together, using a common assessment and accessing specialist assessment as and when required. Learning disability nurses could work with parents with learning disabilities in a community nursing role, or specialist roles in children and family services, working with primary care or maternity services. The values-based approach that the learning disability nurse demonstrates in the way that they work in partnership with a parent with a learning disability will impact on that individual's experiences with other professionals.

Growing older with a learning disability

Critical reflection 7.9

- Write down some of the words you associate with growing older.
- How do you think those terms might be applied to people with learning disabilities?
- Are there differences?

At this stage in life, there may be people living independently, while others may have families of their own, some people may live at home with relatives. There will also be people who have lived in supported living or residential settings for most (if not all) of their adult lives. These environments may have staff who are highly skilled in meeting the needs of people with learning disabilities but less aware of meeting health needs of an ageing population. People with learning disabilities growing older will experience many of the same age-related conditions as all older people, however, this might be more apparent at a younger age. Hermans and Evenhuis (2014) refer to 50 as being the onset of ageing in people with learning disabilities. Due to the increasing likelihood of complexity, the level of support required may intensify as the person ages.

There may be additional complexities or multi-morbidities that present individuals with additional challenges as they age. Flood (2016) described the use of medication for older adults in residential care, identifying the complexity and potential risk of addressing needs in this group. From a nursing perspective it is important that the level of skill in medicine administration is fully appreciated. There are issues relevant to people with learning disabilities and particularly older people that must be understood when administering medication. Communication, swallowing difficulties, the potential for toxicity and complications of polypharmacy, as well as unrecognised adverse effects need to be carefully managed. Flood's (2016) study highlighted multiple methods of medication administration in one group of people and potential risks and hazards influenced by a number of factors. Working in partnership with doctors, speech and language therapists and pharmacy is key to reducing the polypharmacy and overuse of medication for people with learning disabilities. In England, STOMP (Stopping Overprescribing of People with Learning Disabilities) is an agenda being taken forward to raise awareness of the need to ensure the correct therapeutic approaches in the use of medication (NHS England, 2018).

There are often communication and access challenges as well as difficulties for some practitioners in differentiating between the presentation of a person with a learning disability and signs of dementia or other mental health issues, sometimes people experience diagnostic overshadowing. Assumptions can be made that changes in behaviour, personality or presentation are attributed to ageing. Gates (2011) described the outcomes of focus groups with people with learning disabilities and their families to ascertain their views on the future health and well-being needs for the population. The value of a specialist workforce understanding the needs of elderly people with learning disabilities was highlighted and a warning that the two groups should not be 'lumped together' (p 19). As learning disability nurses and healthcare professionals we are learning more about the ageing needs of people with learning disabilities as people live longer than ever before. You are in a position to promote living well in the later years of life and ensuring access to appropriate services at the right time by working in partnership with people, their families and service providers will be important in making this happen.

Understanding the need for people to have an AHC, continue to have their hearing, vision and teeth assessed as well as other routine screenings is important to promote equality across the lifespan. The promotion of healthy ageing for people with learning disabilities does not just belong to learning disability nurses or learning disability services. People have a right to access mainstream services as any other member of the population does. There may be roles for primary or acute liaison learning disability nurses with key responsibilities to facilitate access and promote reasonable adjustments ensuring that people receive access to effective healthcare in as timely way as possible. You will need to develop strong links with district nurses, specialists in diabetes, skin integrity, or dementia as well as members of the MDT such as physiotherapists, speech and language therapists and occupational therapists.

Perhaps the biggest concern for some people with learning disabilities and their families is the current lack of social care provision for an ageing population, with the correct environments (including ground floor living). Learning disability nurses and colleagues in community learning disability teams provide excellent input into what services should be needed in the future and how they should look but often are not in a position to make this happen, there needs to be joint working with a social worker early on and having upfront, difficult conversations about long-term accommodation with the person and their family is important.

Dementia

There is a high association between Down syndrome and development of dementia. A longitudinal study following up 77 women with Down syndrome aged 35 years and older suggested a 95.7 per cent presentation by the age of 68 (McCarron et al, 2014). While the generic dementia pathway would likely mean a referral to memory clinic, there are significant barriers for people with learning disabilities in accessing an assessment this way, for example, communication barriers, lack of experience in communicating with or assessing the needs of people with learning disabilities, inexperience in understanding day-to-day presentation of the person and potential for diagnostic overshadowing, presuming a deterioration or normalising a presentation due to lack of knowledge related to the individual.

Generic services may not be knowledgeable or experienced in the evidence-based assessment tools for people with learning disabilities. There may also be active exclusion of people with learning disabilities in these clinics. Learning disability nurses have skills and knowledge in assessment of dementia and can work in partnership with mainstream services to facilitate access, increase awareness and develop practice. Often, however, learning disability services have developed their own dementia pathway with multidisciplinary assessment and contribution. Each member of the MDT can contribute to the comprehensive assessment of the individual and this process is likely to be coordinated by the learning disability nurse.

End of life care

Some people with learning disabilities can be ready to face the challenge of talking about death and dying, while some professionals may find this more challenging to approach, feeling ill-equipped or lacking in skills to raise sensitive topics (Hopes, 2016). What is important from a learning disability nursing perspective is to recognise that while the person may not have the words, language or ability to verbally communicate their thoughts and feelings, they are able to perceive and understand changes from the environment, the way people around them behave and that there is something different. We should seek to understand the communication needs of the person and to manage information in ways that the person can understand. Does the person have a previous experience of death, a pet, a family member, a favourite TV programme, if not death, do they understand loss? The breaking bad news model from Irene Tuffrey-Wijne (2012) gives examples of stages in preparing people for bad news, knowing where they are in their experience and understanding and how people who support them can engage them in discussion and understanding.

There may be specific problems for people with learning disabilities due to healthcare inequalities which can mean challenges with access to specialist palliative care. Adam et al (2020) highlighted that there are specific needs relating to physical needs, psychosocial and spiritual needs, and information and communication needs for people with learning disabilities and their families. These are often unmet and barriers persist relating to staff knowledge, training and experience, the ability to assess and understand the communication needs of people with learning disabilities and the delivery of equitable care. Many of the studies that have considered palliative care needs of people with learning disabilities have captured the views of healthcare professionals or family members rather than people with learning disabilities (Adam et al, 2020).

Foo et al (2021) further demonstrate this with a study on specialist palliative care staff who did not consistently talk with people with learning disability about their dying and death. This was influenced by experience, relationships, values and perceived capacity of the individual. Improvements relating to the experiences of people with learning disabilities at the end of life are needed. Graham et al (2020) recommend the development of a new role for people with learning disabilities, learning disability nurses with a specialism in end of life care, this is because of the recognised challenges of achieving a good death for people with learning disabilities. Many people with learning disabilities die without their individual wants and wishes being ascertained and understood. Sometimes families and carers are not listened to when care is being delivered and sometimes their views are ignored. Foo et al (2021) describe a 'conspiracy of silence' in the end of life care for people with learning disabilities, the common perception being that this will be too distressing for people with learning disabilities to cope with and process (Tuffrey-Wijne et al, 2010).

It is sometimes challenging for the learning disability team to identify the best time to refer onto other services. Developing links with the palliative care team is very important in order to make sure that a range of preparations can be made and that the teams and carers who support people with learning disabilities are prepared for the future. You can familiarise yourself with a range of resources on the palliative care for people with learning disabilities website (PCPLD) that empower people and their families to be able to approach end of life in an informed and proactive way with opportunities to talk about their thoughts and feelings, wants needs and wishes. Learning disability nurses can facilitate support from other skilled professionals who can address the challenging aspects of enabling a good death and dying with dignity.

Chapter summary

Exploring the role of the learning disability nurse across the lifespan is an empowering affirmation of the variety of opportunities to make a difference and work in partnership with people throughout your career. There are many ways that you can optimise health and reduce restrictions for people with learning disabilities. Working together with the person, their family and other professionals to increase awareness and access to rights-based approaches will be part of your daily practice, regardless of the roles you undertake. You can be fundamental in supporting changing attitudes to valuing individuals and recognising their worth. You can bring strength to others in the way that you demonstrate advocacy and uphold the responsibility of seeing people with learning disabilities as individuals with unique strengths and needs at all stages of development. As a registered learning disability nurse you have transferable skills and are well equipped to work with service users presenting very different needs at all stages of life and in a range of settings.

FURTHER READING

Bigby, C and Beadle-Brown, J (2016) Improving Quality of Life Outcomes in Supported Accommodation for People with Intellectual Disability: What Makes a Difference? *Journal of Applied Research in Intellectual Disabilities*, 31(2): 182–200.

Doukas, T, Fergusson, A, Fullerton, M and Grace J (2017) Supporting People with Profound and Multiple Learning Disabilities. Core and Essential Service Standards. [online] Available at: www.pmldlink.org.uk/wp-content/uploads/2017/11/Standards-PMLD-h-web.pdf (accessed 21 April 2022).

Lenehan, C (2017) These Are Our Children: A Review by Dame Christine Lenehan. Director. Council for Disabled Children. London: Council for Disabled Children. [online] Available at: https://assets.publishing.service.gov.uk/government/uploads/system/uploads/atta chment_data/file/585376/Lenehan_Review_Report.pdf (accessed 21 April 2022).

National Commissioning Board (2019) Guidance: Commissioning Accommodation and Support for a Good Life for People with a Learning Disability. [online] Available at: www. ldw.org.uk/wp-content/uploads/2019/03/Guidance.pdf?msclkid=daf04c52c31111ec8 af762701b9c1d74 (accessed 23 April 2022).

NHS England (2015) Building the Right Support. [online] Available at: www.england.nhs.uk/ wp-content/uploads/2015/10/ld-nat-imp-plan-oct15.pdf?msclkid=bb546f69c31111ec9 663694e31428b10 (accessed 23 April 2022).

RESOURCES

The Health Profile for Children and Young People [online] Available at: https://phw.nhs. wales/services-and-teams/improvement-cymru/our-work/learning-disability-health-improvement-programme/health-profile/health-profile-for-children-and-young-people/ (accessed 23 April 2022).

Maushe, E (2020) Blog: Caring for women with learning disabilities. Nursing and Midwifery Council. [online] Available at: www.nmc.org.uk/news/news-and-updates/blog-caring-for-women-with-learning-disabilities/ (accessed 8 June 2022).

Mencap Sexuality Research and Statistics [online] Available at: www.mencap.org.uk/learn ing-disability-explained/research-and-statistics/sexuality-research-and-statistics?mscl kid=954f5015c31311ec86bc716b0d638ecd

Parents with Learning Disabilities [online] Available at: www.iriss.org.uk/resources/insig hts/parents-learning-disabilities?msclkid=80573312c31411eca53ef3a2624f8d31 (accessed 23 April 2022).

Working together with parents: network information for parents with learning disabilities [online] Available at: www.bristol.ac.uk/sps/wtpn/forparents/ (accessed 23 April 2022).

8   A public health approach

Chapter aims

This chapter introduces you to the principles of public health and explores the importance of this approach in reducing the health inequalities and inequities experienced by people with learning disabilities. It then considers how, as a learning disability nurse, you can use this an approach to inform and develop your practice.

Professional standards and expectations

The importance of a public health approach to nursing practice is evidenced by the Standards (NMC, 2018a) where one of the seven 'platforms' is focused entirely on *'Promoting health and preventing ill health'*. It is not possible to detail all the individual outcomes here but the overall descriptor for Platform 2 states:

> *Registered nurses play a key role in improving and maintaining the mental, physical and behavioural health and well-being of people, families, communities and populations. They support and enable people at all stages of life and in all care settings to make informed choices about how to manage health challenges in order to maximise their quality of life and improve health outcomes. They are actively involved in the prevention of and protection against disease and ill health and engage in public health, community development and global health agendas, and in the reduction of health inequalities.*

WHAT DO WE MEAN BY A PUBLIC HEALTH APPROACH?

Marks et al (2011) suggest that defining public health is a 'contested' issue and illustrate this by providing examples of a range of different definitions used by the WHO. However, while these definitions may vary slightly, there are common themes that run through them namely that a public health approach is concerned with coordinated actions at a societal level, that are focused on reducing inequalities in health through preventing disease, promoting health and prolonging life. The most frequently cited definition encompasses many of these elements stating that public health is '*... the science and art of preventing disease, prolonging life, and promoting health through the organised efforts of society*' (Acheson, 1988).

These actions at a societal level may take many different forms and include, for example, the development and implementation of legislation and policies, targeted programmes of health promotion, public awareness campaigns and monitoring of disease occurrence. Before reading further complete Critical reflection 8.1.

Critical reflection 8.1

- Identify examples of different types of public health actions by completing the table below.

Type of public health activity	Examples
Policy or legislation	
Health promotion programmes	
Public awareness campaigns	
Monitoring disease occurrence	

A clear example of public health action that encompasses many such activities can be seen in the response to the recent Covid-19 pandemic where a coordinated effort (at an international level) was required to reduce the spread of disease and to reduce its impact. In terms of policy and legislation, emergency laws were introduced which (for example) restricted our movements and social contact while also requiring us to undergo testing and self-isolation if testing positive or being in contact with someone who tested positive. At a policy level it became necessary to review policies and procedures to prevent cross infection and hence the requirement to use personal protective equipment (PPE) was introduced. There were several public awareness campaigns to support these measures focusing on areas such as hand hygiene, the use of masks and the need to socially distance. As vaccines became available then awareness campaigns focused on increasing the uptake of these were mounted. Throughout, the measures introduced were reviewed, and key to decision-making were data regarding the incidence of infections and their outcomes.

In deciding which measures need to be taken at a societal level it is, therefore, important that reliable, accurate and timely data is available to inform decision-making. An understanding of demography and epidemiology is thus central to understanding public health (generally) and is relevant to the health and well-being of people with learning disabilities and the role of the nurse in promoting this.

○ **Demography** is concerned with the statistical study of populations and their characteristics such as age, gender, ethnicity, sexuality, genotype, lifestyle factors, employment status and socio-economic status. In health terms these are important considerations since such characteristics may influence health risks, status and outcomes. For example, the health needs of young children are different to those who are aged over 70, the health needs of women and men differ, and unemployment can both arise from, and give rise to, poor health.

○ **Epidemiology** is the study of how often diseases occur within populations and why. Within epidemiology there is a focus on patterns of morbidity (ill health and disease) and an interest in both the prevalence of diseases (how many people in a population have the condition) and incidence (the number of new cases of a condition within a population). So, for example, in relation to diabetes data may be sought both in relation to the number of people who have diabetes in the population (prevalence) and the number of new cases of diabetes that are diagnosed in a particular time period (incidence). By looking at trends in such data it then becomes possible to not only understand what type and level of provision needs to be put in place to support those currently living with diabetes but also to consider future needs, factors that are influencing the trends, develop interventions to reverse or halt any negative trends and assess the effectiveness of such interventions. In addition to morbidity the public health approach is also concerned with patterns and causes of mortality (deaths) with a focus on causes of death, demographic influences on patterns of death and avoidable/premature deaths.

When demographic and epidemiological data are considered together it then becomes possible to consider how factors such as gender, age and ethnicity impact on patterns of health, disease and deaths and, through doing so, to highlight where inequalities in health may exist. For example, Marmot et al (2020) reviewed health in England and concluded that in the ten years since publication of the Marmot Review (2010) increases in life expectancy had stalled for the first time since 1900, that life expectancy follows the social gradient (with most deprived populations having the shortest life span), and that in the 10 per cent of most deprived areas life expectancy had fallen for women during this period. It can thus be seen that both socio-economic factors and gender impact on health status.

Some differences in health status are to be expected – for example, rates of breast cancer will be higher in women, rates of dementia are higher in older people and some people will be predisposed to certain conditions due to their genetic makeup. Such differences might, therefore, be viewed as inequalities since they are differences which are largely unavoidable. Whitehead (1991), however, distinguishes between inequalities and inequities where the latter are potentially amenable to change and hence (if they continue) they are unjust and unfair. So, for example, it may be inevitable that women are more likely to have breast cancer (an inequality) but if the outcome of a cancer diagnosis is influenced by the timeliness and quality of treatment, with women in one geographical area receiving quicker and more effective treatment, then this is an inequity which can and should be eliminated. Identifying and addressing both inequalities and inequities in health lie at the centre of public health.

PUBLIC HEALTH AND PEOPLE WITH LEARNING DISABILITIES

Internationally there is evidence that people with learning disabilities, as a group, experience many inequalities and inequities in health (Krahn and Fox, 2014). It might therefore be expected that a public health approach would have been a central element of learning disability policy, practice and research for some time. However, this has tended not to be the case and there are several reasons for this.

Within learning disability nursing (as within wider support systems for people with a learning disability) a person-centred approach is central to our work and there is a focus on ensuring that individual needs are both identified and met. In contrast, a public health approach focuses on populations rather than individuals and hence there may seem to be a tension between public health and learning disability nursing. However, as you will see later in this chapter, the two are not only compatible but are complementary since if you are to identify and meet the health needs of those you support you need to understand what influences their health and well-being, what risks they face and what actions are required to enhance their health.

As discussed above, gathering and interpreting demographic and epidemiological data are central to a public health approach. However, as will be seen below there are challenges to gathering such data in relation to people with learning disabilities which have limited adoption of a public health approach to identifying and meeting the health needs of people with learning disabilities.

Nonetheless, despite these challenges it is essential that a public health approach is adopted, and these challenges are addressed. As Liao et al (2021) observe, if we do not have a good understanding of the disease epidemiology experienced by people with learning disabilities then they may be exposed to underdiagnosis, misdiagnosis, inappropriate medication and missed opportunities for health promotion and disease prevention. Issues of demography and epidemiology in relation to people with learning disabilities will, therefore, now be explored.

Demography and people with a learning disability

To gather accurate and comprehensive demographic data it is essential that we can clearly identify the population of concern. In relation to people with learning disabilities, however, this can be difficult. For example, there may be a hesitance to assess and diagnose very young children until the nature and extent of any developmental delay is clear. Some families and individuals may be reluctant to accept the 'label' of learning disabilities meaning that they may not be known to, or supported by, formal services. While children and young people may be assessed as having additional learning needs (and hence receive specialist educational support) they may have a very mild learning disability and may not meet the eligibility criteria to access adult learning disability services and therefore 'disappear' from official statistics. Older adults with learning disabilities may move to live in generic care homes for older people (rather than specialist learning disability facilities) and hence they also fall out of learning disability statistics. Data may also be collected by various agencies and bodies in slightly different ways and using different criteria thus making it difficult to collate an accurate picture.

Hatton et al (2016), for example, observed that it was not possible to provide a definitive record of the number of people with learning disabilities in England but, drawing data together from a range of sources, they estimate an overall prevalence of 2.5 per cent. However, they also note that the rate drops 'precipitously' from 2.5 per cent among children in education to 0.6 per cent among adults aged 20 to 29. This reflects the point made above regarding people being 'lost' to the system upon leaving school.

In relation to adults, Hatton et al (2016) observe that it is possible to take three different approaches to estimating such figures, namely:

1. the number of adults using learning disability services;

2. the number of adults known to learning disability services or GPs;

3. the estimated number of adults with learning disabilities in the population.

They suggest that GP registers are likely to be the most comprehensive source of data since other services may be used on a more intermittent basis. However, Glover et al (2019) argue that the identification of people with learning disabilities within GP registers is also known to be incomplete. Hatton et al (2016) thus estimate that even this source is likely to represent only 23 per cent of adults with learning disabilities in the population meaning that there is a 'hidden majority' of 77 per cent who are unknown to services and who are hence unlikely to appear in official statistics. There is thus a difference between the administrative prevalence (those known to services) and the true prevalence.

In relation to data regarding the number of people with learning disabilities it is also important to remember that much of the data we have is drawn from high-income countries such as the UK, the US, Australia, Canada and the Netherlands. However, where data does exist then it suggests that there is a higher prevalence of learning disabilities in low- and middle-income countries and the need for improved data to inform development of appropriate support has been advocated (Maulik et al, 2011).

Critical reflection 8.2

Take time to consider the implications of the 'hidden majority' of adults with learning disabilities for their health and well-being.

- How might health services (generally) and learning disability services (specifically) seek to ensure that their health needs are identified and met?

THE HEALTH OF PEOPLE WITH LEARNING DISABILITIES

The challenge of gathering accurate demographic information in relation to people with learning disabilities means that gaining accurate epidemiological information can also be difficult. This is compounded by the fact that people with learning disabilities often have undetected and therefore untreated health conditions. The reasons for this are many and include that individuals with learning disabilities may not recognise that they have signs and symptoms of ill health and that they are unable to report it to others and hence seek assistance. Those who support them may also not recognise and that an individual is unwell and therefore do not assist them to seek medical help. When help is sought then they may be met with negative or discriminatory attitudes which include diagnostic overshadowing where any changes to an individual's behaviour are attributed to their learning disability rather than being recognised as possible indicators of ill health. Potential health problems which are leading to such changes are therefore not explored meaning that they remain untreated. All these barriers to accessing appropriate and timely healthcare mean that often people with learning disabilities encounter delays in their health needs being recognised and consequently there are corresponding delays in the provision of any treatment sometimes leading to poor outcomes.

Case study 8.1

Adam Peters

Adam Thompson is 42 years old, loves football and going to his local football ground to watch his favourite team. During the football season he usually attends all home matches with his brother and enjoys meeting friends in the bar afterwards. He is very sociable and enjoys meeting other people.

Adam has Down syndrome and lives at home with his parents where he often helps them around the house with various tasks. Recently, however, he has been reluctant to help and often appears to have difficulty doing things he usually does with no problem. He has also been reluctant to go to football matches with his brother and, on the one occasion that he did go along, he became very agitated and hit out at his brother when they were trying to walk up the steps to find their seat in the stands.

Such behaviours are very out of character for Adam and his brother has heard that people with Down syndrome can develop dementia at a young age. He is worried that this may be happening to Adam and takes him to the GP who agrees that this may what is occurring and agrees to refer him for tests. While waiting for tests, however, a family friend asks if Adam has ever had his sight tested. The family can't remember this happening and so decide that it might be a good idea to take him to the opticians.

The opticians found that Adam needed to wear glasses and once these were obtained and worn his behaviour returned to normal. The next time he went to see the football be bounded up the steps to their seat as he could see where he was going and was not anxious.

Krahn (2019) highlights that people with learning disabilities are often invisible in national systems of health surveillance as when such data is gathered there is often no additional question included asking whether an individual has a learning disability. It is therefore not possible to identify whether any of those whose data is included have a learning disability and to compare their data with the wider population. Krahn (2019) further argues that it is not sufficient just to base our health interventions for people with learning disabilities on data obtained from the general population since their health needs and life circumstances are often more complex. A failure to obtain information regarding the health needs of people with learning disabilities and to compare this to data concerning the wider population also means that it is not possible to identify and act upon any inequalities and inequities.

It is, therefore, essential that we identify and understand the health needs of people with learning disabilities since a failure to do so can mean that they are at risk of underdiagnosis, misdiagnosis, inappropriate treatments and missed opportunities for preventative healthcare (Liao et al, 2021). Positively, despite the challenges outlined above there is an increasing body of knowledge. Limitations have been noted in relation to this literature such as a failure in some studies to include data regarding race, ethnicity and other factors known to impact upon health (Krahn and Havecamp, 2019) and the need to question data in terms of who it represents and who is missing has been identified (Krahn, 2019). Nonetheless, it is important that the knowledge that is available is used to improve the health of people with learning disabilities. It is not possible to explore it all here, but an overview of key areas will be provided.

Physical health

A Spanish study found that certain physical health conditions were more prevalent among people with learning disabilities (compared to the wider population), namely urinary incontinence, oral problems, epilepsy, constipation, obesity, skin problems, thyroid problems, chronic bronchitis or COPD, cataracts, heart disease, underweight, stokes and liver disease (Folch et al, 2017). They also found that some conditions were less prevalent such as arterial hypertension, arthrosis, hypercholesterolaemia, allergies and asthma.

More recently a systematic review of 77 papers sought to synthesise data regarding the incidence and prevalence of physical health conditions in people with learning disabilities (Liao et al, 2021). They found that the highest reported prevalence rates related to epilepsy, ear and eye disorders, cerebral palsy, obesity, osteoporosis, congenital heart defects and thyroid disorders. However, they note that prevalence rates varied widely across studies which may be attributable to variations in the population under study and differences in the severity of the learning disability. They found that among people with some genetic conditions these conditions occur more frequently – for example, people with Down syndrome are at increased risk of congenital heart defects and thyroid disorders. Comparisons are also drawn with the wider population, and it is noted that asthma and diabetes occur more frequently among people with learning disabilities while others such as non-congenital circulatory conditions and solid cancers occur either at the same rate or less frequently. The latter, however, they suggest may be due to under-detection.

When comparing the findings of Folch et al (2017) with those of Liao et al (2021) it is interesting to note that the former suggests that asthma occurs less frequently among people with learning disabilities while the latter indicates it occurs more frequently. Such differing findings reflect differing methodologies, and it is important to note that Liao et al (2021) is a systematic review, synthesises findings from several studies and thus might be viewed as stronger evidence.

Mental health

Historically there was a tendency to think that people with learning disabilities did not experience co-existing mental health conditions and that any symptoms exhibited were either part of their learning disability, or that they were due to behaviours that challenge. However, evidence now indicates that they experience the same range of mental health conditions as the wider population (Mazza et al, 2019).

In their systematic review and meta-analysis Mazza et al (2019) reviewed 22 studies and found that a third of people with learning disabilities in these studies met the diagnostic criteria for a co-existing mental health condition. Mood disorders and anxiety were the most prevalent conditions. They also found similar rates among those with mild, moderate and severe learning disabilities but lower rates among those with a profound learning disability. In relation to the latter, it may be that it is more difficult to recognise and assess mental ill health among those with profound learning disabilities since they are less likely to be able to verbalise any symptoms and hence are reliant upon others observing for any changes in mood and understanding the significance of such changes.

Hatton et al (2017) undertook a secondary analysis of data from the *Understanding Society* study to determine the prevalence of mental health problems among adults with and without learning disabilities, and to explore the impact of the social determinants of health on any differences. They found that people with learning disabilities are at significantly greater risk of mental ill health but that such differences may be attributed to their poorer living conditions than their learning disability per se. This reinforces the need to consider how social determinants of health impact on the health and well-being of people with learning disabilities and contribute to the health inequities they experience.

One condition that is known to occur more frequently in people with learning disabilities is dementia and this is often attributed to the occurrence of early-onset dementia among people with Down syndrome. However, one study that included adults with learning disabilities with and without Down syndrome found that, overall, the prevalence of dementia among people with learning disabilities is up to five times that of the wider population (Strydom et al, 2013). They therefore suggest that regular screening may be useful to promote earlier detection and intervention.

Multimorbidity

Multimorbidity is where an individual has two or more long-term health conditions. Often these conditions require treatments such as medication but the effects and side effects of one treatment may interact with those used to treat other conditions and give rise to further conditions through side effects. For example, someone may require long-term treatment with antipsychotic medication for mental health problems but the medication they take may increase their risk of diabetes and can also lead to other health issues such as constipation.

Multimorbidity is common among people with learning disabilities. While the incidence of multimorbidity increases with age (as with the wider population) it often begins at a younger age for people with learning disabilities. For example, in one study of people with learning disabilities aged 50 and over it was found that 79.9 per cent were experiencing multimorbidity with 46.8 per cent living with four or more long-term health conditions (Hermans and Evenhuis, 2014). Rates were found to be highest among those with severe/profound learning disabilities and those with Down syndrome (Hermans and Evenhuis, 2014).

Mortality

While life expectancy of people with learning disabilities has increased over the past few decades (Coppus, 2013), they continue to have reduced life expectancy when compared with their non-learning-disabled peers. For example, a systematic review undertaken by O'Leary et al (2018) identified that across the 27 papers they reviewed, deaths in people with learning disabilities occurred, on average, 20 years earlier than in the wider population. This suggests that people with learning disabilities are at increased risk of premature and potentially preventable deaths but to seek to reduce such inequities it is essential that mortality data is gathered to identify both causes of death and factors that contribute to such deaths (Reppermund et al, 2020). Mortality studies are also necessary to assess the effectiveness of policies and interventions designed to reduce mortality, and to assess inequities over time by comparison to the wider population (Stirton and Heslop, 2018).

There are, however, challenges in gathering accurate mortality data regarding people with learning disabilities since they are not always identifiable within general mortality datasets (O'Leary et al, 2018). One way of obtaining such information would be to collate it from medical cause of death certificates but the presence of a learning disability is not always recorded on such certificates (Stirton and Heslop, 2018). Indeed, learning disability should never be the cause of death but it may be an underlying cause which can also be recorded. A lack of consistency in completing medical cause of death certificates has also been noted and one factor contributing to this is that the person completing the certificate may not be aware of the medical history of the deceased (Stirton and Heslop, 2018). They may thus not be aware that the deceased had a learning disability and the presence of a learning disability may not be an underlying cause of death and hence not recorded.

Studies where the deaths of people with learning disabilities and the factors contributing to these deaths have, therefore, been undertaken. For example, the Confidential Inquiry into Premature Deaths of People with Learning Disabilities (CIPOLD) (Heslop et al, 2013) reviewed the deaths of 247 adults with learning disabilities and 58 comparator cases of adults without a learning disability. As well as the stated cause of death the factors that led up to their death (such as recorded health concerns, hospital admissions, living circumstances) were also reviewed. They found that 42 per cent of the deaths of people with learning disabilities were found to be premature and the most common factors found to contribute to this were delays in diagnosis or treatment, problems with identifying and meeting needs.

More recently the Learning Disabilities Mortality Review (LeDeR) programme in England has undertaken reviews of the deaths of people with learning disabilities and has published both annual reports and action from learning reports (LeDeR, 2021a, 2021b). In their most recent report (LeDeR, 2021a) it is noted that the reporting period covered was unusual in that it covered the Covid-19 pandemic and a significant increase in reported deaths was noted during the first wave of the pandemic between March and May 2020. Due to the unusual circumstances of 2020 and the fact that reporting deaths to the LeDeR project is not mandatory the study team urge caution when making comparisons with data from previous years. They found that at the time of death 46 per cent of adults had seven to ten long-term health conditions. However, while preventable medical causes of death among adults with learning disabilities had remained stable at 24 per cent between 2018 and 2020, there had been a slight reduction in the treatable medical causes of death from 41 per cent in 2018 to 39 per cent in 2020. Nonetheless, when compared with the wider population people with learning disabilities remain three times more likely to die from an avoidable medical cause with most of this excess risk being due to treatable medical causes of death.

Different mortality studies use different methodologies which can make comparison between studies challenging. Therefore, it is important to look across studies in a systematic manner to try to identify mortality rates, causes and recurring themes. The systematic review of early deaths and causes of death undertaken by O'Leary et al (2018) not only identified a 20-year gap in life expectancy between people with learning disabilities and the wider population but also that some groups of people with learning disabilities are impacted in different ways. The presence of a severe learning disability and existing co-morbidities increased the risk of premature death and the gap between life expectancy of women with learning disabilities and their non-learning-disabled peers is greater than that between men with learning disabilities and their non-learning-disabled peers. In terms of cause of death, respiratory and circulatory diseases were the most common cause of death while deaths due to cancer were fewer than the wider population and the cancer profile differed from the wider population (O'Leary et al, 2018).

Factors impacting on health

As can be seen from the preceding sections there are many factors that can impact on the health of people with learning disabilities. The nature and level of an individual's learning disability can influence their health status and health risks. For example, individuals with Down syndrome are at increased risk of congenital heart disorders, hypothyroidism and early-onset dementia, and people with profound or multiple learning disabilities are 6.4 times more likely to die between the ages of 18 and 49 than someone with a mild learning disability (LeDeR, 2021a).

The earlier discussion regarding mortality also identified that while life expectancy of all people with learning disabilities is lower than the wider population, the gap between women with learning disabilities and their non-learning-disabled peers is greater than that between men with learning disabilities and their peers (O'Leary et al, 2018). Gender thus impacts on the health of people with learning disabilities and gives rise to disparities between people with learning disabilities.

In addition, while it was noted earlier in this chapter that while race and ethnicity impact on the health inequities experienced by people with learning disabilities (Krahn and Havercamp, 2019) few studies have focused on this area. However, Magana et al (2016) compared perceived physical and mental health status, obesity, and diabetes of Latino and Black adults with learning disabilities in the US with that of their non-disabled peers and with that of their white peers with learning disabilities. They found that Latino and Black adults with learning disabilities had poorer health outcomes compared with their white peers and that they had poorer outcomes than their peers from the same racial and ethnic group.

Within England, LeDeR (2021a) note that the number of deaths reviewed relating to people with learning disabilities from Black and minority ethnic groups is few. Nonetheless, they highlight the following increased likelihoods of death between the ages of 18 and 49 (compared with white adults with a learning disability):

- 9.2 times more likely for those with Asian/Asian British ethnicity;
- 3.9 times more likely for those of mixed/multiple ethnicities;
- 3.6 times more likely for those of Black/African/Caribbean/Black British ethnicity.

Race and ethnicity need, therefore, to be a focus when planning and implementing public health initiatives and further research is needed to improve our understanding of the impact of race and ethnicity on the health of people with learning disabilities.

Overall, the available evidence suggests that, in terms of health status, we should not view people with learning disabilities as a homogenous group. This has implications for how we target and design interventions to reduce health inequities.

PUBLIC HEALTH INTERVENTIONS AND PEOPLE WITH LEARNING DISABILITIES

Given the limited visibility of data regarding the health of people with learning disabilities within national public health databases (Krahn, 2019) it is perhaps unsurprising that there are calls for the health service and other organisations to be more aware of, and responsive to, the public health needs of this group (Mafuba and Gates, 2013). Nonetheless, there are some key public health developments that have focused on addressing these needs. The mortality reviews discussed above are one example of such a development.

As has already been mentioned in this chapter people with a learning disability may have many undetected, and therefore unmet, health needs. A key public health development focused on people with a learning disability aimed at addressing this issue is the annual health check (AHC). This is an NHS Directly Enhanced Service (DES) which aims to identify, at an early stage, any unmet health needs, to ensure appropriate treatments, to establish trust and to promote continuity of care (Royal College of General Practitioners, 2021). The check is usually conducted by a GP, a practice nurse, or a combination of these two professionals and covers physical, mental and behavioural health. It should include both discussion and questioning and clinical observations (such as weight, blood pressure, urinalysis). Where relevant it should also include syndrome-specific checks where people with that syndrome are known to be at increased risk of certain health conditions. For example, people with Down syndrome should be offered a thyroid function test due to an increased risk of hypothyroidism and all those over 40 should be assessed for symptoms of dementia given the risk of early-onset dementia.

By undertaking such checks on an annual basis, it provides not only an assessment at a point in time but also (in the case of repeated checks) it enables comparison of results between one check and another. This may be helpful in identifying trends in (for example) weight which may be indicative of underlying health problems or present a risk factor in terms of future health. Annual checks can also be very important to identify changes in mental health status and to identify conditions such as dementia at an early stage.

The AHC should also provide the opportunity for adults with a learning disability to discuss issues of concern regarding their health, to receive health advice and should result in a health action plan (HAP). This document should detail health needs, how they are to be addressed, how support is to be provided and by whom, and when they will be reviewed. It should be co-produced, and the individual should have a copy of their HAP. For further information regarding AHCs and to access resources to support such checks please see RCGP (2021).

Of course, health checks can only be of value if they are attended and the most recent data available for England indicates that during the period 2019–20 only 57.8 per cent of eligible people with a learning disability attended for a health check (NHS Digital, 2021). While encouragingly this number shows a statistically significant increase from 51.6 per cent in 2015–16, it still indicates that over 40 per cent of people with a learning disability are not receiving the potential benefits of an AHC. Moreover, even when an AHC is attended, the quality of such a check may be variable and the extent to which it results in a HAP that is supported and monitored is unknown. There is thus a need for further research in this area.

Nonetheless, from the research that has been undertaken it is evident that AHCs do identify previously unidentified health needs and lead to interventions (Robertson et al, 2014), and that while overall they do not prevent emergency hospital admissions, they do reduce preventable emergency admissions for ambulatory care conditions (Carey et al, 2016).

Another example of a public health intervention focused on improving/protecting the health of people with a learning disability has been seen in the context of the Covid-19 pandemic. Here, initially, people with a learning disability were not viewed as a high priority population to receive the Covid vaccination. However, after pressure from third sector organisations and families this decision was changed. Nonetheless, simply stating that they *can* receive the vaccine does not mean that people with a learning disability *will* receive it. For example, some may be needle phobic, some may not be able to cope with attendance at mass vaccination centres and others may not physically be able to attend such centres. In this context learning disability nurses provided support to make sure reasonable adjustments were in place to support access and, where required, arranged specialist clinics for people with a learning disability (see, for example, Whitehouse et al, 2021).

THE ROLE OF THE LEARNING DISABILITY NURSE

Mafuba and Gates (2013) argue that community learning disability nurses are involved in a range of public health activities including health surveillance, health promotion, health facilitation, health prevention and protection, health education and healthcare delivery. Such activities, however, are not confined to just community learning disability nurses since (for example) those working in assessment and treatment units will be involved in health surveillance and healthcare delivery, those working in schools are likely to be involved in health promotion, and those working in prisons may be focused on (ill)health prevention and protection. This is consistent with Platform 2 of the NMC Standards (2018a) outlined at the beginning of the chapter in that it reflects the range of activities delivered across the lifespan and across a range of settings.

It is beyond the scope of this chapter to discuss all aspects of the public health role of the learning disability nurse. Nonetheless, some key areas will be explored, namely health promotion, health needs assessment, the promotion of self-management and advocacy.

In considering these areas (and others) there are also two key elements of practice that are important to remember. First is the role of the learning disability nurse in ensuring that reasonable adjustments are made to enable equity of access to public health initiatives. This may involve ensuring that information is available in formats that people with learning disabilities are able to understand and that they are provided with support to understand it. It may involve changing aspects of policies and procedures such as providing longer appointments or specific targeting to promote greater uptake of screening procedures. It may also involve making adaptations such as pre-visits and desensitisation programmes. Learning disability nurses are well placed to make these adjustments in their personal practice, to raise awareness among colleagues of the need to do likewise and to provide them with support to adapt their practice.

The second element of practice that needs to inform your public health role is what is referred to as 'Making Every Contact Count' (MECC). According to Public Health England (2016), MECC is:

> an approach to behaviour change that uses the millions of day-to-day interactions that organisations and individuals have with other people to support them in making positive changes to their physical and mental health.

> MECC supports the opportunistic delivery of consistent and concise healthy lifestyle information and enables individuals to engage in conversations at scale across organisations and populations.

Through their day-to-day interaction with people with learning disabilities learning disability nurses are ideally placed to identify and take opportunities to provide those they support with the information and skills they need to make positive changes to their lifestyle to improve their health. This might, for example, include taking opportunities that arise to give information about a healthy diet and taking exercise. It might include having discussions about the importance of reducing smoking or ensuring concordance with medication. It might also include providing prompts to access AHCs or screening services. In addition, it is important to remember that as a learning disability nurse you also have regular contact with families and carers who play a key role in supporting people with a learning disability in relation to their health. It is therefore important that you also make these contacts count and use these opportunities to pass on knowledge and skills that will assist them to better support the health of those they care for and thus help to improve their health.

Critical reflection 8.3

Think about contacts you have had recently with people with a learning disability and their families or carers.

- What opportunities were there to make every contact count to promote better health and well-being?

- How will you make sure you use such activities to best effect in the future?

Health needs assessment

To effectively meet the health needs of people with a learning disability, learning disability nurses need to have the knowledge and skills to identify such needs and to prioritise them. This will be achieved when working with individuals, but it is important to be aware of frameworks to support this and of the need to also consider the health needs of groups and populations when seeking to develop services and support.

The HEF (Atkinson et al, 2013) was developed to assist learning disability nurses with identifying the impact that key determinants of health inequalities are having on the individuals they support, to plan appropriate interventions and then to assess the effectiveness of such interventions through reassessment. The aim is to reduce the adverse impact of such determinants. It covers five key determinants, under which are 29 indicators:

1. social determinants – for example, living conditions, employment and safeguarding;

2. genetic and biological determinants – for example, medication, long-term health conditions and crisis planning;

3. communication difficulties and reduced health literacy – for example, difficulty in recognising and communicating health needs and in understanding health information;

4. personal health behaviours and lifestyle risks – for example, diet, exercise and substance use;

5. deficiencies in access to and quality of health provision – for example, organisational barriers, consent and health promotion.

In relation to each of the 29 indicators the situation of an individual is assessed in rela-tion to the impact that each is having on that individual on a five-point scale ranging from no impact to major where major is likely to have a significant and possibly prolonged impact on their health.

Having completed a HEF assessment with an individual it is then possible to display the results visually so that a clear picture can be seen which determinants are having the greatest negative impact and hence where interventions should be focused.

An evaluation of the use of the HEF in Scotland (Duff, 2018) demonstrated that interventions from learning disability nurses reduced the negative impact of the determinants of health on people with a learning disability across each of the five determinants. Across the five determinants an average of a 10 per cent reduction in impact was noted but the reduction in the genetic and biological determinant was 16 per cent. Duff (2018) suggests that this may be the area where learning disability nurses are best equipped to intervene but also notes that they have a positive impact across all domains.

The HEF assessment also records demographic and epidemiological information regarding individuals, such as their age, gender, ethnicity and health conditions. As was noted earlier in this chapter such characteristics are important when seeking to under-stand the health and health inequalities of people with a learning disability. The HEF has the facility to aggregate this data at a community or population level and so it can support identification of the health needs and characteristics of a population which can assist service planning and policy development. As Duff (2018) notes, the information gathered in Scotland has provided health boards with data that identify trends and gaps and provide an evidence base for service improvement and public health initiatives.

Health promotion

Health promotion activities seek to prevent and manage disease at three different levels.

1. Primary – this is concerned with seeking to prevent disease and keep people healthy.

2. Secondary – this is concerned with seeking to identify health problems that people may be unaware of and includes screening programmes.

3. Tertiary – this is concerned with promoting recovery or preventing further deteri-oration when disease or ill health has occurred. This includes promoting effective management/self-management of long-term health conditions.

As a learning disability nurse, you will work at each of these three levels with both individ-uals and groups to promote better health and well-being for those you support.

At a primary level you might, for example, be involved in the development of a tailored programme to assist individuals or groups that you support to increase their phys-ical activity and improve their diet. Through doing so you will hopefully assist them to enhance their current physical health, but also prevent longer term health issues such as obesity, diabetes and reduced mobility. You might also be involved in the development and delivery of sexual health promotion or interventions to promote mental health and well-being. The example of promoting the uptake of Covid-19 vaccinations has already been discussed above but as a learning disability nurse you should also be aware of other vaccination programmes such as the annual flu and pneumonia programmes and promote these to those you support. This is particularly important given that respiratory conditions are a leading cause of death for people with learning disabilities.

At a secondary level you might be involved in supporting individuals to access main-stream screening programmes. While people with learning disabilities (as with the wider population of specified ages) are eligible for breast, cervical and bowel screening they may experience many barriers to accessing such services. For example, they may not be able to understand information sent to them about such tests, other people may decide that testing would not be appropriate for them (eg it might be thought to be distressing); they may be unable to make or attend appointments, or they may not understand the importance of such tests. However, as a learning disability nurse you can address all these barriers through providing education for the individual with a learning disability and their carers, providing information in an accessible format or developing desensi-tisation programmes to overcome anxiety. Promoting uptake of AHCs is also an important element of secondary prevention.

As has already been stated in this chapter, people with a learning disability are at increased risk of certain long-term health conditions such as epilepsy and often experi-ence multimorbidity whereby they simultaneously experience several long-term health problems (Hermans and Evenhuis, 2014). Such conditions require careful management since where there are multiple health problems there are usually multiple treatments and the medication or other treatment prescribed for one may adversely impact on or give rise to another condition. As a learning disability nurse, you will therefore often be involved in tertiary prevention as you assist with monitoring long-term conditions and medications. You may also be involved in liaising with several health professionals and specialists to ensure co-ordination of care. However, a key aim of health policy is to enable people with long-term conditions to self-manage such conditions and nurses have a key role to play in facilitating and supporting this (Evans et al, 2017).

Self-management approaches enable people with long-term health conditions to under-stand their health behaviours, their condition(s) and to develop strategies for managing such conditions daily (Maslin-Prothero and Finney, 2011). Evans et al (2017) suggest that the following principles need to be applied when seeking to promote self-management.

○ There should be knowledge of the condition(s) and how progress should be monitored.

○ There should be active participation in decision-making processes and the planning, implementation and evaluation of self- management should be negotiated.

○ There should be partnership working between the individual, their families/ carers and health professionals to identify and agree outcomes.

○ The individual should feel confident to manage all aspects of their daily lives and to access and use support services.

○ Healthy lifestyles and behaviours should be adopted.

Promoting self-management means that all nurses need to develop positive relationships with those they support respecting their knowledge and experience of their condition while also being confident to provide evidence-based advice and information (Evans et al 2017). As a learning disability nurse, however, there are likely to be additional considerations such as the extent to which an individual can understand their condition, its implications and how it can best be managed. You may, for example, need to consider carefully how information is provided to ensure that is it in an accessible format and delivered at an appropriate pace. It may be necessary to repeat information and it is essential to check for understanding. It may also be necessary to develop systems to provide prompts for activities such as visual reminders or phone prompts to (for example) assist with medication management.

It may also be the case that an individual is able to self-manage some aspects of their condition but not others, and it is important that you adopt a strengths-based approach identifying where they are able to take responsibility for managing their health condition and where they will need support. Where support is required then ensuring that their family and carers have the necessary knowledge and skills to provide this and as a learning disability nurse you will be involved in supporting not only the individual but also those who provide care and support for them.

Critical reflection 8.4

- Read through the case study below and decide how you would support Sally to self-manage their diabetes. You should apply the principles discussed above and think not only about the immediate situation but also about seeking to prevent/reduce long-term effects.

Case study 8.2

Sally Arthur

Sally Arthur is a 45-year-old woman with moderate learning disabilities. She lives with two other women of a similar age in supported living where they are supported by staff on a 24-hour basis. Sally volunteers once a week at a local charity shop, attends a cookery class at a local college and enjoys going to bingo. She also loves her food, and her favourite activity is going out for coffee and cake. Over the past couple of years, however, she has put on considerable weight and staff were concerned that she seemed to be getting very lethargic and had started drinking a lot of water saying that she was thirsty all the time. When she went for her AHC the GP was concerned and ran some tests that revealed that she has diabetes. She was advised that she needed to start medication, modify her diet and take more exercise. Sally knows that she has diabetes but doesn't really understand what this means except that she is meant to eat healthy and take tablets. The staff who support her also do not have a good understanding of diabetes and how they should support Sally to manage her condition.

Advocacy

Advocacy is a key role of the learning disability nurse, and this aspect of the role has been directly linked to reducing health inequalities and inequities (Scottish Government et al, 2012). However, when you think about advocacy you probably think about either supporting individuals with a learning disability to advocate for themselves or (where this is not possible) speaking on their behalf to ensure that their needs and views are heard, and their rights are upheld. Such advocacy at an individual level is certainly important in terms of the public health role of the learning disability nurse. For example, you might be involved in advocating on behalf of an individual you support to receive a particular treatment or to have reasonable adjustments put in place to ensure they can access a health-promoting activity. However, your advocacy role should not be confined to advocacy at an individual level alone.

As a learning disability nurse, you may identify that, at a local level, you have several people you support who have a similar health need. For example, it could be that there is a need for improved education in relation to personal and sexual relationships. However, to develop such provision it will be necessary to secure organisational support, resources, and funding to secure premises, refreshments and to cover travel costs. In such a situation you will need to advocate for the group and this advocacy role may involve activities such as presenting evidence of need, costing the intervention and negotiating with key stakeholders. The information provided earlier in the chapter about demography and epidemiology will be helpful to you in developing a case based on evidence of need.

Sometimes, however, to effect change to reduce health inequalities and equities action is required at a policy or legislative level. Think, for example, of how the introduction of AHCs for people with learning disabilities has required the introduction of a specific policy and funding. The National Collaborating Centre for Determinants of Health defines public health advocacy as:

> a critical population health strategy that emphasizes collective action to effect systemic change. It focuses on changing upstream factors related to the social determinants of health, and explicitly recognizes the importance of engaging in political processes to effect desired policy changes at organizational and system levels.
>
> (NCCDH, 2015)

By suggesting that advocacy should focus on 'upstream' factors it places a specific focus on targeting those factors that lead to health inequities rather than simply responding to the consequences of such factors. It states that engaging in political processes is an essential part of such advocacy and you may feel that being political is not part of a learning disability nurse's role (see Chapter 12 for further information regarding this). However, it is only by engaging with such processes that we can effect positive change to improve the health and well-being of those we support. The types of activities you might, therefore, get involved in as you progress through your career include:

○   raising awareness of factors that negatively impact on the health and well-being of people with learning disabilities;

○   providing evidence of need;

○   presenting this evidence to policymakers;

○   becoming part of a committee or working group that is charged with developing policies;

○   commenting on proposed policies (either as an individual or as part of a professional organisation) during periods of consultation;

○   implementing policies and monitoring their impact.

Chapter summary

This chapter has introduced you to the concept of public health and the importance of the public health role of the learning disability nurse. It has explored some of the challenges of adopting a public health approach in relation to people with learning disabilities but has stressed the importance of addressing these challenges to reduce the health inequities they experience. Finally, it has provided some examples of how you, as a learning disability nurse can adopt a public health approach within your practice and work with others to effect change.

FURTHER READING

Hardy, S, Chaplin, C and Woodward, P (eds) *Supporting the Physical Health Needs of People with Learning Disabilities*. Brighton: Pavilion Publishing.

This book will provide you with further information regarding the physical health needs of people with learning disabilities.

Heslop, P and Hebron, C (eds) *Promoting the Health and Well-being of People with Learning Disabilities*. Switzerland: Springer.

This book provides you with an overview of approaches to supporting people with learning disabilities to improve and maintain health and well-being.

RESOURCES

National Development Team for Inclusion (NDTi): www.ndti.org.uk/change-and-development/learning-disability (accessed 21 June 2022).

This website contains several projects focused on improving the health and well-being of people with learning disabilities.

Scottish Learning Disabilities Observatory: www.sldo.ac.uk (accessed 21 June 2022).

This website contains a range of evidence regarding the health and well-being of people with learning disabilities.

9 Supporting those whose behaviour is described as challenging

Chapter aims

The aim of this chapter is to explore the role of the learning disability nurse when working with those whose behaviour is described as challenging. Key concepts are explored within the context of nursing. There are clear reasons why learning disability nurses are well placed to understand behaviour described as challenging. Nurses have the skills for the assessment and planning needed, as well as health monitoring and liaison with other professionals. On occasion the relationships that are often developed and sustained with families and people with learning disabilities means there may be times when it is appropriate for the nurse to coordinate the teams and services involved. Behaviour is a message and it is our job as learning disability nurses to seek to understand that message. There is also space for reflection on the ethical considerations for learning disability nurses when undertaking behavioural assessment and intervention.

Professional standards and expectations

The NICE guidance (2015) relating to individuals with learning disabilities and challenging behaviour

NICE (2018) focused on service design and delivery for those with behaviour described as challenging

The positive behaviour support (PBS) coalition provides a competency framework which is useful to understand the nurse's role and education needs in relation to delivering PBS

The NMC (2018a) standards of proficiency are clear that all registrants need to understand PBS and have skills in relation to de-escalation and responding to behaviour described as challenging

BEHAVIOUR DESCRIBED AS CHALLENGING

It is essential to be aware of the connotations when we talk about challenging behaviour. Originally used as a term to highlight the challenge a person provides to a service to do better (Blunden and Allen, 1987). The term challenging behaviour has sometimes been used put the blame onto an individual rather than spending time to understand the complexities around how the behaviour developed. The 'challenge' is for us to provide the best environments and support to improve people's experiences and quality of life. When this is effective, behaviour described as challenging should naturally reduce. It is essential that you are non-judgemental in your practice and seek to understand the reason why a person exhibits behaviour you find challenging.

Critical reflection 9.1

Spend some time reflecting on the last time you met someone described as challenging.

- What were the positive and negative words you heard about them?

- Do you think the people who were describing them valued the person and had insight into the behaviour?

- When you met the person, did they match your expectations?

Challenging behaviour is not a diagnostic label and is not something that belongs to the person. Behaviour that challenges is often learned and continues to occur due to environmental factors. If we want to reduce the likelihood of challenging behaviour occurring we have to think about the environmental changes that might be needed. Ideally, within your practice you will promote and provide environments that minimise the risk of behaviour that challenges and maximises quality of life (for the individual and those around them). You will need to recognise a variety of factors that can contribute to behaviour change. For some people specialist behavioural assessment may be indicated; however, there may be the possibility that some environmental changes can be made, and your role as a nurse can involve leading on this.

Throughout this chapter we use the term 'behaviour described as challenging' or the description 'people who have behaviour described as challenging'. This may seem long-winded and repetitive; however it is important to minimise the use of labels and focus on the individual. Behaviour described as challenging can increase risks to the individual (The British Psychological Society, 2018). They may be more likely to experience abuse, isolation, exclusion, restrictive practice, harmful or degrading treatment etc. Good practice is to think about the person first and be clear about the behaviour being described as well as the impact on the person and those around them. You will also note that within this chapter, there are a number of seminal references, many behavioural theories are long established and based on developmental or psychological research, hence older references to support the points made.

CHILDREN

Learning to adapt your behaviour and understanding social rules and expectations is typical in development. Parents may have little knowledge or experience of child development or behavioural management and may rely on the way they were managed as children when they displayed behaviour others found difficult. For typically developing children, this is likely to be ok. Some behaviours that children develop can be managed with time, consistency and through understanding child development, for example, biting as a toddler. Most behavioural issues improve as a child develops. When children are learning about the world, growing and developing, they may use behaviour that parents want to discourage and some approaches can be used typically without specialist input. For children with learning disabilities or developmental delay different approaches will be needed. Greene (2005) describes this in a very user-friendly way: 'people who can behave, will'. Meaning that those who have the skills to meet the demands of the environment, make their needs known and manage things for themselves will do that. Behaviour described as challenging can be more time-consuming, require more energy and leave the child feeling exhausted; it can be an inefficient way to have needs met.

McGill (2021) identifies that

> *children without learning disabilities display challenging behaviour during the 'terrible two's,' but then develop communication and social skills which enable them to get what they want and need. Many children with learning disabilities do not develop these skills and are left with the same needs as other children but are much less able to get them met.*

This can mean that the behaviour becomes functional and continues to be used to have needs met. Parents of children with learning disabilities can find this a stressful time because they are likely to be dealing with a range of other issues. Some of these children may have health needs, or need higher levels of supervision and support, their behaviour might mean that accessing nursery or babysitters can be more difficult. Parents will have other issues to balance such as other children, employment, relationships and their own health and mental health needs.

Early intervention

Ideally, there would be a range of services and supports at an early stage which would allow for the early intervention approach towards behaviour described as challenging. The earlier a family is able to access assessment and intervention, the more likely that the impact will be managed at an early stage. Not all areas have access to skilled children's, MDTs that can become involved at an early stage. There have been recent reports and more focus on the damage to children and young people from inappropriate use of seclusion, restraint and other restrictive practices. The RRISC group highlights a number of case studies where children and young people have not had the appropriate support for behaviour (The Challenging Behaviour Foundation, CBF and Positive and Active Behaviour Support Scotland, PABSS, 2019). This is an ongoing campaign to improve childhood experience and reduce restrictive practice.

WHAT BEHAVIOUR MIGHT BE DESCRIBED AS CHALLENGING?

Challenging behaviour as a social construct means that people define what is challenging based on how we expect people to behave in society, creating an understanding of what is challenging and what is not. Some behaviours are acceptable in some places and not others, for example, shouting or swearing might be ok at a football match but not in the school assembly.

Many things people do may be described as challenging, regardless of whether or not the person has a learning disability. People may be demanding, interrupt others, invade personal space, not cover their mouths when they cough etc. Some people will find these traits very challenging. Culturally you may find some behaviour which would be challenging in one aspect of life is accepted or encouraged in another. Emerson's (2001) definition explores this:

> culturally abnormal behaviour of such an intensity, frequency or duration that the physical safety of the person or others is likely to be placed in serious jeopardy, or behaviour which is likely to seriously limit use of, or result in the person being denied access to, ordinary community facilities.

This reminds us to think about the context in which the behaviour occurs and to understand the limitations the person might experience as a result of their behaviour.

Some behaviours typically considered challenging might be:

o   hitting self or others;

o   biting self or others;

o   shouting, swearing, screeching, spitting;

o   damaging property, the environment;

o   playing with saliva, faeces, regurgitating food.

This is not an exhaustive list, but gives a sense of behaviour directed internally (self-biting), externally (damaging property) and a range of things which on their own may seem to vary in severity. However, this must be considered with caution. A person who shouts daily might find that they are as limited and impacted on by their behaviour as another person who regurgitates their food monthly. That is why it is essential to assess the behaviour in line with a recognised definition, which considers frequency, intensity and duration as well as context and impact (Emerson, 2001). Sometimes you will see descriptions such as violent or aggressive, when referring to an individual's behaviour, we will explore throughout this chapter why these are unhelpful words to use.

Some individuals develop a range of behaviours to communicate different things at different times. Some people will have a very limited repertoire of behaviour and will use the same things to communicate a multitude of needs. There are some behaviours, which may not immediately seem challenging and can be left unassessed and not understood for a long time. Typically this is in people with profound and multiple learning disabilities who self-injure; this may be teeth grinding, eye poking, hand biting, self-hitting etc. The behavioural needs of those with profound and multiple learning disabilities might not be addressed due to the internal impact of the behaviour, or in environments when there are other more outwardly challenging individuals. When there are a range of other complexities related to their care needs, for examples, posture, hygiene, nutrition or epilepsy the behaviour might be overlooked. However, to deliver holistic, person-centred care there should always be a consideration to behavioural needs.

You will find that those with behaviour described as challenging can sometimes be dehumanised in ways. They have labels and reputations ascribed to them and they can have experiences, which challenge our value system. There have been many occasions in my practice where I have been warned, watch out she bites (while the person is standing next to me) or, careful he hits out. I have also heard people described as a 'runner' a 'smearer' and other disrespectful and harmful terms. You have a role to play in supporting accurate and meaningful recording and descriptions of behaviour. You may also need to challenge values, attitudes and beliefs of the people and services supporting the person. This can be an incredibly emotive topic, everyone thinks they know about behaviour and how to manage it! Make sure that the descriptions you use are observable.

Violent and aggressive do not describe what a person does. These are emotive labels applied to an individual, which give you a sense of how the person is viewed and understood. They can also mean different things to different people. What I consider aggressive and what somebody from a different community, culture or background might consider aggressive may look very different. Daniel was described as 'trashing' his bedroom, on observation some pillows were on the floor and a poster had been ripped from the wall. When Morgan's mum described him 'trashing' the kitchen, cupboards were off the hinges, the back door had been kicked until it broke and cups and plates were smashed after being thrown at the wall. The tolerance and expectations, experiences and motivations of the people describing the behaviours in this way may be very different.

As a nurse leading behavioural assessment, you need to provide resources, tools, recordings and reports that allow others to understand the issues and the inferences being made. This means using clear and specific descriptions. Sally was not aggressive towards John. Sally gritted her teeth and raised her hand, as if to hit John on the head. Jack was not challenging in the environment; Jack slammed his hands on the desk and said 'I'm going to throw this chair at the wall'. You must give a clear picture of the behaviour, and this makes sure that those recording and reporting the behaviour are clear on what they are being asked to measure. You will be able to analyse the information easily if clear and agreed descriptors have been used. Only by doing this can you ensure that the behaviour can be measured.

Self-injury

This behaviour can be distressing to observe and while supporting a person who displays this level of behaviour you may find that you struggle to understand how and why the behaviour is happening. You must always try to understand the function of the behaviour. Why does X need to self-injure? You can support a safe environment, teach skills to others to minimise harm and support a level of observation that is engaging and supportive rather than custodial and intrusive.

There may be specific situations, which affect the likelihood of self-injury such as times of day or year, particular noises, phrases, people or events. Being sensitive to a person's history and capturing this in a respectful and person-centred way is important to your role and relationship.

RULING OUT UNDERLYING CAUSES OF BEHAVIOUR CHANGE

When George had Covid the first thing that the team supporting him noticed was a change in appetite, he seemed distressed when eating and pushed his food away. He seemed to be seeking specific tastes and used his pecs book to request his most preferred food and drink items. They took his temperature fist and then supported him to have a PCR test. This returned positive. George was supported to self-isolate and staff wore masks and PPE when in close proximity. Nobody else in the environment contracted Covid and the staff were confident that they had supported George from a physical health perspective. It might have been different if they had considered the new behaviour to be challenging rather than an indicator of a physical health change.

When in pain people with learning disabilities:

○ might find this difficult to describe or describe it in ways that are difficult for others to recognise;

○ can become hypo- or hypersensitive to the experience;

○ may communicate pain by changes in their behaviour, look out for changes in vocalisations;

○ they may withdraw and be less motivated to engage in activities or regular routines;

○ might not be as motivated to eat or drink;

○ might have a change to their sleep patterns or they may seem restless.

Whenever there is a change in a person's behaviour we should always seek to rule out an underlying health condition, this can be incorporated into a full functional assessment to help understand the behavioural presentation and inform future planning for the person's needs. Involving parents and carers in the process is essential to having a complete picture.

Physical health

It is essential that physical health factors be ruled out when a person starts to display behaviour described as challenging. You will need to understand the person's health status, experience and demonstration of illness or medical issues. You will need to know if the person had an AHC or other physical health investigation. You will need to liaise with other health professionals to ensure that you consider the individual's health needs and access issues.

o   Joe starts to push away his plate at mealtimes, he usually enjoys food and staff have tried to encourage all of his favourite items. He has barely eaten for the last three days and screamed and threw his ice cream today. Joe's sister said she thinks he might have toothache.

o   Raheem stayed in bed this morning, when his mum tried to get him up for school he pulled the covers up over his head and waved her to go away. This is quite unusual and his mum brought the ipad up to his room to encourage him to get up, he slapped it away and covered his ears. His mum decides to try some paracetamol because she thinks he might have a headache.

o   Lucy will wring her hands and rub them against her teeth in the build up to her period, this can cause redness and sore patches, sometimes breaking the skin. The team, supporting her ask her GP to prescribe mefenamic acid, as they are concerned about how distressed she becomes. They encourage Lucy to use hot water bottles, warm baths and comfy clothing around the time of menstruation, Lucy is supported to request these items.

There continue to be misconceptions related to how people with learning disabilities feel and display pain. A significant contribution to this relates to the paucity of research in this area for people with learning disabilities, who may be excluded from trials and the development of the evidence base due to a variety of reasons. The difficulties with communication and exhibition of behaviour which to others is unusual or difficult to understand can mean diagnostic overshadowing happens, the persons presentation is attributed to the fact they have a learning disability or have displayed behaviour described as challenging. Increasingly though, there is exposure of poor quality care and treatment of people with learning disabilities who are not afforded the fundamental assessments of their needs. Nursing observations and monitoring of signs and symptoms of deterioration and change are essential in promoting positive outcomes for people with learning disabilities.

There have been situations where people have been described as exhibiting pain-related behaviour 'for attention'. This needs to be assessed and understood in the bigger picture of somebody's life, asking 'Why does X need to do that to get attention?' how can we work with them to understand this? what else can we improve in this person's life so that they have meaningful, appropriate and beneficial ways of getting attention instead?

Sensory influences on behaviour

People with learning disabilities are more likely to experience sensory impairments than the general population, it is important to consider these needs in relation to presentation of challenging behaviour because there are opportunities to enhance health and quality of life, through thorough assessment.

The sensory experiences an environment provides can influence behaviour. This might be about how bright or noisy a place is, what it smells like and feels like. Some people may be over or under stimulated by the environment which might lead to sensory seeking or a need to escape. There may be specific alterations that need to happen to an environment to meet a person's needs. This might be about making physical changes, creating space, using soft closers on doors to prevent banging, replacing strip lights due to the brightness or humming noises they present. However, there may be environmental changes that include teaching skills to an individual and allow them ways to make their needs known and having them met. An example could be: if strip lights bother one person they might be taught to put on a cap in a room where the light makes it difficult for them to concentrate rather than turning off or changing the lighting and impacting on everyone's experience.

Eyesight

People with learning disabilities can experience higher than the general population level of sight problems but are much less likely to have access to appropriate eye care. Eye care needs can be overlooked for people with learning disabilities, particularly where there is a reliance on others being able to identify and respond to the need. The estimated prevalence of eye problems was explored by Emerson and Robertson (2011) finding that adults with learning disabilities were ten times more likely to have a sight problem than other adults, and six in ten would need glasses. There is evidence that self-injurious behaviour or other behaviours described as challenging may occur due to eye-related pain, changes in vision and challenges in communicating (de Winter et al, 2011). You will be able to support a person to prepare for and attend an optician appointment, the person does not need to be able to read or speak to be able to have an eye test. The benefit from a good eye assessment can be life changing for the individual, they may have been in pain, anxious, confused and socially limited due to their eyesight. A learning disability nurse may be able to support the person to wear glasses or contact lenses as prescribed and this may then lead to a reduction in challenging behaviour.

Case study 9.1

Geraint's eye problems were noticed by his teacher when he was approximately six years old, his eyes were often red and sore looking, he was often rubbing his eyes and sometimes hit his temples. The school nurse became involved and they made sure that he was supported to attend the optician and subsequently hospital appointments where he was found to have a condition that distorted his vision. This was due to unusually shaped corneas, which could make his vision blurry and cause headaches. Geraint's parents worked with the school to increase the time that he would tolerate wearing glasses but as he got older he needed to have specific contact lenses to change the shape of his corneas. Geraint would become very distressed when these were applied, he found them painful and he would scream and cry when his mum approached him to prompt him to put them in.

> ## Critical reflection 9.2
>
> - What support as a learning disability nurse could you give to Geraint and his family to address these issues and make the process easier for them?
>
> - Who should be involved in the plan you develop?

Hearing loss

People can be born with hearing loss or there can be deterioration over time. A study from McClimens et al (2015) identified undetected prevalence of hearing loss for people with learning disabilities and that the level of hearing loss can be more severe in those with learning disabilities than in the general population. Mainstream testing might overlook the specific needs of people with learning disabilities. The implications of hearing loss and problems for people with learning disabilities can be far reaching, people may mask their problems, but this can have other consequences for participation, inclusion and mental health and well-being.

Mental health deterioration

In the past, there has been a view that those with learning disabilities do not experience mental health issues. We know now, there is an increased prevalence of mental health problems among people with learning disabilities, compared to the general population and there can sometimes be challenges in assessing the mental health needs of people with learning disabilities. You will learn skills related to this during the pre-reg nursing programme.

Behaviour described as challenging is not a mental illness although some people with a mental health condition may display challenging behaviour. You may need to conduct mental health assessment to help your understanding of the person's presentation and consider the best way to support them. You will have specialist skills as a learning disability nurse which mean that the potential for diagnostic overshadowing can be ruled out.

Medication

According to Public Health England, every day approximately 30,000 to 35,000 adults with a learning disability are taking psychotropic medicines when they do not have the health conditions the medicines are for (NHS England, 2016b). We know that children and young people are also prescribed them. There is no evidence base for medication purely for challenging behaviour. As with all medication there can be harmful effects on learning and cognitive abilities and inappropriate use may be particularly detrimental to those with a learning disability. NICE (2015) identifies that there can be a role for antipsychotic medication if other appropriate interventions have failed, where the risk to the person or others is severe and if treating any co-existing health problems does not improve behaviour.

It is essential that monitoring and review of medication is undertaken. The short-term side effects of antipsychotics can be extremely unpleasant, and the long-term side effects potentially serious. Within a behavioural assessment, you must consider the impact of any medication that the person uses, when was this last reviewed and are they concordant with the prescription. There are many examples of people with learning disabilities being prescribed medication and being unable to safely administer for various reasons. This needs to be considered when you are working with a person, do they know how to take their prescribed medication and are they able to. People with learning disabilities, relatives and carers must be provided with adequate information about psychotropic drugs and their side effects, and need to be informed of the availability of other support and management strategies.

Pain

Some people with learning disabilities might experience pain as part of their condition. Specific issues might be related to syndromes where there are muscular or joint-related difficulties. If a person is non-verbal then they may exhibit behavioural changes, which indicate pain. You may observe them to be withdrawn, holding a strange body posture or avoiding touch, food, drink, personal care etc. In other people you may see behaviour that might be described as challenging, screaming, crying, self-harming, biting, hitting parts of their own body or hitting out at others for example.

Some people with learning disabilities can find it very difficult to connect the painful feeling with a source of pain. They may not have the language to describe the body part or the communication skills to accurately explain symptoms. This can be frustrating for the person and those attempting to manage the issues.

It is important to recognise that the original cause for a new behaviour can be pain related. However, over time the pain may be treated and the source identified but the behaviour might remain as this may have been reinforced by other maintaining factors, for example, attention when hitting themselves.

You must make sure that people do not suffer pain, unnecessarily, because of others judgements about how the person might communicate or be experiencing pain. Using a pain profile or assessment can be helpful to support those who don't know a person with learning disabilities well to understand what a person looks and sounds like when they are in pain as well as how they might behave. Pain pictures can be helpful and highlight the importance of nursing observations and making an evidence-based assessment and description of pain-related presentation.

QUALITY OF LIFE

It can be difficult to define and measure quality of life. Sometimes the term might be used to describe an internal state, for example, how happy or satisfied a person is deemed to be. The concept might also be used to describe how engaged a person is, for example, activities or experiences the person has. There may also be times when we use this to understand the broader determinants of health such as housing, education, employment, social status and income. You will be able to support a person to describe the things that help them to have a good quality of life and also increase opportunities which enhance their quality of life and this is what really matters. How does a person describe the things that are important to them? What do they say they want and need in life and how do they measure success? The relationship that you develop with people with learning disabilities will be invaluable to how these questions are asked and answered. You will have specific skills and knowledge that allow you to synthesise this information with the wider assessment and knowledge gained, so that you can be clear about what the person wants and needs.

When we seek to make behavioural changes we should consider what the impact of the change will be on the person's quality of life, behavioural change should strive to positively impact on this. Quality of life could be considered an outcome measure related to behaviour change. By understanding, assessing and implementing approaches for behaviour described as challenging, you will seek to address quality of life issues.

Critical reflection 9.3

- Take some time to explore quality of life measures: think about how they relate to your life and the lives of people you know who have a learning disability.

UNDERSTANDING AND MANAGEMENT OF BEHAVIOURAL RISK

Function

All behaviour has meaning, it happens for a reason. We all use our behaviour as a way of communicating and it achieves something for us. Functional assessment is a way of working this out, using a series of behavioural assessments that help us understand why the person needs to use behaviour in the way that they do. The setting events, antecedents and consequences to behaviour are identified through assessment and then hypotheses are made about what maintains the behaviour and therefore why it happens. The nurse can take part in the assessment or lead the work. This depends on where an assessment is happening and how data is being collected.

In order to understand function it is helpful to consider the three-term contingency of antecedent, behaviour and consequence, based on Skinner (1953). You may recognise this from behavioural assessments you have been involved in as ABC. ABC charts are a helpful tool to use within behavioural assessment. They can record incidences, capturing descriptions of what the behaviour looks like (the topography) and the events preceding and following the behaviour. You will take part in completing the ABC chart, post-incident and analysing a group of ABC charts in order to identify patterns and plan interventions.

Setting events

These are the things that make a behaviour more likely to happen, and there can be many setting events such as being tired, hungry, thirsty, unwell or environmental-related issues. On their own they do not always mean challenging behaviour will occur; however, the more setting events in place the more likely that somebody's behaviour might be 'triggered'. In conducting assessment you will seek to identify the setting events and minimise the likelihood of them leading to an incident of challenging behaviour. Either by changing the way you support the person at that time, for example, reducing demands or reviewing other things which may increase the likelihood of the behaviour happening.

These are sometimes called slow triggers or distant antecedents. Generally meaning the conditions under which the behaviour described as challenging is more likely to occur and which have a delayed impact on the presentation of the behaviour.

Antecedents

These are the things that occur directly before the behaviour happens. This might be the person being told that they cannot have or do something they want, having something end unexpectedly, an unwanted demand or unexpected event.

These might also be called fast triggers: specific events that reliably occur just before the behaviour happens, having an immediate effect on the presentation of the behaviour. Examples of fast triggers include:

○   being asked to do a complex task;

○   being asked to do too many tasks in one go;

○   being rushed or hurried;

○   being interrupted during a favoured activity or event;

○   having something unexpectedly cancelled.

Consequences

The consequence is what happens after the behaviour. This might be how people respond, for example, giving attention, or a preferred item or minimising environmental demands.

When our granddaughter is watching cartoons and the adverts begin, she starts to whimper, giving us the early indication that she might cry. Her grandad immediately reaches for the 'skip ad' button which stops the whimpering and the adverts. Her behaviour is likely to be repeated at the next adverts as her whimpering has been reinforced by a return to the cartoons. This behaviour may then go on to be generalised to other situations where she wants something (a tangible) or to avoid something.

Personal and environmental factors

Behaviour described as challenging is socially defined and is best understood as an interaction between the person and their environment. Personal explanations may encompass biological factors, for example, there are some specific conditions highly associated with behavioural challenges: Prader-Willi is one. When people have this condition, there is a biological reason why they do not feel full or satisfied after eating and they will seek out items to eat, often leading to obesity. When restrictions are placed in the environment and attempts made to stop the person seeking food then behaviour is likely to be challenging. Environmental factors might relate to the physical or emotional environment, the characteristics that make the environment nurturing or controlling for example. If a person has a specific communication need, for example, they rely on Makaton, and there are few Makaton users where they live then the environment is likely to contribute to the behavioural presentation if the person is frustrated and becomes upset when trying to communicate their need. Other examples of personal and environmental factors include the following.

1. Personal characteristics such as: ACEs, past experiences and trauma, thoughts and emotions, mental and physical health, level of intellectual impairment, pain, anxiety, being tired or hungry. A person's skills and abilities, for example, communication, adaptive behaviour, self-care skills, ability to express needs etc.

2. Environmental factors, for example: how hot, noisy, overcrowded, small or boring a place is. How easily the environment facilitates access to the things a person wants and needs. How able an individual is able to get away from things they do not like, who else they share the space with and their characteristics. The environment also includes how people treat and communicate with the person, the things they have to do, how much help they get and the quality of staff interaction etc.

Smoothing the person-environment fit (Lewin, 1951) is essential to make sure that the person's needs can be met and to reduce the likelihood of behaviour described as challenging. This needs careful consideration when designing interventions and support plans. An options appraisal (as described in Chapter 6) might be useful to help think through the potential challenges of implementing an intervention where there is not a smooth fit.

There is very rarely a single cause for the reason that anyone develops behaviour described as challenging. As you have explored, behaviour can develop because of factors within the environment and due to internal (personal) factors. Emerson (2015) states that: '*there is strong evidence that some of the key factors causing challenging behaviour can be changed, and when changed can lead to marked reductions in challenging behaviour*'.

The environment

This refers to everything in and around us. The environment is made up of people, places, equipment and resources. Behaviour described as challenging is influenced by how people respond to and reinforce behaviour. When the behaviour described as challenging has impact on getting things, getting away from things or receives more attention than other behaviours then the behaviour is more likely to reoccur.

Case study 9.2

Siobhan Logan is one of four children, she is 11 years old and is a twin. Her sister Megan does not have a learning disability. Megan and Siobhan have been in the same classes throughout primary school but they now attend different secondary schools. Siobhan has started to do things at home which her family is struggling to understand. Siobhan's mum is a homemaker and her dad is a bank manager. They have very traditional roles in the family and they eat dinner at the same time every day, which Mrs Logan prepares. At the dining table Mr Logan likes to ask the children about their day. Since starting secondary school Siobhan has started to tip drinks or salt onto Megan's food 2–3 times a week. This has caused upset and disruption to the whole family and her parents cannot understand why this is happening. They have asked for some support to help understand her behaviour.

You go to visit the family and meet Mrs Logan, she describes her frustration at the difference in the levels of independence Megan and Siobhan are able to have and repeatedly explains how high achieving her other children are. This is a very important point for you to think about in the assessment. You decide to do some mealtime observations as this seems to be a key point of challenge for the family.

When you observe the routine, you notice that Siobhan is barely spoken to during the meal. The other children are asked to talk about their day and before Siobhan is asked there is an incident of spoiling her sister's meal which takes the attention off Siobhan and causes much fuss and chaos in the kitchen.

Critical reflection 9.4

Reflect on Siobhan's story.

- Why might this be a new behaviour?

- What are the environmental factors influencing this? What are the distant antecedents/slow triggers?

- What are the immediate antecedents or fast triggers?

- What further assessment will help you and the family understand Siobhan's behavioural needs and presentation?

HYPOTHESIS OF FUNCTION

When working with somebody with behaviour described as challenging you will need to assess and find out: what does the person get or avoid by performing the behaviour? People with learning disabilities will only use behaviour in these ways when there are deficits in their environment and the things that they want and need are not freely available to them. You do not need to hit your head to get somebody to acknowledge you when you enter a room, sadly some people with learning disabilities have learned that they do.

The most common way of describing functions of behaviour are identified as: tangible, sensory, escape and attention.

- **Tangible:** they do the behaviour to get something – an item, a walk, a cup of tea, a TV programme, a favourite toy or activity

- **Sensory:** somebody does something because it gives them internal sensory feedback, for example, eye poking – see lights and potentially release endorphins; this can be the most difficult behaviour to impact on through intervention as the behaviour is self-rewarding/self-stimulating and does not need items or other people to be performed (masturbating, playing with faeces, regurgitating food, eye poking, head hitting, hand biting).

- **Escape:** the person uses the behaviour to get out of doing something they find difficult or aversive, for example, pushing away work or food items because the environment is difficult, hitting others to make them go away when they are asking you to do something difficult.

- **Attention:** the behaviour is used to get or maintain social attention. In a group home if somebody is sitting quietly and appearing settled they may be more likely to be left alone, without attention, the person who slams doors or throws items is highly likely to be given attention. Wanting attention is not a bad thing, we all need to feel recognised, wanted, valued and loved etc. Imagine walking into work or placement this morning and nobody said hello?

RECOGNISING RESTRICTIVE PRACTICE

There are some behaviours that can make a person's day-to-day life difficult. Sometimes people may do things that hurt themselves or hurt other people. That can make it difficult for them to have a good quality of life and may put them at risk of experiencing things that we would not want to happen to us, for example 'restrictive practices' which might mean being stopped from doing or having things by the environment, equipment or people in the environment. People who you support as learning disability nurses need to have confidence that their rights will be upheld. People deserve to have support in safe and person-centred ways, practice must be pro-active and values based in the approach. The Royal College of Psychiatrists and the British Psychological Society (RCP and BPS, 2016) identify that:

behaviour can be described as challenging when it is of such intensity, frequency or duration as to threaten the quality of life and/or the physical safety of the individual or others and is likely to lead to responses that are restrictive, aversive or result in exclusion.

Central to help avoid and reduce behaviours that challenge is understanding and recognising restrictive practice. There are clear power imbalances in many situations for people with learning disabilities and sometimes the staff and supporters of people may come to abuse their power. This may not be intentional. They may find ways of managing a person's behaviour, which is about reducing damage to the person or the environment but inadvertently creates other issues. Sometimes cultures can develop where abuse of restrictive practice is overlooked and other issues can develop.

There are many examples of the use of physical restraints to prevent self-injury, such as arm splints or helmets, which create a dependence with the use. Often used to prevent severe injury the introduction of equipment can cause more issues for the individual as it does not seek to understand the source of the issue and teach alternatives. Instead providing a quick fix. The person who has been hitting their head, communicating a need within the environment is now prevented from doing so. This means they may start to use other behaviours to communicate their need.

You will acknowledge that there are occasions where restrictions are used within services to keep people safe and to support de-escalation of behaviours. In services there are consistent messages that these instances are only as a last resort and used to keep people safe. However, we cannot get away from the challenge of how we do this and the ethical dilemmas we face. It is essential that we remember 'restrictive practice is making someone do something that they don't want to do or stopping someone from doing something that they do want to do' (Skills for Health, 2014). Environments with high levels of restrictive practice can indicate abuse and environments, which are unpleasant to live in, are also likely to be unpleasant to work in (CQC, 2021). The nurse's role in recognising restrictive practice and providing leadership in reducing restrictive practice must be embraced. NICE (2015) is clear that restrictive interventions are only used as the last resort.

Overuse of medication

Medication can also be a restrictive practice, where medication is used inappropriately, without an appropriate diagnosis or with a deliberate sedative rather than treatment approach. There are times when this might be appropriate, and considered to be in a person's best interest, for example, an anaesthetic to allow for a necessary treatment; however, there are examples of overprescribing or inappropriate prescribing. There are many examples of people being prescribed antipsychotics without an associated, diagnosed mental health condition. The campaign in England: Stopping Over Medication of People with Learning Disabilities (STOMPwLD) (NHS England, 2016b) focuses on reducing the use of medication prescribed with the aim of reducing challenging behaviour while recognising the appropriate alternatives of psychological or other interventions (The British Psychological Society, 2018).

It may sometimes be appropriate to consider the use of antipsychotics but this should be after other approaches have been attempted, for example, psychological interventions or in situations where there has not been a response to treatment for mental or physical health issues. Antipsychotics might also be considered when the risk from the behaviour to the person or others is severe (eg physical attempts to injure others or self-injury).

You might find in your nursing practice that there are people who believe medication can be the answer; the issues related to training, resourcing and understanding of underlying factors can lead to an over-reliance on medication. There are no specific medications licenced for challenging behaviour, in your role you will need to be clear and educated in relation to this in order to enhance others understanding.

THE NURSE'S ROLE IN POSITIVE BEHAVIOUR SUPPORT

At the heart of NICE (2015) recommendations for working with those with behaviour described as challenging is a phased approach to assessment and intervention, based on the principles of positive behavioural support (PBS). Positive behaviour support is a values-based, recognised approach to increasing quality of life for people with learning disabilities who display behaviour described as challenging. 'Over the last three decades, [PBS] has increasingly become the model of choice in supporting people whose behaviour poses challenges to services' (PBS Coalition, 2015). PBS is considered by many in the field, to be the most evidence-based approach to behaviour described as challenging and underpins policy across Wales and the UK.

While PBS is increasingly being promoted as best evidence-based practice, it can be misunderstood. PBS is not regulated in terms of how organisations can say they deliver the approach. This can be challenging for you as nurses who might be heavily involved in the assessment of behaviour but not the day-to-day delivery of intervention. There are providers who report that they deliver specialist, PBS and in actuality, there are hidden, abusive practices in closed cultures. The learning disability nursing profession need to be alert to the potential for inappropriate use of restrictive practice and bullying, degrading or inhumane approaches to care and treatment. Positive behaviour support (PBS) is a person-centred approach to helping people with a learning disability who might use behaviours which challenge. It involves understanding the reasons for behaviour and looking at the person as a whole and finding new ways of supporting the person. It focuses on improving quality of life and teaching new skills to replace the behaviour which is described as challenging. The British Psychological Society (2018) is clear that *'it is inherent with the practice of PBS that a broad range of professionals are required to support the implementation of PBS that truly meets the needs of those with challenging behaviour'* (p 1).

One of the most important things that you need to consider as a nurse supporting a behavioural assessment is the role of the mediators. These are the people who are responsible for delivering the plans. The carers, family members or supporters who will have a key role in implementation and you are likely to have a detailed understanding of their skills and needs. It is essential that you take on board their views. Sometimes they will be the people who are talking about the issues and the impact of the behaviour. They may not realise that they might have to make changes, sometimes people think the issues lie solely with the person with a learning disability and do not understand the role they play in influencing presentation of behaviour. You will need to communicate, negotiate and clarify the approaches to supporting the person with behaviour described as challenging to be clear that everybody is on the same page. The PBS Coalition (2015) sets this out in the competency framework, emphasising the importance of the mediators and environment the person is in, understanding their role in taking forward the plan. The mediators will have a role in completing documentation and reviewing information, you will need to support their knowledge and understanding of this. Sometimes where there are challenges for families you will need to be creative in supporting data collection. Making daily contact to complete behaviour charts may be one way to do this.

Case study 9.3

You have been working with a family for four weeks, they have five children living at home, two dogs and a rabbit. The environment is quite impoverished, neither parents work and the house is very busy. Cameron is the youngest child, he has a learning disability and Autism. Cameron is 7 and he is slim, non-verbal and always seems hungry. He loves to watch colourful cartoons and can request preferred items using a PECs book. In the four weeks you have known him you have observed a number of bruises on his knees and face. His parents tell you that he drops down hard onto his knees and punches himself in the face. You have left scatterplots and behaviour monitoring forms in the home but the parents have not written anything down. You are becoming increasingly concerned about the family's ability to work with you and address Cameron's needs.

Critical reflection 9.5

- Make a list of the concerns you have after reading this case study.

- What might be preventing the family from recording his behaviour?

- Can you think of alternative ways to support the family in the assessment?

- How will you address some of your concerns, who else will you need to involve in this?

SPECIALIST TEAMS

A specialist team may have a role in conducting a comprehensive assessment or supporting those particularly at risk. There may also be clinicians in specialist teams who act as consultants and support others to develop their behavioural approaches.

Specialist teams are often multidisciplinary and so as a nurse it could be that you work directly within a team to conduct assessment and intervention. Ideally, the team will be part of a wider specialist service and will have relationships with other professionals to support the ongoing implementation of interventions and reviews. Team members often work with those who care for and support the person to develop an understanding of behavioural function. Teams will also consider how those who support the individual can interact with them in ways that will reduce the likelihood of behaviour becoming challenging. Training, consultation, direct work and role modelling are other elements of the specialist team who often hold detailed knowledge of the person and their needs. Teams are often small and can have referral systems which rely on shared understanding of the severity and complexity of behavioural presentation.

RECOGNISING THE IMPORTANCE OF THE QUALITY OF THE ENVIRONMENT

From a learning disability nursing perspective, you are likely to be involved in assessment and understanding of need, which helps individuals to communicate the challenges they face. You will have specialist knowledge about the development of behaviour, the importance of communication and the requirements to make changes for the individuals benefit rather than the service.

Understanding the factors that contribute to challenging behaviour helps us to understand how to change the support or the environment to better meet and fit the person's needs. The likelihood of a person displaying behaviour described as challenging often depends on the quality of the service or environment they are in. McGill et al (2020) describe an environment, which can be associated with reduced frequency and severity of challenging behaviour as a 'capable environment'. The factors, which contribute to the environment as being capable rather than challenging, can be attributed to the system the person functions in and the direct delivery of support from staff.

According to McGill et al (2020), there are 12 key areas that either have an impact on reducing the likelihood of behaviour or have a positive impact on the person and other's quality of life.

1. positive social interactions;
2. support for communication in all aspects of the person's life;
3. support to participate in meaningful activities;
4. consistent and predictable environments that commit to personalised routines and activities;
5. support related to the involvement of family and friends, establishing or maintaining these relationships;
6. opportunities for choice are provided, clear communication is used to support choice making;

7. more independent functioning is encouraged, opportunities are provided to develop skills;

8. the way personal care and health is supported is dignified and personalised;

9. the physical environment is acceptable and provides for individual needs;

10. staff are mindful and skilled and able to lead on capable practice;

11. support is arranged and delivered within the wider understanding of challenging behaviour;

12. care delivery recognises the need to ensure quality and safety (as well as other things) from an individual and support perspective.

The more of these standards that are present in the environment, the more likely it is that service users are living a good life. In your role, it might be necessary for you to support the environment working in partnership with the setting to understand how able they are to meet needs. By developing these professional relationships, you will have a sense of how capable the environment is, including these standards in your assessments and reviews will help you monitor and feedback your views on the placement.

THE POSITIVE BEHAVIOUR SUPPORT PLAN

The positive behaviour support plan follows the assessment and should be developed co-productively.

A PBS plan should always set the scene with a pen picture of the individual, describing their skills and attributes and the things that are important to them.

Case study 9.4

Sam's pen picture

Sam is 24 years old. He is 5ft 8in tall and weighs 11st. He has dark blonde hair and blue eyes. He loves going for walks in the countryside or seaside, he enjoys pottery, live music and visiting his family. He is often described as very caring towards others, has a great sense of humour and perseveres with things he enjoys. Sam is good at art, he loves to paint scenes and views, he is meticulously tidy, likes things to be in their proper place and he knows the names of famous pieces of classical music and their composers. He enjoys talking to people about all of these topics and most of all likes to share his interests with his favourite people – his mum Sue and his dad Dave, his brother Jonathan and his housemate Molly, who he describes as his best friend. Molly and Sam often cook together with support to plan the recipes and buy the ingredients; Sam mostly enjoys washing up and tidying away afterwards.

Critical reflection 9.6

- Thinking about the pen picture, how do you feel when you read this?

- Is this what you expected to read about somebody with behaviour described as challenging?

- From a nursing perspective how might this prepare you for meeting and supporting Sam?

The PBS plan is multicomponent and draws on a range of psychological theories, models and approaches to promote an enhanced quality of life for the individual, ensuring that their needs are met and that there is a reduction in the likelihood of challenging behaviour (British Psychological Society, 2018). There will be a range of sections which help the reader to understand the person's needs, nurses can work together with the person to develop the plan. The plan can be written in an accessible way so that there is shared ownership and agreement on how it will be implemented.

The plan will be based on a comprehensive behaviour assessment report and is likely to include the following sections:

o background information including the pen picture and current medication;

o personal characteristics;

o strengths and needs;

o motivational analysis, listing preferred activities, items, people and places (preferred reinforces);

o the behaviours of concern, the identified risk factors and the relationship between behaviour;

o identified gaps in support and mediator analysis which helps identify the strengths and needs of the people who will implement the plan;

o conditions under which behaviour described as challenging is less likely to occur;

o summary of current and previous approaches towards the behaviour described.

A PBS plan should focus on the pro-active and preventive strategies, including teaching new skills. Strategies to avoid crisis will be built in (antecedent management or ecological manipulations) and recommendations on how to keep people safe must be made. If the safety plan or crisis management incorporates restrictive interventions then these must always be the least restrictive. There must also be a clear plan on how to reduce restrictive practice going forwards.

You need to be clear that people delivering the interventions understand how to avoid restrictions and use proactive approaches. There may be cost, resource and other implications of implementing the PBS plan. Education and training needs for mediators will have to be considered.

Chapter summary

Behaviours described as challenging can have long-term implications for a person's relationships, care experiences, treatment and quality of life. Those who are labelled challenging are more likely to experience abusive practice, restrictions and out of area placements (Emerson and Einfield, 2011).

The learning disability nurse will play a key role in the support of individuals, families, teams and services to understand and respond to behaviours described as challenging. There will be barriers that you might need to overcome in behavioural practice; the views of others and perceptions of why behaviour happens. In your professional practice you must always: think person-centred, conduct personalised assessment, consider the views of the person and those who support them, work together with the person, their mediators and providers and develop plans which focus on increasing quality of life, reducing restrictive practice and teaching skills.

Developing your knowledge and understanding is key to making improvements in the lives of others. There are many professional programmes focused on developing positive approaches to challenging behaviour, this ranges from one-off modules to master's programmes. There will be something to meet your needs as you develop confidence and skills in working with those whose behaviour is described as challenging.

FURTHER READING

Gore, N J, Sapiets, S J, Denne, L D, Hastings, R P, Toogood, S, MacDonald, A, Baker, P, Allen, D, Apanasionok, M M, Austin, D, Bowring, D L, Bradshaw, J, Corbett, A, Cooper, V, Deveau, R, Hughes, J C, Jones, E, Lynch, M, McGill, P, Mullhall, M, Murphy, M, Noone, S, Shankar, R and Williams, D (2022) Positive Behavioural Support in the UK: A State of the Nation Report. *International Journal of Positive Behavioural Support*, 12(1): i–46.

NICE QS101 (2015) Learning Disability: Behaviour that Challenges. [online] Available at: www.nice.org.uk/guidance/QS101 (accessed 30 November 2021).

Seligman, M (2011) *Flourish*. London: Nicholas Brealey Publishing.

RESOURCES

All Wales Challenging Behaviour Community of Practice Padlet: https://padlet.com/Impro vementCymru/CoPChallengingBehaviour?msclkid=6d345946c31511ecaf0b440bcc9db 172 (accessed 23 April 2022).

The All Wales Challenging Behaviour Community of Practice is the largest and most established COP in the UK. This link provides a range of materials, including recordings of the meetings to help you understand the function and work of the COP.

Challenging Behaviour Foundation: www.challengingbehaviour.org.uk/?msclkid=7d913d98c 31311ecb3a38ac6de11bb40 (accessed 23 April 2022).

The challenging behaviour foundation hold a plethora of resources which are written in user friendly ways and incorporating the voices of people with learning disabilities and their families.

Hill's Perma Model: A Scientific Theory of Happiness: www.bild.org.uk/wp-content/uploads/2021/03/The-PERMA-Model-Booklet-Update.pdf (accessed 23 April 2022).

Hill's Perma model focuses on the components that make up wellbeing and authentic happiness, a model that helps us think about the lives and experiences of people with learning disabilities.

An Introduction to PBS: www.bild.org.uk/resource/an-introduction-to-pbs/ (accessed 23 April 2022).

The introduction to PBS is very accessible and summarises the key points of positive behaviour support and why it is important in our practice.

Section 3

Advancing practice

10 Innovation in practice

Chapter aims

The aim of this chapter is to demonstrate approaches to innovation in learning disability nursing introducing relevant concepts in the context of quality improvement. Use of language will be explored throughout the chapter, as well as the cultures and models that you can use to develop services and practices. Improving the quality and safety of patient care is at the core of nursing practice. You need to question why you do what you do, and explore if you can do better (or not). This chapter explores the need to adopt a creative and innovative approach to practice, recognising that learning disability nurses have a key role in making change happen. It includes identifying areas for change, managing change and evaluating the impact of innovation. Resources and links are provided to support you.

Professional standards and expectations

The process of revalidation (NMC, 2019) encourages all nurses to think about outcomes and the way you apply nursing models within practice, this includes setting goals, carrying out evaluation and undertaking review.

The Health and Care Standards (2015) have seven themes focused on good quality, safe care. There are specific measures for practice relevant to innovation in practice. Providing evidence against the standards helps in the measurement of progress, for example, quality improvement, research and innovation and listening and learning from feedback.

ADOPTING A CREATIVE AND INNOVATIVE APPROACH TO PRACTICE

Learning disability nurses have a proud history of innovations that put the individual at the centre of nursing care, key worker roles, named nurses and delivery of person-centred care are just some examples of this. Changing practice is driven by a desire to improve the experiences of those they support and their acquisition of health outcomes. Undertaking improvement work not only supports personal development but can also contribute to professional practice. There have historically been challenges in demonstrating the evidence base to support learning disability nursing. Strengthening the Commitment (Scottish Government et al, 2012) reinforced the need for learning disability nurses to share and develop best practice in order to advance the profession. It is important to make time within your practice to reflect on what you have achieved, to think about the skills you used to approach challenges and consider how this can be shared with others. Reflection is also important for revalidation (NMC, 2019) and evidencing your growth in professional practice is a specific requirement.

Responding to challenges often requires creative thinking; it is important not to predetermine your approach or believe that you alone must find a solution. Creative moments occur when you talk with others about the work you are doing, the challenges you are facing and question the status quo which often lead to collective problem-solving (cohort thinking or echo chambers). Collective discussions in virtual or face-to-face ways can help with creativity, learning lessons and sharing experiences, for example, in a professional nurse forum, or special interest groups. There may be communities of practice at a local, national or international level that offer this space. It is important to be open-minded and recognise the potential prejudgements or bias you might have to a way of doing things. Being curious can be particularly helpful when there is a problem to solve or a sense of '*being stuck*' (Jones et al, 2019). Syed (2016) describes how innovations are context-specific, meaning that, the time and place where the problem occurs leads to a particular response. Innovation comes from a desire to solve a problem, sometimes it comes from failure and often a solution to a problem seems very simple in hindsight (as do many things).

Within your professional practice there will be many occasions where you need to use influence. Many learning disability nurses blog or use other social media such as, Twitter or Facebook, recognising their responsibility as role models and leaders within the profession. Having a public platform gives opportunities to share the more positive aspects of the learning disability nurses role. The purpose of developing a professional, social profile is generally to raise awareness, morale and to inspire others to act as role models and to celebrate what we do. The ultimate purpose is often to raise the profile of people with learning disabilities and learning disability nursing to inspire others into the profession.

Often the experiences of people with learning disabilities are highlighted when things have gone wrong. The public are more likely to hear of when people with learning disabilities have experienced poor or abusive practice, when standards have not been good enough or when people have needlessly died. This was present during the Covid-19 pandemic, where inequalities were exposed; in access to healthcare, vaccines, escalation of treatment and disproportionate deaths. The negative experiences, unfair treatment and discriminatory practice can contribute to the challenges that learning disability nurses feel in their professional pride and identity. There are times when the more innovative and creative approaches to nursing practice can feel discredited by those who might be sceptical about the future of the profession or taking improvement forward. Being positive and creating new opportunities, contributing to professional and service development does not mean that you are naïve to the wider issues and the continued challenges for people with learning disabilities in our society today. As professionals, leaders and role models in learning disability nursing we have an obligation to promote a positive image of the people that we work with, and our profession. Innovating with new ideas, methods or creative approaches are some of the steps to achieving this.

EMOTIONAL INTELLIGENCE AND INNOVATION

In clinical practice, there may be occasions when you ask why people do things the way they do? When you think things are going well for you, you do not always see a need to change things. Sometimes people will be emotionally invested in the way things are done, and they may feel safe and secure in the predictability and routine. Fresh eyes and new roles can bring a dynamic for change into an environment that has been happy doing things the way they have. When you think things are going well, you do not always see a need to change things. Asking questions can make people feel uncomfortable and suggesting change might make people feel defensive, leaving people feeling that they are not doing their best, which hits at the heart of being a nurse. Change can be difficult; you must be emotionally intelligent in the way you propose and introduce change. There will be a need for others to be seen and heard during the change process.

Empathy is expected within the nursing profession and you will base many of your behaviours on how you perceive others are thinking and feeling. Mansel and Einon (2019) state that empathy is paramount for great leadership. When you want to make a change, share good practice or suggest a different way of doing things, as a leader you will need to demonstrate empathy, compassion and self-awareness in how you approach this. The reflective practice embedded in nursing prepares you for some of the skills you need to drive the profession forward. There may be times, when leading on changing practice that you need to be vulnerable and to demonstrate this actively. One way of displaying vulnerability in the change management process is to express confusion openly. Confusion is an uncomfortable feeling, but all learning takes effort and being in a state of confusion can be personally motivating, as you seek to solve a puzzle and learn more about how you understand an issue. As you seek to understand and learn deeply, you will problem-solve and gain new insight and ways of thinking about issues. Brown (2021) highlights that courageous leadership can mean not shying away from confusing information or data, at the risk of appearing wrong, but acknowledging exploration of new problems for solving.

When you broach the topic of improving practice, there may be a perception of conflicting agendas. Improving care and saving money may not seem compatible to your teams, but there may be some scepticism about the motives for change. However, often you will find that efficiencies or cost savings are not the goal of an improvement, but occur as a side effect of the approach to improving quality. It is also important to understand that while you are thinking about demonstrating value, this does not have to be purely financial; there are other benefits to changing practice. It is important to think about access, quality, workforce and finances in that order, if you have achieved the first three aspects at the right level then the finances will '*fall out*', as they say.

The language of change

There is much literature published on the technology of innovation and various tools and models have been applied over time to help structure and measure change. Some common terms used in change language used to describe motivators, behaviours and traits, which influence how innovation is adopted, are outlined in Table 10.1. The terms are collated based on Health Foundation (2015a), Barr and Dowding (2019), Local Government Association (2013) and Ledderer et al (2020).

Critical reflection 10.1

- Think about the terms in Table 10.1: have you heard these applied in practice?

- Are there other change terms you are familiar with?

- What are the factors that you think influence a learning disability nurse in accepting or embracing change?

Table 10.1 Key terms for making change and improvement

Nudges	Provides information, for example, how others are moving forward, detail on how to move forward, puts building blocks in the environment to create a default position, for example, 'we all do this'. This promotes behaviour change (widely used in public health).
Shoves	Puts barriers in place that make the less healthy/less preferred (organisationally) choice less attractive, creates a disincentive for not choosing the preferred approach
Smacks	Provides a punishment for non-compliance with a promoted option.
Change agent	The person who has power to make the change, commanding, moulding and guiding (Sullivan, 2012)
Opinion leaders	People who are respected and valued and are highly influential in the environment. They may not be senior people, they may not be in leadership roles, but their buy in will impact on how others respond.
Change champions	Those who are able to champion the change, they may have a stake in the change or particularly knowledge about the change issue.
Innovators	Creative and connected people who are willing to take risks and introduce change.
Early adopters	The people who are first to accept, embrace or work within the change
Early majority	Take time to adopt the innovation, most people fall into this category.
Late majority	Often suspicious about the innovation and adopt much later, sometimes because they have to!
Laggards	Might be hostile to the ideas of change and dislike it. Often the last to adopt change and may cling to tradition. Sometimes by the time the laggard has accepted and adopted the change, others have moved onto a new way of doing things.
Rejectors	Might challenge or sabotage the change and will be open about their dislike of change.

MANAGING CHANGE

There are many ways that you might be involved in change. You might need to lead on changing a process, for example, managing transitions for service users between environments or implementing a new policy, which involves changing the way that observations are conducted and recorded. Organisational change may include things like looking at staffing establishments, developing new roles, integrating services, changing shift patterns, implementing a government policy such as the Nurse Staffing Act (2016) or the reducing restrictive practice framework (Welsh Government, 2021b). Within nursing you will develop skills, learning to adapt and cope with change at multiple levels, some of which you will take a lead on, feel involved in and be aware of. Sometimes change will be imposed, perhaps at a national level, this might be because of scandals, changes in government, updated policy, research or other sources of evidence. You may need to use your skills to bring others on board with the change, influencing how change is accepted and embraced, alleviating concerns or fears.

From a personal perspective, one thing you will need to consider is whether you have the right skills to get the best out of people. You will need to listen to people and take on board their views, sometimes these might be in conflict with your own. There might be challenge and disagreement, questions and conflict when working through ideas and solutions. You will need to learn to embrace this and accept that you will not always have the same opinions as others but that an agreement has to be reached, even if that means agreeing to disagree.

McGregor (in Kurt, 2021) suggested that managers hold beliefs about the way people are and their assumptions would determine the way that they treated people. People were categorised according to whether they were considered to be Theory X or Theory Y, explored in Table 10.2.

Table 10.2 Theory X and Theory Y

Theory X – workers prefer to be treated in a way that allows them to avoid responsibility	Theory Y – employees want responsibility and are intrinsically motivated to do a good job
• Employees are lazy and do not like their jobs • Employees need direction and lack motivation • Workers need to be punished or rewarded to ensure that they do what needs to be done • Workers lack ambition, desire for growth and do not have goals	• Employees take pride in their work and are happy to accept new challenges • People can work in a self-directed way, they do not need to be micro-managed • Workers will feel internally satisfied if they are able to contribute • Workers are keen to be involved in making decisions

(Adapted from Kurt, 2021)

> ### *Critical reflection 10.2*
>
> * When you read through Table 10.2, did you recognise thoughts about your colleagues? What were they?
>
> * What can you learn from the categories of Theory X and Theory Y?
>
> * What kind of management style would you adopt if you worked with a Theory X person?
>
> * In what ways can understanding this model help you to manage change in a better, more person-centred way?

You might have found some of the components of McGregor's theory challenging or perhaps outdated; however, it is likely that you will find reflecting on these points useful. By understanding how McGregor's model presented a Black and white approach in Theory X or Theory Y you can also think about the shades of grey that make up things such as personality, human behaviour, mood, interest, pleasure, motivation and aspirations and how this contributes to an employee's ability to innovate.

McGregor's model should help you to recognise that one size does not fit all; it is important to recognise the skills and attributes of your team and find ways to get the best out of them. People may have a preference for how they conduct themselves at work, but in daily practice this will be impacted on by a range of factors. Taking a holistic approach to understanding colleagues is important, just as you would with people who use services and their families. There are a range of competing issues that impact on how your colleagues or team members will behave in the workplace. Some people will relish data analysis, presentations, leading and chairing, others might like to provide information and evidence that allows their colleague to build information, reports or assessments. There are some parts of all jobs that people will have to do; it is important that we test and stretch people but also balance this in a way that is satisfying and fulfilling to them. Finding creative ways to support people means finding out what is important and valued by them.

SHARING AND LEARNING

The Royal College of Nursing (RCN, 2021) draws together many examples from across the UK in the Connecting for Change report of learning disability nurses in new and innovative roles. The review from the RCN also highlights there are a range of forums where innovation can be shared. Improvement programmes may be taking place at a service, regional or national level. One example of this is the HEF (Atkinson et al, 2013) which was developed by learning disability nurses to provide a specific tool to measure outcomes. The HEF focuses on measuring the impact of interventions delivered by learning disability nurses and recognises the gaps in tools and models specific to learning disability nursing practice.

NHS Fab stuff (Fabstuff, nd) is an online collaborative where active sharing and networking is encouraged. Individuals will upload their summary papers, posters and reviews of improvements made in practice. Making data count is one of the campaigns that is promoted on the website, very much focused on the use of existing data and spreading awareness of how to maximise this in teams, health boards etc. This is important to think about, as one of the potential barriers you will experience will be that people feel that innovation will be time-consuming. If you can reassure those involved in the development that there will not be a demand on them as existing data will be accessed then they may be more engaged in the process. People who are doing the job, day to day are more than likely going to be the people who can tell you what needs to change and why. As you progress in your career and development, it is very important that you remain close to practice. You need to appreciate the daily challenges and demands faced and grasp how these are addressed.

Reflect on a time that you were involved in a change, who were the people who helped make this successful, what did they do?

Critical reflection 10.3

- How would you define innovation?
- Think about the leaders in learning disability nursing. Reflect on and outline how you see them innovating practice.
- How do they garner support or influence others in taking forward change?

The Learning Disability Senate, UK Learning Disability Nurse Consultant Network, Learning and Intellectual Disability Nursing Academic Network and LD Consortium are just some of the groups where leaders in learning disability practice come together to develop professional practice, debate and explore issues and contribute to research and development. These groups are visible on social media, on website platforms and members regularly come together in virtual and face-to-face ways to progress the agenda for people with learning disabilities and their families.

There are a number of organisations that offer funding for innovative projects, evaluations and research in practice; there are repositories of good practice projects on sites such as The Queens Nurse Institute (QNI), The Burdett Trust and The Royal College of Nursing (RCN). An application can help purchase equipment, fund dedicated staff time, access training or develop resources needed for a creative idea or innovation. There will be people where you work, who are able to guide and support you with developing business cases and proposals. Ensuring that you are well prepared with bids, giving yourself enough time to gather the data that you need is important; there are often tight timescales to adhere to and sometimes opportunities are announced at short notice.

Barriers and enablers of change

There are things within your organisations that will enable you to take forward innovation. However, where these are not present they can pose significant barriers. Understanding the processes and structures, the resources and key leaders in your service will help you when you have an idea you want to progress. Some of the barriers and enablers are outlined in the next few paragraphs.

Cultures

Cultures develop and grow and can take years to form and although often the word is often perceived negatively, this is not always the case. However, workforce culture can create environments that are reluctant to change, accept new ideas or new people, this might mean they are very difficult to improve. People assimilate and ascribe to a culture, sometimes without knowing they are part of something that can be difficult to understand by outsiders. Nurses will identify nursing solutions when faced with a challenge, other professionals will think of their training, knowledge and skills to help them understand and address an issue. How supportive, collaborative and inclusive the culture of your workplace is will have a huge influence on how able you are to take forward improvement (Jones et al, 2019).

Critical reflection 10.4

- How would you describe your professional culture?
- Think about what being a nurse means to you. How do you identify with other nurses?
- What does this mean for how you engage with other professions?

Leadership

Leadership should be present at all levels, when introducing change you need to feel that you are supported by people who understand and embrace improvement work. Barr and Dowding (2019) describe this, management and leadership need to be effective for successful change. Visibility, critical thinking and relationships are identified by Moore (2020) as some of the leadership qualities needed in nursing. The attitudes and values of others are important in setting the tone and creating a culture that is reflective, learns and embraces problem sensing (Jones et al, 2019). There should be people within your organisation who have been invested in from a quality improvement perspective and are able to support others in this work. This includes service users and their families.

Critical reflection 10.5

- Reflecting on your processes for co-producing work with service users and families, where are the opportunities for them to influence improvement work?

In terms of your own leadership skills, there are sensitivities to be aware of. You must be mindful that when you are seeking to improve, others might perceive this negatively. This may be because people feel that other previous efforts are being discounted or criticised. You may invest time and effort into spreading an innovation, but unless others are able and choose to adopt it, there will be limited impact. There will be some people whom you work with who are eager to embrace or lead on change, and others will need more time, evidence and support for them to adopt or accept change.

What is important is that as a leader for change, you set out your expectations and create a safe environment in which teamwork, inclusivity and continuous improvement is embedded.

Critical reflection 10.6

- What do you think a safe environment looks like?
- What are the features in your workplace that support you to share and spread ideas?
- What are the things that make you shy away from raising ideas or making suggestions?

Workforce

Workforce needs must be understood, people should feel empowered and able to identify concerns and ideas. Investment in making sure that staff have an understanding of the concepts of improvement and innovation fosters a culture ready for change. You may find that this has not always been prioritised; people may not be on the same page. If the workforce leans towards risk aversive or paternalistic approaches, they will naturally be less inclined to try new things. You will need to recognise these issues in areas that you are supporting. When you place a priority on improvement, sharing the vision with the workforce is important, having a communication strategy is essential. Where there have been investments in the workforce, opportunities must be provided for using these skills. Giving others an opportunity to lead on change can be empowering and motivating. Understanding who is interested and skilled to be involved in development opportunities will be essential in your professional practice. Scott (2017) describes the importance of knowing the strengths and skills in your team and finding ways to nurture and grow that.

Critical reflection 10.7

Think back to the chapter on leadership.

- What have you taken away from the ideas raised in relation to professional practice?
- What are the leadership skills you identify in yourself and how do you see the interface between leadership and innovation?

Infrastructures

Infrastructures are not always as capable as you might need them to be when you start to think about delivering on improvement. Sometimes you will have to manage with what you have, but often there will be ways of addressing these challenges. Communications teams, information technology supports and operational managers will have access to resources that can support you. Find out about the quality improvement forums and networks within your areas and build relationships to help you tap into existing skills and resources. There must be sufficient resource and time set aside to allow for planning, idea generation, data collection and analysis and implementation. This might mean that you have to have some up-front conversations about the challenges you identify and the support you need.

Governance structures

Governance ensures adherence to an overall strategy, provides context to activities, captures performance indicators and reinforces accountability. Think about the processes you have in your organisations, do you know what happens to the data you produce in your daily work, who analysis and acts on the information? From a nursing perspective who represents you within these processes, how much communication do you see which reflects what happens within your team, division, service group, region etc how are you able to influence this?

LEARNING DISABILITY NURSES DEMONSTRATING VALUE

We do not introduce change for change sake. Change for some can feel very difficult, unsettling and time-consuming. Listening to people and finding out what things in the workplace or system they find challenging will help you to identify potential improvements. Capture feedback, seek views of those who use services and those who provide them. In your role you will need to think very clearly about what change you are trying to make and how you will know when you have achieved it. If you want to have improved outcomes, you will need to clearly understand a baseline and what an outcome means now. You can understand this by observing, listening and immersing yourself in the environment and culture.

A parent once said that she could tell what experience her child would have in hospital after walking 15 steps onto the ward (NHS England, 2017). The 15-step challenge has been adopted in many areas of practice and can be used as a benchmark for a service experience.

Critical reflection 10.8

Next time you visit an area, or walk into your own workplace, stop and think about the following.

- How welcoming is the environment?

- How safe does it feel?

- How much did you feel it was caring and involving?

- How well organised and calm did it appear?

- How would you give feedback to the environment?

- If you were the nurse in charge, how would you want to receive feedback of this nature?

The Good Practice Project (Department of Health, 2013) identifies a number of innovations across a range of environments and services for people with learning disabilities. The way that the paper describes how the panel selected good practice examples for publication gives a wonderful insight into values, dignity, respect and quality. The panel describes thoughts on a variety of approaches where the language was not quite right, where the attention to the needs of people who used services did not seem to be a priority or perhaps was secondary to the outcome of the improvement. There are descriptions of how there were some tokenistic approaches taken or examples that might not have been in the best interests of people who use services.

The quality of the good practice projects was measured with respect to:

o   how much they had been co-produced;

o   how much the capabilities of people with learning disabilities had been at the forefront of the project;

o   what the project did for building community capacity;

o   the collaborative approach towards integration;

o   how committed the project was to personalisation.

Critical reflection 10.9

Read one of the good practice examples from the Department of Health (2013).

- Thinking about the quality checking measures above, how would you describe the project against the five bullet points.

- What will you take away from reading about the projects?

Think about a service innovation you are aware of in your organisation.

- Do you know what costs are involved in this?

- Have you been included in any communication on what the innovation is hoping to achieve?

- Who do you think will benefit from this service innovation?

Learning disability nurses have continually adapted and innovated, the way that people with learning disabilities live in society has changed significantly throughout the last century and there continue to be evolving roles for professionals working in the field. Rose (2021) recognises one of the challenges for learning disability nursing is the small numbers of nurses in the field undertaking a broad range of roles. There is positivity in thinking about the diversity in the roles of learning disability nurses but the variation can impact on how we define the role of the nurse, measure impact and realise a pathway for professional development and progression. One way that you can influence the understanding of the role of the learning disability nurse is through the demonstration of value. This means that you need the skills, techniques and resources to allow you to evidence impact, recognise steps to improvement and to be able to negotiate with stakeholders on driving forward change.

The Royal College of Nursing (2018) Demonstrating Economic Value Programme gives an opportunity for nurses to consider the skills needed to apply economic principles to their practice. McMahon and Hoong Sin (2013) describe how the purpose of an economic assessment is to influence decision makers. Understanding who the decision makers are and how to influence directly or indirectly is one aspect of this. You may also need to think about how to further develop those relationships, where the gaps are in your partnerships and how you might need to target specific groups? Being clear about the outcomes you hope to achieve (short, medium and long term), how they will be measured as well as who will benefit from the outcomes is essential. In being clear about the intended outcomes you can consider the actions you will need to take to achieve them. There will be people within your organisation who are skilled in developing business cases, progressing change and project management. Linking into these corporate functions will be helpful for you in developing the idea and learning from others experience.

Understanding and identifying costs of care delivery means being really clear about all of the aspects which contribute directly or indirectly to how the service is delivered. Some examples of direct costs from McMahon and Hoong Sin (2013) include staff, premises, materials, training and travel. There can sometimes be arrangements in place, which are not aligned to a specific budget stream. This might not be questioned until there is a threat identified to how this can be delivered, for example, a company providing free resources ceases to trade. Indirect costs may be related to arrangements for sharing spaces, where training is provided in exchange for use of equipment, printing costs or tea and coffee! Sometimes companies might provide materials for free, or other costs may be covered by a partner organisation.

Critical reflection 10.10

Jane is a community nurse, running a health promotion group looking at bowel management and prevention of constipation. The sessions run monthly for half a day with 25 attendees, they are currently advertised via email and on posters in day services and other local authorities and health providers. The sessions are delivered in a community centre. The room is given free of charge because Jane also delivers the basic life support training for the staff yearly. Jane provides tea, coffee and biscuits; she brings the equipment with her, which she stores in her office base 15 miles away.

- Identify the components from the example that would provide a direct or indirect cost if the community centre was no longer able to allow Jane free use of the room?

Case study 10.1

In engaging with stakeholders about a new build for a Child and Adolescent Mental Health Team (CAMHS), children and young people were clear that they wanted a bright and interesting waiting room with access to things that would keep them entertained while they waited. Senior managers within the consultation period were insistent that there should be no waiting room, as no child should have to wait; the service needed to be more efficient and work in a timely way to meet needs. There had to be a solution to this that addressed the concerns of the senior managers but also met the needs of the children and young people. A rigid view that '*no one should wait*' didn't help and seemed naïve to the clinicians involved, who could identify many unforeseen circumstances where appointments could be delayed or run over. Before the service could take forward any further development, discussions to consider the underlying issues and complexity of the clinician and service user experience had to take place.

A key role of the learning disability nurse is promoting and increasing independence. Supporting an individual to self-manage and meet their own needs is motivating for them, increases their confidence and builds skills. It also can mean less need for direct support for some individuals. Adopting strategies that have been effective in other parts of the service might be effective if reasonable adjustments and context-specific adaptations are made.

The Welsh Government has introduced Patient Initiated Follow Up (PIFU) as an alternative to offering traditional follow-up appointments. This is part of 'Transforming the way we deliver outpatients in Wales: A strategy and action plan 2020 to 2023' (Welsh Government, 2020a). The proposal means people being 'Seen on Symptoms' rather than routinely being invited to outpatients for reviews. There were a number of drivers leading to this change, such as clinical experience, service user feedback, recognising changing population need and stagnant models. In order to take this forward for a learning disability population there are a number of things to think about.

> *Critical reflection 10.11*
>
> - Do you think the PIFU approach might be appropriate in increasing independence and empowering people with learning disabilities?
>
> - What might the barriers be to adopting the PIFU model in a specialist learning disability service? Think about health literacy, communication factors and health inequalities.

People with learning disabilities may not have the ability to recognise when their needs have changed and that they need to make contact with a team supporting them, they may be reliant on others to help them recognise these needs, it is important that a service led decision to introduce an innovation such as PIFU considers the challenge of implementation. There could be risk of disengagement, missed deterioration, reduced health and well-being and it is essential that only those with the assessed skills and capacity to recognise a changing need are put forward to be supported on a PIFU pathway.

PATHWAY DEVELOPMENT

Pathways in our clinical practice can be helpful for a number of reasons:

- to improve adherence to guidelines;
- to reduce variations in practice;
- to allow for measurement and comparisons;
- to improve outcomes and overall quality of care;
- to reduce costs.

Pathways can help people with specific conditions, needs or diagnosis understand the transitions they will go through during a clinical experience. Pathways also give clarity on steps needed to achieve a desired outcome. Clinical pathways have been around for some time but continue to evolve and develop in order to meet needs and maintain best practice against the evidence base. A pathway is best described as an identified order of clinical interventions, written and agreed by a group of stakeholders with clear and appropriate timescales to guide process. There may be a clinical document that holds information that is more complex, to empower the person and their family to understand the choices available to them in their care journey it is most helpful if the pathway is presented in a visual way.

When developing pathways there are can be challenges of bringing people from lots of different backgrounds and experiences together. There may be professionals or family members with unrealistic requests or expectations, with standards of practice that do not match service user experience or service standards.

Some of the things that need to be in place to develop and implement a successful pathway are:

o   a committed organisation;

o   pathways included in quality improvement programme;

o   strong senior, leadership and medical commitment;

o   development is inclusive across professional groups;

o   service users are involved in development and review;

o   based on best evidence and includes outcomes;

o   variation analysis is undertaken and used to make changes;

o   ongoing support – education, training, reflective practice;

o   all staff involved complete the pathway.

The King's Fund (Naylor et al, 2016) identifies elements needed to take forward the development of pathway-based approaches to care. Table 10.3 considers some of these. The values described fit with the expectations of learning disability nurses throughout their professional practice.

Table 10.3 Skills and resources to take forward pathway work (adapted from Naylor et al, 2016, p 13)

Professional attributes	System attributes	Role of service users/ carers
• Taking the 'whole person' perspectives • Communication and consultation skills • Negotiation and collaboration • Leadership	• Co-ordination of care • Proactive care • Values-based approaches	• Peer support and self-management • Support for family and carers to participate • Collaborative decision-making • Seen as partners

The 'five whys' is a popular approach of understanding challenges, through repetitive interrogation of information to explore the cause-and-effect relationships underlying a particular problem. The approach can be used in advance of change or during the change process. The five whys might be used to unpick issues or to narrow the focus of a project. If you decide to adopt this approach it is imperative that you create a safe space, agree ground rules and encourage openness and honesty within the process. Asking and repeating the question 'Why?' can help to determine the root cause of a problem or issue in practice. Each answer the respondents provide will help you to formulate the basis of the next why? The five in the name relates to anecdotal evidence about the number of repetitions needed to resolve the problem. The five whys do not only uncover immediate issues related to care delivery, but use of the questioning can also help to understand issues at a macro and micro level, for example, due to organisational or team processes.

DRIVERS FOR CHANGE

Drivers are the pressures that lead to the need for change; these might be felt internally or externally. Understanding drivers and unintended consequences helps you to think about the implications for you and your service delivery.

The PESTLE (Table 10.4 adapted from Aguilar, 1967) is one tool that can help you work through the external drivers which will impact on how successful a change will be. Bush (2019) explored the future of the NHS through the use of the PESTLE, considering factors such as Brexit, austerity measures, the ageing population, access to technology and other factors which were considered to be threats or enablers in healthcare delivery.

Table 10.4 The PESTLE

The PESTLE	Areas to think about as you work through an idea for change
Political	The position of the government, the impact of foreign policy, political relationships and status. Taxation priorities, the plans for investment in health and social care.
Economical	This can relate to how able the organisation is to compete for a skilled and capable workforce, the wages and opportunities that the service provides. This will also relate to the economic pressures on the service in terms of delivering safe and effective care. Consider costs and income to the service you work in.
Social	Expectations of responsive and person-centred practices. The use of social media and increased public awareness and expectations. The impact of Covid-19 on mental health and well-being. Societal inequalities and impact on health.
Technological	Increasing move to online appointments, challenges for people with learning disabilities, access, skills, resources. Networks not always linked up, systems between health and social care may not be synced.
Legal	Court of Protection, Mental Health and Mental Capacity Acts. duty of care, duty of candour, risk of litigation, human rights framework, the Equality Act.
Environmental	Expectations on organisation's to be environmentally responsible, challenges for the NHS to manage recycling, single-use equipment and infection prevention control standards.

Think back to the CAMHS waiting room example. How do you think Covid-19 would impact on those discussions?

The NHS Confederation (2020) draws together a number of innovations through Covid-19 and highlights the factors that contribute to their success. One of the key phrases used during the consultation on innovation was the concept of *building the plane as we flew*', this reflects the way that innovations were rapidly developed, in real time, in service delivery and care and treatment of patients. This is representative of the first step of Kotter's (2014) change model, focusing on ensuring others appreciate the urgency of the need for change. The use of digital technology grew rapidly in 2020, and innovations that had been difficult to embed prior to the pandemic had more successful uptake.

Prior to Covid-19, you may have attended meetings where delegates attempted to remotely dial in. Often this presented challenges, the connection, the equipment, the failure of others to remember to include the remote participants, being able to indicate that there was a contribution to make etc. A key driver for changing this, making sure everyone could be included and that technology met the demands, was in March 2020 and the fact that we had to stay home, travelling was against rules and footfall had to be reduced. Now, many of us would not contemplate making the long journeys that we did previously for face-to-face contact. For people with learning disabilities and their families, however, a range of issues need to be considered related to use of technology and resources. This is highlighted by the NHS Confederation (2020) suggesting that it is important to recognise the challenge for some disadvantaged groups regarding digital literacy, when promoting online services. While online and video consultations might work very well for some individuals, for others they are completely inappropriate.

> ## *Critical reflection 10.12*
>
> - Take a moment to reflect on why use of technology might be difficult for some people with learning disabilities and their families. Write down your thoughts.

The All Wales delivering healthcare to people with learning disabilities padlet (Gwellent Cymru/Improvement Cymru (nd) draws together a range of materials aimed at increasing the uptake of the AHC. The identified problem recognised poor uptake of the AHC in Wales. One solution to addressing this was a co-produced development of an educational resource, aimed at health professionals, GP practices and people with learning disabilities. This freely accessible resource draws together key themes in bilingual presentations with structured lesson plans. This is a freely accessible resource, there is a feedback mechanism which allows for the resources to be reviewed. The delivery of the pack relies on joint working, the practice needs to identify their learning needs and link to the local community learning disability team who will organise a session to deliver the learning. Typically, this is difficult due to the volume of demands on primary care and during Covid the use of technology has been a lever in delivering the pack.

USING A MODEL FOR CHANGE

There are many models of change and selecting a model will depend on a variety of factors. This may be influenced by your knowledge and experience, whether there is a preferred approach in your organisation and the nature of the proposed innovation. It is important to think about the change you want to make before choosing a model.

Lewin's change theory

Lewin's (1951) theory is one of the earliest frameworks developed and describes three stages: 'unfreezing, movement and refreezing'. This reflects recognising and understanding a need for change, implementing a different way of doing things and embedding the change as 'normal practice'. Lewin's change theory is widely used in planning change and recognised factors which can drive or resist change, this is often useful as there are frameworks which help unpick this detail.

The RAPSIES model

The RAPSIES change model (Goppe and Galloway, 2017) has seven steps, incorporating all aspects of change (see Table 10.5). It recognises that, due to the complexities involved – the environment, the participants as well as the role of the change agent – change processes do not follow a linear route.

Table 10.5 The RAPSIES Framework

The model			Practical implementation
Step 1	R	Recognition	Is change needed, why?
Step 2	A	Analysis	Where does change need to take place and who will be involved in making change happen?
Step 3	P	Preparation	Identify the change agent. What resources are needed? Education needs, etc what are the predicted outcomes?
Step 4	S	Strategies	Clarity on how the change will be brought about.
Step 5	I	Implement	The change is made
Step 6	E	Evaluate	Feedback is gathered from those involved, how do they find the change, are intended outcomes being met?
Step 7	S	Sustain	How do you ensure that the innovation is embedded in practice and change has taken place?

PDSA cycles

One widely used model in the NHS is the Plan, Do, Study, Act (PDSA) cycle (NHS Improvement, 2018) (see Table 10.6). This model starts by acknowledging the need for change and subsequently planning for it (Drake, 2020). An initial PDSA is completed and then this becomes the first step in an ongoing process. Additional cycles are then carried out introducing small tests of change. Using small tests to change and learning from ideas that do and do not work can mean that there is learning in action and opportunities to adapt throughout

There are three questions which guide the use of the model.

1. What are you trying to accomplish?

2. How will you know that the change made is an improvement?

3. What change can be made that will result in improvement?

Table 10.6 Plan, Do, Study, Act

Plan	Do	Study	Act
Develop a plan for the test and data collection	**Carry out the test (on a small scale)**	**Learn from the test**	**Carry out the next cycle**
State the aim – what question do you want to answer. Be clear on what you expect to happen. Develop a plan: What do you need to do? How will you do that? When and where will the plan be carried out? What data will you collect?	Take the action and put the plans in place. Collect data. Record the processes, note the unexpected problems and findings. Start to analyse the information.	Work with your team to analyse the results and compare them to your predictions. Reflect together on: What happened? What went well? What didn't go so well? How do you and the team feel? Summarise the learning from the reflections.	Draw on your learning from the last test. Are there adaptions you will make? Will you adopt the change at a larger scale? Do you need to abandon this change idea? Make a plan for the next PDSA.

Putting this into practice: people with learning disabilities who may be vulnerable do not always have opportunities to learn about safeguarding and could be vulnerable if they do not know they have a right to express their experiences. People should be given opportunity to learn and know how to raise their concerns.

Aim: to work with a small group of people with learning disabilities in understanding concepts of safeguarding using accessible information

Questions and predictions:

Will there be potential side effects? There will need to be care taken to empower people but also make sure understanding is assessed and that people and those supporting understand the consequences of new knowledge.

Is this a valuable use of time? The work can be empowering for service users and increase skills, awareness of safety and improve quality of managing safeguarding issues.

Might people be triggered or traumatised from the experience of exploring the issues? Care will need to be taken to ensure that people are supported and if there is distress or disclosures suitably trained individuals involved in the project will offer direct support. Following each teaching session a debrief, using mindfulness-based approaches will be undertaken.

→

Plan	Do	Study	Act
Areas will be approached where there have been recent safeguarding referrals. Teams from those areas will be asked to volunteer for the pilot The accessible safeguarding video will be used over a six-week period (developed by people with learning disabilities in a self-advocacy group). Information will be gathered on the value of the videos and impact on individual's presentation.	Data will be collected on how people engage with the videos. An accessible questionnaire will be used to gather information at the end of each session. Mood and presentation of the individuals will be monitored during the week.	Will there be potential side effects? People have been thoughtful after the sessions, asking questions about content there have been no disclosures or allegations made. Is this a valuable use of time? Staff have reflected that this feels worthwhile and rewarding. Might people be triggered or traumatised from the experience of exploring the issues? The mood monitoring and support sessions give people the opportunity to reflect in the moment on the experiences.	An adaptation will be made. Each video will be summarised and described in an accessible worksheet so that the service users have a summary to work through while watching. This will then be used to understand the learning from the videos.

EVALUATING THE IMPACT OF INNOVATION

Sometimes the change will not go to plan or will take much longer than expected and that might be ok, you may learn things that you hadn't expected to. This should be built into the findings and reporting on change process.

It is important when attempting change that evaluation is built in, this is essential to be able to learn, spread and maximise impact. There should be discussion at the beginning of a project on how it will be evaluated. This will be based on what you and the stakeholders want to learn. For example, does a colour-coded medicines chart reduce drug errors? If evaluation is not done well it can damage the credibility of an innovation and limit the effectiveness of the approach and measurement of the outcomes.

Sometimes evaluation is done continuously, throughout a process, this means if something is not working, it can be adapted in real time. Often there is before intervention data collection and post-intervention data collection, The Health Foundation (2015b) cautions that these kinds of evaluations can give misleading results; they may not take into account other unaccounted for change. Before and after studies are also limited in that the results cannot be generalised outside of the context of the study.

Why do we evaluate?

The main reason that we use evaluation is that it can help us in the development of a deep understanding of the best way to make improvements (The Health Foundation, 2015b). In evaluation we make comparisons on the way things have been done and can be done. The use of evaluation can help us understand how and why something has been effective (or not). We may also have to use an evaluation in order to attract or maintain a level of funding. When a new service or team is designed to address a need, there may be a short-term period of funding to support the initial start-up and then evidence is gathered to decide whether to make this part of a substantive approach. Are the resources, finances, time and outcomes justified? An evaluation helps us to understand this: for example, evaluation of how the introduction of an intensive support affected emergency admissions to an assessment and treatment unit.

Evaluations can also help others. Maybe by giving others an opportunity to be heard; service users, families and staff can give their perspectives on an experience. If something works well on a small scale and in a specific area, a good evaluation will consider a range of questions that help others in similar situations identify whether this is an innovation, they can adopt. There are lots of factors which might indicate no, because context, culture and local issues might not be right at the time for the innovation to take place. This might be related to the way that the idea is introduced, developed and cascaded within a new environment. Also, it may be that the change was invested in the original setting, because something needed to be done to achieve a better outcome. Attempting to pick up that idea and embed it in a new setting where there is not an investment in the improvement might mean this is not successful.

How is evaluation different from other measures?

There are many ways of evaluating. The method will depend on the type of intervention being evaluated. There are not set standards or guidelines which are predetermined, as with audits. Evaluations can be creative and should be designed specifically for the innovation. It needs to be clearly aligned to the initial question and will bring in different measurement tools dependent on the parameters of the intervention being evaluated. It may include a variety of methods and can draw on existing data that is collected within other processes, for example, audit, this can be a good way of ensuring that those involved in the improvement do not feel challenged to produce more data. You may need to encourage or negotiate on participation in your improvement because your colleagues or peers may perceive that being involved may be burdensome on their time etc. If participants think that there are minimal asks in terms of data collection then they may be more willing to support. Mansel and Einon (2019) capture this when a level of frustration is expressed by clinicians on the demands of completing audits, data collection and reports.

STAKEHOLDERS

One of the main things that you need to take into account when managing a change process is your stakeholders. There may be some challenges and difficult conversations. Ideally you would like these things to take place within a culture of learning and understanding and you will need to lead this. Discussing strategies for making change within the clinical environment can be helpful, because you are able to create a vision and consider practical implications in the moment. It may not always be possible, sometimes change needs to happen because lessons have been learned and things have gone wrong. That may mean there is defensiveness, perception of blame and 'being changed'. There might be colleagues who feel they are doing 'the best they can, with what they've got'. It may feel like a very personal challenge to a professional if they perceive that there is a challenge to how they do what they do. Being clear about expectations, making agreements together and involving people as much as possible is important in minimising the impact of this.

Education and persuasion might be necessary to drive forward the change. Giving people time and space to understand the rationale, learn about the tactics and practice using tools can be helpful. Hearing from others who have learned through the process of change might be helpful, inviting guest speakers to the area, providing workshops, online resources or question and answer sessions can be built into the project. You might want some of these things to be very structured and others more fluid, dependent on the dynamics of the team or group and the pace at which the change process is taking place. Some people may want to discuss issues one to one and having designated space for this can be helpful, offering those opportunities to hear concerns, reflect back and agree on participation will be important.

Sustaining change

Sustaining change is a recognised challenge, Silver et al (2016) describe the effort needed to continue with improvement work after the initial momentum has been garnered, or the project outcomes have been achieved. The importance of selecting tools that will support sustained improvement needs to be considered at the outset. You will need to build consideration of these into the project planning and the implementation stages, they will be refined as the project progresses. The use of visual tools, such as a performance dashboard, a process control visual display or other real-time tracking measures can help in keeping the improvement on team's agendas. Introducing standard work which supports clinicians to follow specific steps, recognising their responsibility to completing tasks and where others are responsible in the process can support sustainment. The use of these tools embedded in culture will improve quality, experience and sustain momentum for change.

At a time when there is acknowledgement of the challenges in recruitment to learning disability nursing and retention in healthcare as a whole, it is essential that we do not lose the enthusiasm for creativity within the profession. The pre-registration nursing programme build on service improvement and innovation throughout the three years, planning the seed for professional practice and creating opportunities to embrace innovation and research. Valuing the contribution of learning disability nurses to service development may sometimes mean undertaking less traditional elements of quality improvement and formalising more innovative approaches. You will need to develop your confidence and competence to plan, implement, measure and sustain change (see Table 10.7).

Table 10.7 Steps to building your confidence in innovation

- Ask questions about the problems you see in practice.
- Listen to the feedback you hear from service users, families and colleagues.
- Share your ideas with colleagues.
- Find out where you can connect with people. What forums are there for sharing ideas, working together, accessing supervision and support?
- Contact your organisation's library; often a summary of relevant research and articles are circulated on a regular basis.
- Stay in contact with your HEI, there will be many opportunities to support future learning for student nurses and you can become involved in research and development, curriculum design, sharing good practice and simulation based-education.
- Use social media: Twitter chats are one way that communities can be brought together to explore areas of interest – @theQCommunity and @WeNurses are two Twitter groups where members share ideas and support innovative practice
- Share information. When you participate in a learning activity think about how you will disseminate what you learn. Virtual ways of working make this much easier. A webinar, a Teams talk, a Q&A session can be easily arranged and fit into a short 'lunch and learn' slot.
- Join a community of practice.

Chapter summary

Making change happen will stretch your skills and competence, it can be challenging and rewarding. Throughout your professional practice it is important that you embrace these challenges and see them as opportunities for learning and development and improving the experience of people who use services. Knowing who the key leaders are in and outside of your organisation is important for you as you hone your skills in professional practice and change management. There are recognised challenges in sustaining change and it is essential that you think about how you can motivate others at all stages, communication is key and relationships are essential. This chapter has provided opportunities for taking time to reflect and recognise the skills and behaviours that facilitate change, from a personal and relational perspective. You will not make change alone, support others who will implement change and ensure there is psychological safety within the process.

FURTHER READING

Gregory, S, Headrick, L A, Barton, A J, Dolansky, M A and Madigosky, W S (2018) *Fundamentals of Health Care Improvement: A Guide to Improving Your Patients' Care,* 3rd edition. Oak Brook, IL: Joint Commission Resources.

NHS Improvement (2018) The Learning Disability Improvement Standards for NHS Trusts. [online] Available at: www.england.nhs.uk/wp-content/uploads/2020/08/v1.17_Improvement_Standards_added_note.pdf (accessed 3 April 2022).

RESOURCES

Fabstuff: A Social Movement for Sharing Health & Social Care Ideas, Services and Solutions That Work: https://fabnhsstuff.net/ (accessed 9 June 2022).

Fabstuff is a website that hosts innovative ideas from practice; clinicians and teams can upload their improvement ideas and projects.

Gwellent Cymru/Improvement Cymru (nd) Darparu Gofal Iechyd i Bobl ag Anableddau Dysgu/ Delivering Healthcare to People with Learning Disabilities: https://padlet.com/Improve mentCymru/DeliveringHealthcareLD (accessed 9 June 2022).

The delivering health care to people with learning disabilities padlet brings together a range of resources and lesson plans to support clinicians in primary care to develop knowledge and understanding of the needs of people with learning disabilities.

11 Leadership

Chapter aims

This chapter introduces you to some key approaches to leadership, some of the challenges you may encounter when undertaking a leadership role, and the importance of organisational culture. You are encouraged to reflect on your own development as a leader. Throughout, specific reference is made to your role as a learning disability nurse and importance of effective leadership in ensuring person-centred, appropriate, timely, safe and quality support for people with learning disabilities and their families.

Professional standards and expectations

The NMC Standards (NMC, 2018a) state that nurses provide leadership in the delivery of care across a range of settings and in an interdisciplinary context. Indeed, an entire platform (Platform 5) within the Standards document is focused on *'Leading and managing nursing care and working in teams'*. Within this a range of related competencies are identified, including the following.

- *5.1 understand the principles of effective leadership, management, group and organisational dynamics and culture and apply these to team working and decision-making*

- *5.5 safely and effectively lead and manage the nursing care of a group of people, demonstrating appropriate prioritisation, delegation and assignment of care responsibilities to others involved in providing care*

- *5.6 exhibit leadership potential by demonstrating an ability to guide, support and motivate individuals and interact confidently with other members of the care team*

- *5.12 understand the mechanisms that can be used to influence organisational change and public policy, demonstrating the development of political awareness and skills.*

WHY IS LEADERSHIP IMPORTANT?

Critical reflection 11.1

- Before reading further, note down what you think leadership is and why you think it is important. You may want to return to these notes at the end of the chapter and to reflect on whether your thinking has changed in any way.

The importance of leadership is often highlighted when there are failures in care with a lack of leadership being noted in the reports of inquiries into such failures. For example, when looking back on 50 years of NHS inquiries Powell (2019) notes that, while these focus on different types of care settings and issues, there are several recurring themes of which one is how a lack of leadership contributed to the failures. This view had also previously been expressed by the King's Fund (2011) who stated that the inquiries highlighted '*painfully and acutely*' what happens when there are failures in leadership and management.

Perhaps one of the most widely known of these inquiries was that which took place into standards of care in the Mid Staffordshire NHS Foundation Trust between 2005 and 2009 (Francis, 2010). This highlighted numerous problems including poor patient care and patient experience, poor management of key issues and poor governance, and a negative culture within the organisation. This culture was found to encompass poor staff attitudes, low staff morale, bullying, acceptance of poor standards, denial and disengagement from management. All these areas suggest a lack of effective leadership and the link between leadership and organisational culture will be returned to several times in this chapter. Perhaps, therefore, it is unsurprising that Sir Robert Francis concluded that addressing this negative culture (which is essential if standards of care are to be improved) would take '*determined and inspirational leadership over a sustained period of time from within the Trust*' (Francis, 2010, Sect 136).

It would be a mistake, however, to conclude that such failures of care and leadership do not occur in settings that support people with learning disabilities. Indeed, as detailed in Chapter 1 the Ely Hospital Enquiry in 1969 exposed an abusive and closed culture of care in a long-stay hospital for people with learning disabilities. From this followed numerous similar inquiries which hastened calls to close long-stay institutions and to move to more community-based provision of care and support. However, despite changing models of care failures and abusive cultures continue to be exposed, and the past decade has seen televised exposes of such care in both Winterbourne View and Whorlton Hall (Willis, 2020). Having reviewed reports relating to Ely Hospital, Winterbourne and Whorlton Hall, Willis (2020) concludes that a common theme running through them is a lack of leadership leading to failures in care. She further argues that where clinical and managerial leadership are lacking then this can lead to a sense of disempowerment among both staff and those they support.

Such inquiries into standards of care are not confined to the UK. In Ireland, a televised expose of care in a unit caring for people with severe and profound learning disabilities led to an enquiry (Aras Attracta Swinford Review Group, 2016). Abusive care, negative staff attitudes and a poor quality of life for residents were highlighted. Change at both service and national levels was called for to promote a social model of care that would safeguard human rights. A lack of leadership was identified as a key contributory factor and the need to strengthen leadership within the service and the need for leadership development programmes at a national level were recommended.

Jukes and Apsinall (2015) argue, therefore, that the current emphasis on leadership in learning disability settings is, in part, a response to these failures in care. If poor leadership is a key factor in poor and abusive care then good leadership is required to effect positive change (Northway, 2019). Indeed, research has shown that practice leadership is a key factor in promoting a positive quality of life for people with learning disabilities living in group homes (Deveau and McGill, 2019; Humphreys et al, 2020).

UNDERSTANDING LEADERSHIP

As Northouse (2019) observes there are many ways to complete the sentence '*Leadership is …*' Indeed, much has been written about this topic both generally and in the context of healthcare and nursing. However, despite the high levels of interest in understanding leadership it is said to remain an '*elusive concept*' about which different commentators offer a range of perspectives (Barr and Dowding, 2016). This section will therefore explore the nature of leadership, some of the leadership theories and approaches that have been proposed, and the relationship between leadership and organisational culture. It will then discuss alternative leadership approaches that are currently being promoted.

The nature of leadership

There are many different definitions of leadership. Indeed, Gopee and Galloway (2017, p 66) suggest that the noun 'leadership' has four possible meanings.

1   *The activity of leading.*
2   *The body of people who lead a group.*
3   *The status of the leader.*
4   *The ability to lead.*

It can thus be viewed in terms of which activities it involves, those who are viewed as occupying positions of leadership and the possible status this confers, and the extent to which those who lead have the necessary knowledge, skills and personal attributes.

Northouse (2019) defines leadership as '*a process whereby any individual influences a group of individuals to achieve a common goal*' while Gopee and Galloway (2017) suggest it is '*a dynamic two-way process based on a leader-follower relationship*'. They further add that leaders need to be visionary, to show others the way forward while anticipating developments and innovating, seeing both the bigger picture and being focused on developing individuals. Despite leadership being conceptualised in differing ways there are key elements that are viewed as central, namely that it is a process, that it involves influence, that it occurs in groups and that it involves common goals (Northouse, 2019). It is, therefore, concerned with working with others to identify and work in a co-ordinated manner towards agreed aims and goals.

Referring to the previous section of this chapter concerning failures in care it can thus be seen that a lack of leadership may lead to a range of issues such as unclear or conflicting goals, a failure to influence others such that they work together in an effective manner and a failure to monitor what is happening (or not happening). Where this occurs in the context of healthcare it can be seen how such issues give rise to poor and abusive care.

One area that gives rise to much discussion and debate is the relationship between leadership and management. Crombie and Garland (2017) argue that while there are differences between the two concepts, they are related rather than being totally separate entities. They suggest that management is focused on ensuring that processes are followed to get things done and the responsibility for this usually lies with key individuals with positions of authority within an organisation. For example, a community nursing team manager or a unit manager within an assessment and treatment unit will be identified as a manager with responsibilities for their area of service provision. As Ellis (2022) observes managers are usually identified by their position and job title. Their role descriptions will often include specific managerial elements such as line management responsibility for others, budgetary responsibility and accountability for health and safety.

Demonstrating leadership skills, however, is an important element of management, and Ellis (2022) argues that nurse leaders in clinical settings need to demonstrate both management and leadership. Consider a nurse manager working within an assessment and treatment unit – while you would expect them to run an effective and efficient service that is well managed it is also evident that to do this, they need to be able to motivate their staff team, promote core values through role modelling and encourage and support the development of their team. In other words, they need to be both a manager and a leader.

However, it is possible that leadership can be demonstrated by people who are not in specific managerial roles. For example, it may be that one person within a team may have developed a specific area of expertise and take a lead in developing a key area of service provision. This could include a situation where one nurse in a community learning disability team has a particular interest in dementia, has undertaken study in this area and therefore both supports other (sometimes more senior) staff when they are providing support for a service user with dementia and co-ordinates training concerning dementia for families and paid carers. It may even be that, as a student nurse, you take a lead on planning care for an individual you support or take the lead on providing a training session for colleagues concerning a topic you have recently researched for an assignment. Similarly, families may play an essential role in leading the co-ordination of care for their family member and people with learning disabilities themselves may take a lead in (for example) delivering education to healthcare professionals.

It has also been suggested that since leadership does not occur in a vacuum understanding the context within which it operates is essential (Thomas-Gregory, 2017).

Ellis (2022) notes that nursing takes place within the context of a range of policies, procedures and guidelines that determine what we do. For learning disability nurses this will include professional policies, national strategic policies focused on the needs of people with learning disabilities and wider healthcare policies. Nurse leaders need to be aware of such directives, act on them and support their teams to do likewise. They also need to be able to influence the development of such policies, an issue that will be returned to in Chapter 12 when political awareness is discussed.

Critical reflection 11.2

Think about the context within which learning disability nursing operates.

- Which key policies and legislation impact on the development of services and provide future direction?

- What are the key aims and goals stated in these documents?

Here you will need to consider not only learning disability-specific policies but also wider policies that shape health and social care. You will also need to consider the country within which you are working since health and social care are the responsibility of the devolved administrations within the UK.

However, these policies, procedures and guidelines are only one element of the context of learning disability nursing. Ellis (2022) argues that values also need to be understood since these provide guidance as to how we should operate. The values that underpin learning disability nursing were explored in Chapter 2 and you might wish to revisit them in terms of their implications for leadership.

A further important element of context that needs to be considered in relation to leadership is the concept of power. If leaders are to influence others and effect change then they need to understand how power operates within their organisation and between organisations. This includes developing an understanding of types of power, where power is located and how this can be influenced. For example, if a community learning disability nursing team leader wants to secure an additional nursing post to ensure they can meet increasing service user need they will need to understand who has the power to make such a decision, what resources will be required, what information they will need to provide to make the case for such resources and the best way to communicate this information. The importance of understanding power and developing political awareness will be explored further in Chapter 12 in relation to learning disability nursing.

Theories of leadership

A range of different theories of and approaches to leadership have been proposed, and these have been categorised in different ways by different authors. For this chapter the typology proposed by Gopee and Galloway (2017) will be used to structure the discussion. They place leadership theories into the following four groups:

1. trait theories;

2. functional theories;

3. behavioural and style theories;

4. contemporary theories.

The first three of these groups are discussed here while the fourth is discussed in the section on alternative leadership approaches.

Critical reflection 11.3

Think about leaders you know and admire – they can be people you have encountered in a work context or in another setting.

- What personal qualities do they possess that you feel make them good leaders?

- Are there any common personal characteristics among the people you identify?

If asked to think of leaders they admire, and the personal characteristics they possess, people often identify characteristics such as integrity, honesty, enthusiasm, initiative. This is the basis for what is referred to as traits theories of leadership, which focus on the personal qualities individuals possess which are said to make them 'great' leaders. Reviewing the research in relation to leadership Northouse (2019) identifies the following major leadership traits – intelligence, self-confidence, determination, integrity and sociability.

This approach has attracted some criticisms such as traits being difficult to accurately define, not all successful leaders possess all traits, possessing few traits does not mean an individual is a poor leader, and it is unlikely to be possible for an individual to possess all the traits identified in the range of research (Gopee and Galloway, 2017). In addition, it is viewed as providing a poor basis for leadership development (since it tends to see leaders as 'born' rather than being 'created') and for failing to take account of the outcomes of leadership (Northouse, 2019). Nonetheless, we can all probably identify certain traits that we believe are essential to effective leadership and Thomas-Gregory (2017) argues that when leadership is discussed in the context of nursing, and great nursing leaders are considered, then description often centres on the traits possessed by such leaders. It thus said to be '*intuitively appealing*' since it reflects a commonly held view that leaders are special and gifted, and people often feel the need to see leaders in this way (Northouse, 2019).

Functional theories, as the name suggests, focus on the functions of leaders rather than on the traits they possess (Gopee and Galloway, 2017). This group of theories is also sometimes referred to as situational leadership and, drawing on the work of Adair (2010), Ellis (2022) argues that the leader needs to attend to three elements of their role – the task, the individual and the team. Their key functions are to define the task, plan how the task will be achieved, briefing the team and controlling the processes (Ellis, 2022). So, for example, as a learning disability nurse leader you might be responsible for defining a change that is needed in practice, planning how and when the change can be achieved, ensuring that your colleagues working with you understand the need for the change and how it will be achieved and making sure that you monitor and support the change.

Underpinning the functional or situational approach is the view that different situations require different leadership approaches and that a key function of the leader is to determine what is required by matching their leadership style to both the strengths and needs of their team and the task at hand (Northouse, 2019). So, for example, a very inexperienced team working on a new and complex project are likely to require different things of their leader to an experienced and established team that are working on a project similar to those they have worked on many times before. However, even where there is a very experienced team there may be a new member who requires more support from the team leader than other team members.

This approach is viewed as having several strengths such as its practicality, that it emphasises flexibility, and that it encourages an approach to team members that recognises their different needs (Northouse, 2019). However, it is also viewed as having limitations such as its limited evidence base, ambiguity in relation to the development needs of team members and for failing to account for demographic characteristics (eg age, gender experience) that impact on the relationship between the leader and their team (Northouse, 2019).

Behavioural and style approaches to leadership focus on what leaders do and how they act (Northouse, 2019). They focus on the day-to-day behaviour of leaders which is developed through education and life experiences to a form, a pattern or 'style' (Gopee and Galloway, 2017). There are some traditional leadership styles which include authoritarian or autocratic (the leader makes decisions and exercises power and control), democratic or participative (the leader seeks the views of all parties, encourages two-way communication and encourages collaboration), permissive or laissez-faire (the leader monitors from a distance and encourages autonomy) and bureaucratic (the leader follows rules and procedures, communication is impersonal and power is exercised by applying rules) (Gopee and Galloway, 2017).

It is likely that you will have encountered many, if not all, of these leadership styles and each may be appropriate in certain circumstances. For example, an autocratic leadership style may be appropriate in emergency situations such as a fire (Crombie and Garland, 2017). However, it may not be so appropriate when seeking to introduce a change in practice that requires all staff to understand why it is needed and how it can be achieved by working together. In this situation a more democratic or participative approach may be more effective.

The NHS Leadership Model (NHS Leadership Academy, 2013) has been developed specifically for those who work in the context of health and social care. It is an evidence-based model that reflects the values of the NHS, builds on previous research and experience and reflects what those who use the NHS are asking for from leaders.

The model comprises nine dimensions (see Figure 11.1) each of which is broken down into different behaviours where leaders can self-assess their level of competence. It is suggested that each of the nine dimensions is important to leadership but, depending on the context in which a leader works, some dimensions may take on greater importance than others (NHS Leadership Academy, 2013).

Table 11.1 The nine dimensions of leadership

Leadership dimensions
1. Inspiring shared purpose.
2. Leading with care.
3. Evaluating information.
4. Connecting our service.
5. Sharing the vision.
6. Engaging the team.
7. Holding to account.
8. Developing capability.
9. Influencing for results.

(NHS Leadership Academy, 2013)

Northouse (2019) argues that the behavioural approach to leadership differs from either the trait or situational theories in that it is not a unified or prescriptive approach. Instead, it suggests that the actions of leaders towards others are focused on both the task and relational levels and that in some situations there is a need to be more task-oriented while in others a relational approach needs to take precedence. A strength of this approach is that it encourages leaders to reflect on their actions and to determine how they may wish to change and develop (Northouse, 2019). Nonetheless, as with other approaches, it is also viewed as having limitations including that the research in relation to this approach is inconclusive and that it is not identified a universal leadership style that can be effective in all situations (Northouse, 2019). Whether a universal leadership style is achievable or even desirable might, however, be questioned given the importance of context in determining the requirements of a leader. Nonetheless, some concerns have been raised regarding what might be considered traditional leadership approaches and the need to consider alternatives has been emphasised.

The need for change

As already noted in this chapter, there are many approaches to, and theories of, leadership and each have their own strengths and weaknesses. However, it is important that leadership is appropriate to the context within which it operates, and it has been suggested that traditional leadership approaches are not well suited to the challenges that are currently facing healthcare. For example, Weberg (2012) argues that such approaches fail to address the complexity of healthcare provision for three key reasons – they focus on linear thinking, they fail to address organisational culture and they are not prepared to support innovation.

In relation to linear thinking Weberg (2012) suggests that healthcare systems have traditionally focused on management rather than leadership and have viewed the leader's role as being to maintain control and stability. However, if we take the example of services for people with learning disabilities healthcare is only one element of this system of support and, to ensure person-centred and coordinated support, health services must work with other agencies such as social services, education and third sector providers. Even within the context of healthcare there can be challenges of co-ordination between specialist learning disability services and mainstream healthcare provision as well as between primary, secondary and tertiary services. This means that maintaining control and stability may be challenging (and possibly inappropriate) since leaders may not be able to directly control key factors and need to work across organisational boundaries rather than within rigid hierarchical structures.

For example, in an assessment and treatment unit it may be that there are residents who need to be discharged to more suitable, long-term community living. However, to achieve this requires somewhere to live and an appropriate support package which, in turn, require commitment from the local authority, a housing provider and appropriate community-based services. None of these is within the direct control of the nurse manager within the unit and hence they will be required to demonstrate leadership through influencing others and working across organisational boundaries to achieve the goal of community living for those they support.

The King's Fund (2011) argues that the ability to work across boundaries, and to persuade others as to the appropriate course of action, is important within the context of contemporary healthcare. Those working in such a manner are often referred to as 'boundary spanners' and Bryson (2017) suggests that such leaders need to:

o   develop and communicate a shared vision that is based on shared values;

o   be skilled in negotiation and influencing;

o   possess emotional resilience;

o   understand how the system works;

o   possess change management skills.

As can be seen from the earlier discussion regarding more traditional leadership approaches and theories, many fail to account for all these leadership attributes and tend instead to focus on stability and control.

The focus on stability and control also means that traditional leadership approaches are poorly prepared to support innovation and yet such innovation is crucial to ensuring that services and supports change to meet changing demands and challenges. Consider, for example, how quickly many services had to adapt the way in which they provided support in the context of the Covid-19 pandemic. More broadly think about the many changes that have occurred in learning disability services over recent decades (see Chapter 1) – without innovation then such developments would not have occurred. West et al (2014) go as far as to say that where the leadership focus is on command-and-control, innovation may be lacking as there is a tendency to scapegoat individuals and a culture where failure is feared.

The second deficit that Weberg (2012) identifies in traditional leadership approaches is the failure to address the issue of organisational culture. For example, if the traits leadership approach is taken as an example it would suggest that the traits of the leader are sufficient to ensure success rather than the organisational culture within which they operate and the impact they may have on this. However, as was highlighted earlier in this chapter, where failures of care have been identified the presence of a poor organisational culture has been highlighted as a contributory factor, and effective leadership proposed as a key recommendation to effect change.

Barr and Dowding (2016) suggest it is difficult to provide an overall definition of culture because it encompasses so many different elements. However, Gopee and Galloway (2017) suggest that organisational culture *'relates to the way in which the collective group of people who belong to an organisation go about their work'* (p 127). This encompasses shared values, norms, beliefs and assumptions (Gopee and Galloway, 2017). When there is a positive culture then (in the context of healthcare) those who work within the organisation will be committed to delivering care that is person-centred, safe and effective and they are likely to demonstrate these values through their practice because they also feel they are valued and respected. However, where there is a negative culture, or a strong sub-culture that does not subscribe to such values, then this will have a negative impact on the care delivered.

For example, Gopee and Galloway (2017) highlight how the second Francis Report (2013) exposed an organisation whose culture was focused on doing the business of the 'system' rather than on patient care and recommended that there was a need to develop a shared culture which put patients first. Similarly, Willis (2020) notes how when the BBC broadcast the programme detailing abusive care of people with learning disabilities at Whorlton Hall the staff were filmed talking in front of a wall that had the words 'rights', 'respect' and 'empowerment' written across it. While there was an explicit organisational statement of these values the behaviour of staff was disrespectful of the rights of residents who were significantly disempowered. This suggests that staff were either unaware that these were the values they were meant to display in their practice or that they deliberately chose not to engage with them.

Critical reflection 11.4

Think about a setting in which you have worked where you feel that there was a positive culture.

- What was it that made you feel that it was a positive culture?
- What role did the leader play in creating and sustaining this culture?
- Could anything else have been done to further strengthen the culture?

Jukes and Aspinall (2015) argue that learning disability nurses have a key role to play in promoting a positive culture within services. Their ability to lead change, collaborate and empower others make them well placed and through setting clear boundaries, effective communication, promoting innovation and being visible, they can effect change. Tee (2017) suggests that all who work in an organisation contribute to the organisational culture but that leaders play a key role in setting expectations, modelling behaviour and promoting what is desired in terms of culture. Indeed, West (2021) argues that *'Every interaction by every leader every day shapes the culture of the organisation'* (p 64).

Leaders cannot, however, do this alone yet in the context of public services the approach to addressing organisational problems linked to culture has often been to bring in *'super-hero'* leaders who are expected to transform the organisation (King's Fund, 2011). Such an approach is, nonetheless, viewed as unsuited to the current context of healthcare delivery (King's Fund, 2011). This then gives rise to consideration of what might be more appropriate ways of supporting leadership in healthcare and to what Gopee and Galloway (2017) refer to as the 'contemporary' theories.

Alternative approaches to leadership

In response to perceived deficits in traditional leadership approaches, several alternatives have been proposed. One example, referred to as 'connective' leadership, is where the focus is on the role of the leader in fostering intra- and inter-organisational relations to achieve organisational goals (Gopee and Galloway, 2017). While this does seem to address the need for leaders to act as boundary spanners (King's Fund, 2011) it is viewed as limited as a leadership theory since other leadership approaches also stress the need for the leader to facilitate interconnections (Gopee and Galloway, 2017).

A second approach is what is referred to as distributed leadership. This is where the focus is on moving away from viewing leadership as being concentrated in the actions of a few senior individuals in an organisational structure to a system that recognises that a range of individuals at different levels within an organisation may bring knowledge, abilities and skills which enable them to take on a leadership role in a particular context or in relation to a particular issue. As Curtis (2021, p 220) observes, within a distributed leadership approach *'No individual should have a monopoly of or responsibility for leadership'* with a co-operative approach being adopted instead.

The King's Fund (2011) supports the need for more *'diffuse'* approaches to leadership as they argue that the health service needs strong leadership from *'board to ward'* – in other words at all levels within the organisation. While few learning disability nurses will be working in a ward setting, the community services they work in are often widely dispersed and hence leadership is required across the various locations in which support is provided. Adopting such an approach, however, requires more than just expecting individuals at lower levels in organisations to take on leadership roles, and needs instead to be understood in terms of both leadership practices and organisational interventions (Turnbull-James, 2011). This means that it requires new approaches to the development of leaders if organisational change is to be achieved, but also that such development needs to be rooted in the specific organisational context in which leadership is to be enacted. It is a dynamic approach that is suited to the complexity of healthcare and means that an individual may be a leader in one situation but a 'follower' in another (Turnbull-James, 2011).

Another leadership approach that has been recently promoted within the context of healthcare is what is referred to as 'compassionate leadership'. Such an approach is based on the premise that responding effectively to the current challenges in health and social care requires '*radical innovation*' and '*transformational change*' which, in turn, requires that staff are freed from bureaucracy and command-and-control. Compassionate leadership is viewed as the key element for creating a culture within which such innovation can occur (West, 2021). As with distributed leadership it requires that all staff are viewed as leaders and that they should be enabled to be the best they can be (West, 2021).

It can thus be seen that compassionate leadership has the potential to both address the issues of organisational culture discussed earlier in this chapter and promoting the innovation identified as essential by Weberg (2012). However, what does this approach mean in practice?

Compassion is said to require four key elements:

1   *Attending – paying attention to others, noticing.*

2   *Understanding – listening to achieve a shared understanding.*

3   *Empathising – responding in an empathetic manner, recognising distress but not being overwhelmed.*

4   *Helping – taking intelligent action to assist.*

(West, 2021)

In relation to leadership these elements need to be present at a variety of different levels, namely the organisation, the team and the individual. For example, at an organisational level it is important that there are mechanisms for identifying when there may be discomfort or distress (attending), ensuring that there are opportunities for views to be shared in a candid and open manner so that issues can be clarified, any response needs to recognise the impact (positive or negative) it will have on others (empathising) and there needs to be visible action (helping).

Case study 11.1

Gemma Lewis has been qualified as a learning disability nurse for eight years and, since qualifying, she has worked primarily in a community setting. Recently, however, she has moved to a new post in a different organisation and is now responsible for leading a team of community learning disability nurses. The service she has moved to is undergoing a lot of changes to respond more effectively and appropriately to the needs of those they support and one key element of this is moving from being a Monday to Friday service to one which is seven days a week.

On taking up post Gemma takes time to carefully *attend* to those she is working with – this includes the team of nurses, other professionals they work alongside and, most importantly, the people with learning disabilities they support and their families. She notices that among the nursing team there is some reluctance to change their pattern of work. She therefore takes time to listen to their concerns but also to listen to why people with learning disabilities and their families feel that they need support seven days a week. Through this she gains an *understanding* of how some individuals and families have experienced crises during weekends and have found it impossible to get support. She also gains an understanding of how, for some nurses, weekend working will be extremely difficult due to their personal circumstances and family commitments while for others there is a fear that they will be unsupported while working at weekends.

Gemma can *empathise* with all these feelings but recognises it is important that people with learning disabilities and their families have access to support. She therefore spends time speaking with her team, acknowledging their concerns but also helping them to understand why the change is necessary. She suggests that they work together to try and find a helpful way forward (*helping*). Through this discussion as a team, they can identify that some team members are happy to work weekends while others would prefer to work during the week and thus agree a rota that suits everyone. They also work out a system for ensuring that all staff feel supported and that the change in working patterns will be regularly reviewed.

The following '*Compassionate Leadership Principles for Health and Social Care in Wales*' have been identified:

- *enable safe, trusting and engaging systems and cultures;*
- *strengthen respect, voice, influence and control;*
- *create environments where collective leadership thrives;*
- *establish the conditions for our workforce to reflect, learn, continually improve and innovate;*
- *manage behaviour positively, openly, courageously and ethically;*
- *develop supportive and effective team and inter-team working.*

(Millar, 2021)

It is the stated ambition that by 2030, in Wales, '*leaders in the health and social care system will display collective and compassionate leadership*' (NHS Wales and Social Care Wales, 2021). Leadership development will, therefore, be focused on promoting the four key elements of compassionate leadership discussed above (West, 2021) to ensure effective leadership (clear vision, alignment and commitment), inclusive leadership (positively valuing difference, commitment to equality and inclusion, clear role), collective leadership (individual and shared leadership responsibility across boundaries) and systems leadership (shared vision and values, constructive and ethical conflict management and mutual support).

These more contemporary theories do appear to respond to the perceived limitations of some earlier leadership theories, but it is important to remember that, as time progresses and there is greater implementation of alternative approaches, then their limitations may also emerge. Moreover, when looking at the traditional leadership approaches, while they have limitations, they also have strengths. However, the context of health and social care is constantly changing and what is perhaps most important is that leaders understand the different approaches and utilise them to best effect – what is appropriate in one context may not be appropriate in another. The next section of the chapter will therefore consider some of the issues that need to be considered when seeking to develop leadership in the specific context of learning disability nursing.

LEADERSHIP IN LEARNING DISABILITY NURSING

Strengthening the Commitment (Scottish Government et al, 2012) stated that 'Strong leadership in learning disability nursing is essential' (p 46) if the profession is to develop and to respond to the challenges it faces in meeting current and future needs. Accordingly, it made the following recommendation:

> Leadership in learning disabilities nursing needs to be strengthened in practice, education, and research settings with robust, visible leadership at all levels, including strategic and national levels.

> (p 47)

It is important to note here that leadership was viewed as being required across settings (practice, education and research) and at a range of levels. While practice leadership is often discussed the areas of education and research are perhaps less frequently focused on. However, without strong learning disability nurse leadership within educational settings then there may be difficulties with the preparation of future learning disability nurses, with continuing education for those already registered, and in ensuring that all nurses (whatever their field of practice) develop an awareness of the health needs of people with learning disabilities and their role in addressing these. Similarly, as was highlighted in Chapter 4, there is a need for learning disability nurses to progress to positions of research leadership to ensure further development of the evidence base and to support translation of this knowledge to inform practice.

To take forward the recommendations of Strengthening the Commitment (Scottish Government et al, 2012) a UK wide steering group was established both to provide leadership for this activity and to act as role models for learning disability nurses by being 'visible, approachable and actively expanding the horizons of learning disability nursing' (Scottish Government et al, 2015). However, despite this commitment to leadership development within learning disability nursing several concerns have been expressed. For example, Gray (2015) argues that there is a need to strengthen leadership, highlighting the fact that many learning disability nurses work in services that are managed by people with little or no experience in the field. He further argues that learning disability nurses working in all settings need to be able to access professional leadership even across organisational boundaries and that this requires identifying and supporting future leaders to develop.

A reduction in leadership roles within learning disability nursing has been highlighted by the RCN (2021). A failure to address this will, they argue, negatively impact on leading rights-based cultures of care, safe and effective practice. Elsewhere it is argued that the potential for learning disability nurses to take on leadership roles is not being fully realised. For example, Savarimuthu (2020) suggests that, in relation to positive behaviour support plans, learning disability nurses are often key to implementation while other professions take the lead. However, he argues that nurses should be empowered to take on this leadership role and to lead research that advances understanding of this approach to delivering support.

There thus seems to be agreement that learning disability nurses are both well placed to take on leadership roles and that the development of this aspect of their role is key both to the development of quality support for people with learning disabilities and the profession. Indeed, Jukes and Aspinall (2015) argue that learning disability nurses should embrace the leadership challenge and become a '*palpable source of development*' in taking services forward. However, such development needs to be supported at both a personal and professional level and the next section will explore how this might be achieved.

Leadership development

In seeking to develop leadership in learning disability nursing there are several things that need to be considered and the first is how, as an individual, you might develop your own leadership skills. If you are a student nurse then taking on a leadership and management role might seem like a future aspiration (Ellis, 2022) but you will be developing as a leader even before you complete your course and become a registered nurse. This will, in part, be achieved through some of the theoretical input on your course as you learn about various aspects of leadership and management. However, there will also be opportunities when undertaking clinical placements to develop as a leader. This might, for example, be through shadowing a more senior member of staff or it could be through supporting a junior student. There might be opportunities for you to take the lead in organising an event such as a student conference or even a student society. Think back to what was said earlier in this chapter about distributed leadership, and you may see opportunities to lead in a particular area.

There can also be more formal opportunities for student nurses to develop their leadership skills. For example, the Council of Deans of Health, in partnership with the Burdett Trust, run a student leadership programme (see Resources for more details). As part of this they offer the opportunity for students to apply for places on their 150 Leaders programme which aims to motivate students to take on leadership roles. The programme comprises several elements.

- ○ The opportunity to be exposed to senior, experienced leaders.
- ○ Reflective practice.
- ○ Understanding and developing emotional intelligence.

- ○ Empowering attendees to think differently and to raise concerns regarding patient safety.

- ○ Network with likeminded people across professions and geography.

- ○ One to one mentorship with a senior leader to share experience, learn from them and to work with them to develop their own future leadership goals.

(summarised from Kolyva et al, 2018)

An evaluation of this programme identified that those attending had gone on to engage in a range of activities including engaging with professional bodies, in strategic meetings, in research, with the media and conference presentations as well as leading in practice (Kolyva et al, 2018).

Critical reflection 11.5

Think about situations in which you have taken on a leadership role. This could be as a nurse or in another capacity.

- What approach(es) did you use?

- What do you feel were your strengths?

- What areas do you need to develop further and how might you do this?

Your experience during your pre-qualifying education will provide a good basis for your future development. However, as a leader it is important that you commit to life-long learning, and this is particularly important as you transition to your new role as a registered nurse and take on a more formal leadership role. Donaldson and Sabin (2017) recognise the importance of this and suggest that there is a need to provide support and to 'scaffold' the development of leadership skills during this period. This, they argue, means that there should be structures in place for the newly registered nurse to support, nurture and critique their leadership skills. Mentorship, supervision and preceptorship all have an important role to play here (Donaldson and Sabin, 2017) and these might be provided both within the employing organisation and externally (see Chapter 12 for further discussion).

There are also some specific programmes that seek to support the leadership of newly registered learning disability nurses. For example, in 2019 The Florence Nightingale Foundation facilitated a programme for learning disability nurses working at Bands 5 and 6 to assist them in developing their leadership roles. An overview of what it was like to participate is provided by Funmi Dasaolu, a Learning Disability Liaison Nurse (a link to her post is available in the Resources section). Similarly, the Foundation of Nursing Studies offer fellowships for aspiring leaders and early career learning disability nurses in England (between six months and five years of qualifying). This programme offers mentorship and coaching as well as personal development planning to assist those attending to realise their aspirations as leaders (see Resources section for more details). The focus is on developing leaders to promote caring cultures of care which, as has been seen earlier in this chapter, is a key role of leaders.

Such programmes may not, however, be accessible to all and, whether you are able to participate in them or not, it is also important that you accept personal responsibility for your leadership development. The importance of personal development will be explored further in Chapter 12 but here is it timely to note the advice provided by Ellis (2022) who suggests there are several strategies that can be employed when seeking to develop yourself as a leader. These include setting yourself incremental goals, active listening, understanding and communication, believing in yourself and being clear about your values, developing emotional intelligence and resilience, and effective time management. He also argues that when developing as a leader it is important not to be afraid of making mistakes since if we accept responsibility and engage in reflective practice this provides useful learning from which to develop.

Critical reflection 11.6

Think about where you want to be in your career in five years' time.

- How do you need to develop your leadership knowledge and skills to achieve this?
- How will you achieve this?

As a learning disability nurse, you will be working in a range of settings and in a context that is constantly changing. You may work for different organisations and across organisational boundaries. You may be someone who moves into senior and strategic leadership positions – and it is important that learning disability nurses put themselves forward for such roles. All these factors reinforce the need to constantly review and expand your leadership skills as you progress through your career.

There is a need, however, to also consider the development of leadership at a collective as well as an individual level if learning disability nursing is to continue to progress as a profession. This requires that there is debate and discussion among learning disability nurses as to how this is best achieved, and professional organisations can play an important role in this process. For example, the RCN (2021) has committed to highlighting the impact of reductions in learning disability nursing leadership positions and to advocating for leadership and career pathways for learning disability nurses. It is essential that all learning disability nurses engage in such debates and that they encourage and support their peers to take on leadership roles.

Supporting leadership development for people with learning disabilities

As has been noted earlier in this chapter current leadership approaches tend not to view leadership as being confined to a few people holding senior management positions. This means that, in addition to leadership being more widely distributed among healthcare professionals, discussion has also focused on how those who use healthcare services can also take on leadership roles.

One of the recommendations arising from the Francis Report (2013) was that there needed to be strong leadership if change was to be realised. As part of the discussions and debates that followed from this the important role of 'patient leaders' emerged. These are individuals who are viewed as supporting the work of healthcare organisations in two key ways (King's Fund, 2013). First, they are identified as being a 'community channel' in that they are externally facing, linked with local communities, and thus bring a wider perspective to issues. They may, for example, be a representative of an external organisation such as a support group for those who live with a particular condition and through that organisation have extensive community networks that they can communicate with. Second, they are seen to have an important role internal to healthcare organisations as they can act as a 'critical friend' ensuring that the patients' perspective is central to strategic discussions and policymaking (King's Fund, 2013). They can thus constructively challenge decision-making or the absence of decision-making from the perspective of those who use health and social care services.

While, in the context of learning disability services, we would not usually refer to 'patients' it is evident that over recent years people with a learning disability have become actively involved in defining strategic priorities, shaping services and supports, and providing feedback concerning the quality of care provided. This has occurred at both an organisational level and at a national level. However, it is also important to recognise that they may have had limited opportunities to access leadership development opportunities and support (Caldwell, 2010). It is thus essential that, when seeking to promote opportunities for people with learning disabilities to take on leadership roles, support tailored to individual strengths and needs is provided. This may be through leadership development courses run by, for example, self-advocacy organisations but it could also be through individual mentorship and coaching.

As a learning disability nurse, you have an important role to play in supporting the leadership development of people with learning disabilities. This may take the form of questioning a lack of their active participation in the leadership of your organisation, creating leadership opportunities, adapting processes to support participation and providing individual support and mentorship.

Case study 11.2

A local learning disability service is currently planning how best to provide education for colleagues working in a primary care setting to enable them to understand the health inequities that people with learning disabilities often face when accessing primary care. Tom Johnson, a community learning disability nurse, has been asked to lead this project. From the beginning he decides that this is a project that should be co-led by an individual who has a learning disability since they are best placed to comment on the experience of people with a learning disability. He therefore presents a case to his line manager as to why this is important and secures some additional resources to pay an individual with a learning disability on a part time basis to take on this co-leadership role. Through a process of interview and appointment Faith Bankole is appointed. Faith is an active member of the local self-advocacy organisation and is very committed to improving healthcare for people with learning disabilities. However, she has had very limited opportunities to take on a leadership role. Tom and Faith therefore work together to identify their individual strengths and how they can best support each other. Faith agrees to help Tom better understand the barriers that she and her peers experience in accessing primary care. Tom agrees to help Faith with things like chairing meetings and making presentations. At first, he takes a leading role in these activities but through support Faith gains confidence and takes on greater responsibility as the project progresses. As the project comes to an end, they both reflect on what they have learnt and the skills they have acquired. Both agree that they have become more confident as leaders and would be looking to get involved in leading more projects in the future.

Chapter summary

This chapter has argued that effective leadership is essential to the provision of quality, person-centred, support and services, and that it is a key role of the learning disability nurse. A range of different leadership approaches and theories have been explored and their strengths and weaknesses highlighted. It must be remembered, however, that in practice it is likely that you will need to draw on a range of different approaches depending on the role you find yourself in and the specific situation. It is important, therefore, that you start to develop your leadership skills from an early stage in your nursing career and that you continue to reflect on these and learn throughout your career. This is essential if we are to promote better services, supports and quality of life for people with learning disabilities.

FURTHER READING

Ashton, J (2021) *The Nine Types of Leader: How the Leaders of Tomorrow Can Learn from the Leaders of Today.* London: Kogan Page.

This book provides you with further information regarding leadership approaches.

Curtis, E A, Beirne, M, Cullen, J G, Northway, R and Corrigan, S.M (eds) (2021) *Distributed Leadership in Nursing and Healthcare. Theory, Evidence and Development.* London: Open University Press.

This book provides you with further information regarding the nature of distributed leadership and its implementation in the context of healthcare.

Sheerin, F and Curtis, E A (eds) (2019) *Leadership in Intellectual Disability Service. Motivating Change and Improvement*. Abingdon: Routledge.

This book explores aspects of leadership specifically in the context of learning disability services.

Taylor, R and Webster-Henderson, B (eds) (2017) *The Essentials of Nursing Leadership*. London: Sage.

This book will enable you to explore the wider context of leadership in nursing.

RESOURCES

Council of Deans and Burdett Trust Student Leadership Project: www.councilofdeans.org.uk/ studentleadership/ (accessed 21 June 2022).

This website contains further information regarding the project as well as publications, blogs and podcasts.

Foundation of Nursing Studies' Learning Disability Aspiring Leaders Fellowship: www.fons. org/programmes/learning-disability-fellowship (accessed 21 June 2022).

This page gives information on the Learning Disability Aspiring Leaders Fellowship.

The King's Fund: www.kingsfund.org.uk/ (accessed 21 June 2022).

This website contains a lot of resources relating to leadership including reports, blogs and podcasts.

NHS Leadership Academy: www.leadershipacademy.nhs.uk/ (accessed 21 June 2022).

This website features details of the various leadership courses that they provide and access to bitesize learning resources.

Nurses and Midwives Talk: https://nursesandmidwivestalk.com/ (accessed 21 June 2022).

The Nurses and Midwives Talk project has interviewed 380 nurses and midwives from around the world (some of them are learning disability nurses). You can register to access the recordings many of which touch upon the subject of leadership.

Learning Disability Nurse Leadership Development Programme: https://legacy.florence-nigh tingale-foundation.org.uk/learning-disability-nurse-leadership-programme-overview-by-funmi-dasaolu/ (accessed 21 June 2022).

This is the link to access Funmi Dasaolu's overview of the programme.

12 Professional development

Chapter aims

As seen throughout this book, the needs of people with learning disabilities are constantly changing. This requires that the services and supports they receive also adapt and change to ensure that such needs are both identified and appropriately met. This, in turn, requires that as a profession, learning disability nursing needs to continue to evolve and adapt to ensure that it remains relevant to those it seeks to support. Chapter 1 explored the history and development of learning disability nursing showing how this has been achieved to date. Going forward, however, its future development is dependent upon you and other learning disability nurses continuing your professional development, whatever career stage you are at. This chapter assists you with this by exploring professional and career development and providing strategies to help you in this process. Through taking personal responsibility for such development, and through working together with others, the profession of learning disability nursing will also progress and develop.

Professional standards and expectations

The Standards of Proficiency for Registered Nurses (NMC, 2018a) state that, at the point of registration nurses, must be able to

> *1.17 take responsibility for continuous self-reflection, seeking and responding to support and feedback to develop their professional knowledge and skills*

Completing your pre-registration education is, however, the beginning of a new phase of learning and professional development as you transition from student nurse to registered nurse. The Standards (NMC, 2018a) thus state that achievement of these proficiencies provides the knowledge and skills required at the point of registration but that these then need to be built upon as registrants gain practice experience *'and fulfil their professional responsibility to continuously update their knowledge and skills'*. The NMC Code (2018b) sets out this professional responsibility by stating that as a registered nurse you must

> *22.3 keep your knowledge and skills up to date, taking part in appropriate and regular learning and professional development activities that aim to maintain and develop your competence and improve your performance*

Such CPD needs to be evidenced as part of the process of three yearly revalidation that all nurses need to engage with to maintain their registration. In addition to requiring registrants to reflect on their practice and the requirements of the Code (NMC, 2018b) revalidation also requires that 35 hours of CPD are evidenced each three-year period. This must include 20 hours of participatory activity defined as any learning that requires 'interaction with one of more professionals'. This might include activities such as attending a conference or course as well as attendance at meetings where (for example) new ways of working are explored. The elements of revalidation will be explored at various points in this chapter and there is also a link to NMC resources in the Resources section at the end of the chapter.

CAREER PATHWAYS

Forty years ago, a learning disability nurse, at the point of registration, would probably need to consider which ward in a long-stay hospital they wanted to work in upon qualification since that is where employment opportunities would have been. While some alternative career opportunities were beginning to emerge at that time, as services began to focus on the need for more community-based patterns of care and support, these were limited. In contrast, a learning disability nurse at the start of their career as a registered nurse today is likely to have a wide range of options. These still include working in residential settings but have expanded to include working in community teams, in schools, in acute hospitals, in prisons and in many more settings. Employment opportunities are also available working in different sectors such as the health service, social care, the independent sector and the third sector. This means that your career pathway has the potential to be very diverse and may lead you into roles you had not anticipated at the point of registration. However, it is helpful to be aware of potential career paths, to consider where you see your future and to plan how you might move towards your future professional goals.

Transition to registered nurse

Completing your initial nurse education, achieving your qualification and transitioning to a new role as a registered nurse is a time of both excitement and anxiety (Donaldson and Sabin, 2017). You will be taking on new responsibilities, possibly working in a new setting, and how you are perceived by both yourself and others will change. A key factor in ensuring a successful transition is the support you receive from others and hence the NMC (2020) has set out principles for preceptorship with a view to providing structured support. They state that

The preceptorship period provides the basis for the beginning of a lifelong journey of reflection, and the ability to self-identify continuing professional development needs, as the nurse, midwife and nursing associate embarks on their career and prepares for revalidation.

(NMC, 2020)

Acknowledging that arrangements for preceptorship vary across the different countries of the UK they identify five principles that can be applied across settings. These are set out in Table 12.1.

Table 12.1 The principles of preceptorship

Principle	Key features
1. Organisational culture and preceptorship	• A *'kind, fair, impartial, transparent, collaborative'* culture that fosters good interprofessional and multi-agency relationships • An understanding of the importance of systems and processes to support and build confidence among newly registered nurses • The approach to preceptorship prioritises mental and physical health and well-being and promotes working within the Code
2. Quality and oversight of preceptorship	• Processes enable all those requiring preceptorship to be identified and there is capacity to provide this support • There is understanding of the need to work within national and local policies • Preceptorship complements induction and operates within a clear governance framework • Preceptorship processes are monitored and evaluated
3. Preceptee empowerment	• Programmes are tailored to the needs of the individual and provide them with the resources required to develop confidence as a newly registered nurse • Preceptees have a nominated preceptor • Preceptees have opportunities for reflection and feedback
4. Preparing preceptors for their supporting role	• Preceptors act as role models, receive support and engage in professional development • Are supportive, constructive, share effective practice and learn from others
5. The preceptorship programme	• Should be timely and aligned to the preceptee's role • Should recognise the competence attained at the point of registration • Should be agreed with the preceptee, vary in length according to their needs/organisational requirements • Should support the preceptee to achieve identified goals within the specified timeframe

(Adapted from NMC, 2020)

As a newly registered learning disability nurse it is important you are aware of these principles and that you work with your employer to ensure that they are upheld as they will support you to develop confidence in your new role. As you progress through your career, however, you will move from preceptee to preceptor, and it will be important for you to use them to provide a framework within which you can support others.

Critical reflection 12.1

Look at the principles of preceptorship set out in Table 12.1.

- If you were responsible for ensuring that these were present for newly registered nurses in a clinical setting what actions would you take?

- What supports would you put in place?

- How would you know if the strategies and supports are effective?

Career progression

Career progression is often an area of concern for learning disability nurses particularly as they may hear from others that opportunities for progression are limited within this field of nursing. However, this could not be further from the truth with a wide range of potential roles and opportunities opening in recent years.

Traditionally career progression has involved following pathways that lead into roles focused primarily on leadership/management, education or research. This has meant that, to progress, practitioners have often felt that they needed to move away from direct clinical care. In relation to learning disability nursing this has also sometimes meant moving away from a sole focus on learning disabilities since (for example) certain management roles require the post holder to manage both learning disability and mental health services due to integrated service structures. Similarly, those seeking to progress a career in education may have had to move away from a focus on learning disability nurse education to take on broader, generic management positions.

However, recent developments have led to the development of new roles that enable practitioners to gain promotion while remaining clinically involved. For example, some learning disability nurses are working as advanced nurse practitioners. Consultant nurse positions encompass elements of leadership, clinical practice, education and research. Similarly, opportunities to take on clinical academic roles that encompass clinical practice and research are beginning to emerge.

Career progression may not, however, always be about promotion and it can mean taking the opportunity to gain experience with working with different service user groups (eg children, those whose behaviour is viewed as challenging, those with complex health needs and those who are ageing). It can also mean gaining experience of working in a range of settings (eg assessment and treatment units, community learning disability teams, special schools, acute hospitals and prisons). Over recent years the range of positions open to learning disability nurses has increased and now we see them working not only as nurses in specialist residential settings or as community learning disability nurses but also as acute care liaison nurses, school nurses, prison nurses and primary care facilitators.

It is also important to note that increasingly the relevance of the skills and knowledge that learning disability nurses bring to their roles is being recognised by other areas of, and specialisms within, health and social care. In several instances this has resulted from learning disability nurses challenging situations where posts have been advertised as being open (for example) to RN (Adult) nurses only. They have looked at the role requirements knowledge and skills sought, identified that they meet such requirements and have applied for such posts. Consequently, there are learning disability nurses holding posts in areas such as dementia care, epilepsy, stroke rehabilitation, hospice care and neurology. This is a positive development but there is the potential for this to reduce the number of learning disability nurses available to work within learning disability services. Hence, there is a need to recognise this diversification of roles in workforce planning and to ensure that additional learning disability nurses are educated and retained to guarantee appropriate numbers are available to identify and meet the needs of people with learning disabilities both now and in the future.

Critical reflection 12.2

Think about the learning disability nurses you know and the range of roles and settings that they work in. You might know these individuals personally or through other mechanisms such as social media or hearing them speak at a conference.

- How do they apply their professional knowledge and skills within their role?

Further education

When considering your career progression, it may be that (depending on your chosen path) you need to undertake further formal academic or professional qualifications. For example, your role and service requirements may mean that you need to become a nurse prescriber. Similarly, if you wish to move into an educational post you may need to undertake a recognised teaching qualification. You may decide that you want to advance your knowledge and skills through applying to undertake a master's level course. This could be in a specific clinical area such as dementia, mental health, safeguarding or advanced nursing practice. It could, however, also be a course focused on an area such as leadership and management.

Courses leading to a master's level qualification will extend your knowledge and skills in relation to research. However, if you feel that you specifically want to pursue a career in research then you might opt to undertake a postgraduate research degree. This might be a Masters in Research, an MPhil or even a PhD. It is also worth noting that there are various routes to obtaining a doctorate. There is the 'traditional' route which requires you to undertake a significant and original piece of research over a period of three to four years full-time study or four to six years part-time study. It is assessed by submission of a thesis (usually 80,000–100,000 words) and a viva. A professional doctorate combines some taught modules with a smaller research-based project. Some universities also offer what is known as a portfolio route to PhD which allows practitioners to draw upon practice-based research projects and to develop a critical overview of these projects demonstrating the original contribution to knowledge.

If considering further formal study, it is worth contacting your local university/universities to see what opportunities are available. However, it is also important to note that many institutions now offer courses that can be studied at a distance which may open different opportunities and possibilities for you.

SUPPORTING PROFESSIONAL DEVELOPMENT

Throughout your career it is a professional requirement that you continue to develop and extend your knowledge and skills. This section will therefore explore some strategies that can assist you in meeting this requirement, namely reflective practice, networking, finding a mentor, CPD and personal development planning. Each of these areas is a requirement of the revalidation process and a strategy that will assist you with meeting revalidation requirements. Together they form a tool kit that you can draw upon to ensure your continued professional development.

Reflective practice

Reflection on your professional practice is something that you will be familiar with from your nurse education course. Indeed, you may have been required to submit reflective accounts as part of your course assessments. However, reflection is not an activity that is confined to your time as a student nurse: it is something that should be engaged with throughout your professional career. As a registered nurse you will be required to complete a minimum of five reflective accounts per three-year period as part of the process of revalidation. It is an important element of your professional development which supports you to evaluate and improve the care you deliver (Nicol and Dosser, 2016). It also enables you to determine what your educational needs are (Ingham-Broomfield, 2020) and thus assists with planning your CPD (see section below).

Ingham-Broomfield (2020) suggests that reflection can focus on everyday events, unusual events, things that have gone well and negative experiences. Traditionally, reflection has tended to be viewed as something that is done after an event, but Nicol and Dosser (2016) suggest there is consensus that it should occur at three points.

1. *Before the event* – thoughts are focused on what your aims are and how you might achieve them. To do this you will need to draw upon your previous experiences (for example, 'have you encountered something like this before?', 'what happened?' 'what learning can be transferred to your current situation?'). You may also draw upon wider evidence (see Chapter 4) and legal and ethical frameworks (see Chapter 2).

2. *Reflection in action* – here you reflect on how you are undertaking an activity or handling a situation. You will be assessing the impact that your actions have, how you feel about this and modifying your approach as required.

3. *Reflecting on action* – after an activity or situation you look back on your performance, assess what worked well and what didn't, identify any learning needs that have arisen, identify any learning that took place and how this might be used in similar situations in the future.

Nicol and Dosser (2016) add that for reflection to be meaningful it is important that you think critically, draw meaningful conclusions and develop an action plan.

There are several tools to assist you with reflection. For example, you are probably familiar with the various models of reflection that have been developed and which you can use as a framework (see Ingham-Broomfield (2020) and the Resources section at the end of the chapter for further information). It is important to reflect as soon as possible after an event, but it may not always be feasible to engage in a structured reflection immediately. Nicol and Dosser (2016) thus suggest keeping a reflective journal and making notes under the following headings which you can then use later as a basis for reflection.

o   *'What happened?*

o   *How did I feel?*

o   *What are the main points?*

o   *What do I need to explore further?*

o   *What are my initial thoughts were this to happen again?'*

If writing in a journal is not possible then an alternative might be to record your thoughts in relation to these questions using the voice memo function on your phone. Whichever method you use remember to observe requirements regarding confidentiality and do not include the names of individuals or services.

Case study 12.1

Jason McCormack has been a registered nurse learning disability nurse for two years. Having worked in a residential setting since registration he has recently moved into a community nursing post in the local Community Learning Disability Team. The team has received a referral from a local GP asking for support for Alex Johnson, a 35-year-old man, who is said to have a mild learning disability and who has recently been diagnosed as having depression. Jason has been asked to visit Alex to undertake an initial assessment and, before he visits, he decides that he should update himself on depression and the various interventions that can be helpful (*reflection before the event*).

Alex lives at home with his mother, and both are present when Jason visits. He has no previous history of depression and therefore Jason asks about how the

→

depression is affecting him and whether they can identify anything that might have triggered it. Jason learns that Alex's father had recently died in an accident, that Alex was very close to his father, and that he used to spend a lot of time with him. His mother feels that his current difficulties are a response to his father's death particularly as he has been unable to speak about it. She also says that she does not know how best to help him or of any services that might support him.

Alex said he went to see the GP on his own, that he didn't tell the GP he saw about his father, and that he was just prescribed medication. He added, however, that he didn't think the tablets were working. Jason explains that it can take a while for anti-depressant medication to take effect. He also says that he has only recently taken up post and that he would like to find out about what local bereavement support there might be to help Alex (*reflection in action*). He agrees to visit again after he has spoken with team members and to agree a plan to work together with him.

When he discusses his assessment with the team Jason learns that the team psychologist has a special interest in bereavement and that she will be able to offer Alex some support. However, Jason also feels that he needs to learn more about bereavement and people with a learning disability (*reflection on action*). He decides to do a literature search, see whether there are any courses available and asks the psychologist if he can meet with her to discuss this.

Reflection can be undertaken as a group as well as an individual activity. For example, as a learning disability nurse you and your colleagues might be involved in de-escalating a situation in which someone you support is getting agitated and is at risk of causing harm either to themselves or others. Using the three stages of reflection suggested by Nicol and Dosser (2016) you might, as a team, agree a plan of action reflecting upon previous experience of supporting the individual, their positive behavioural support plan and the staffing resources you have available. During the activity you will all constantly assess the level of anxiety being shown by the individual, the impact of your interventions and (based on this assessment) will adjust your interventions as required. Once the individual is calm and safe then as a team you might discuss the event to identify what worked, what didn't work and whether anything needs to change in the future. Discussing your reflections as a team can be helpful as while you will all have been involved in the same event you may have experienced it differently and noticed different things. By sharing and discussing these experiences then learning can be maximised and future care enhanced.

Networking

Networking, in the context of nursing, has been defined as

a long-term process of building linkages and maintaining relationships, throughout professional life.

(Jain et al, 2011, p 1)

However, it is the aim of building such relationships that is important. Drake (2017) suggests that networking should be viewed as building relationships to achieve goals and identifies three different types. First, she refers to *operational* networking which involves building relationships which are internal to an organisation. A learning disability nurse working in a community learning disability team might therefore work at developing effective working relationships with other members of the MDT. This will require developing an understanding who does what, how support may be accessed and how the different professions and support staff work together. Your primary reason for doing this will be to ensure that you can offer timely, coordinated and effective support to your service users. However, there will also be professional benefits for the nurse who learns with, and from, their colleagues. It is also worth noting that learning disability nurses often work across services and organisations and therefore operational networking may, of necessity, also include building relationships with key individuals in organisations other than the one in which you are working.

The second type of networking identified by Drake (2017) is what is referred to as *personal* networking where an individual develops links with key contacts outside of their organisation. For example, a learning disability nurse might join a community of practice relating to an area of interest such as positive behaviour support or dementia. Within this context they may be able to meet with and learn from both learning disability nurses working in other services, other professionals, families and people with learning disabilities.

The final type of networking is described as *strategic* networking (Drake, 2017) and this involves activity at higher organisational levels where the focus is on achieving goals through working with and through relationships that are both internal and external to an organisation. For example, a senior learning disability nurse might be involved in seeking to develop an effective discharge policy for people with learning disabilities being discharged from acute hospitals to social care and supported living settings. To do this they will need to work together with colleagues from learning disability, acute care, primary care, social care and housing support services. This will be easier if the nurse concerned has existing links with key people within these services, but even where it is necessary to develop them for a particular piece of work such relationships may be key to the development of future projects when the need arises. For example, if a service is needed for a service user from another organisation, it is often easier to access it if you know who to go to in that organisation and have an existing professional relationship with them.

Networking is viewed as a key skill of the learning disability nurse as it is essential when enabling people with learning disabilities and their families to access the support they need to achieve and maintain health (Hartnett and McNamara, 2021). While this has probably always been the case, Hirst and Irvine (2020) argue that the diversification of the role of the learning disability nurse and the diverse (and often dispersed) settings in which they work has given this element of the role even more importance. Indeed, networking can reduce the isolation that can be experienced when working in dispersed settings (Abdulla et al, 2013). It has a key role to play in enhancing quality of care and support as well as facilitating professional development.

Networking can be achieved using a variety of means. For example, links may be established through activities such as attending conferences, joining professional organisations and through what Drake (2017) refers to as 'connector' relationships whereby you link with others who themselves have a wide network and who then link you with those in their network. This latter approach is often used where one more experienced individual provides mentorship to a junior colleague and, as part of this, they introduce them to key people. Networking can also take place in day-to-day practice through, for example, linking with people you encounter at meetings.

It is important to remember, however, that relationships are two-way, and it is therefore key that as a learning disability nurse you are aware of the knowledge and skills you bring to a professional relationship. It is also important that you have the confidence to share this with others and be open to providing support and assistance to others.

Increasingly, networking is taking the form of 'social networking' through various platforms such as Facebook, Twitter, LinkedIn and Instagram. Interacting with others via social media does require time and commitment to build and sustain relationships with others but, according to Hirst and Irvine (2020), such activity might be 'considered essential' for nurses wishing to keep abreast of best practice and to develop their knowledge and skills. They identify several benefits to joining online networks which include the development of connections with colleagues and organisations, expanding knowledge, being able to share information and best practice and influencing policy at local and national levels. In relation to the latter, for example, you might become aware that a policy is being developed and that a period of consultation has been started. This awareness enables you to contribute to this consultation which you might otherwise have missed. Other benefits that can be derived from engaging with online networks include that it can provide you with the opportunity to link with individuals and groups that you otherwise not have contact with. For example, key professional leaders may be accessible via social media and because contacts take place online geographical distance is not a barrier. This means that it is possible to network at an international level.

Interestingly Hartnett and McNamara (2021) highlight that while networking has always been a core skill of learning disability nurses, it was used to particularly good effect during the Covid-19 pandemic. In this context learning disability nurses used social media to share resources and to organise webinars. This was important since everyone was confronted by a new and challenging situation in which knowledge was changing on almost a daily basis. Also, many people with learning disabilities were being confronted with new and complex information that constantly changed meaning that there was a need for accessible materials to be produced and shared quickly. Learning disability nurses therefore shared information, learnt from each other and supported each other using social media.

Each social media platform has a slightly different focus and way of working but they enable you to 'follow' either individuals or to join a group that shares a common area of interest. Engagement may be through posting items of interest, responding to and commenting on other people's posts and comments, and through engaging in organised discussions. Some Facebook groups and Twitter accounts specifically aimed at learning disability nurses are available and some examples are provided in Table 12.2.

In addition to these you may want to follow key individuals – for example, leaders within learning disability nursing, colleagues working in a similar area of practice or individuals who share a common interest. Remember, however, that it is important to extend and expand your network and so you may (for example) want to follow groups and individuals who focus on other areas of nursing, those who focus on other aspects of support for people with learning disabilities, policymakers and key learning disability organisations and journals.

Table 12.2 Facebook groups and Twitter accounts for learning disability nurses

Facebook:
RCN Learning Disability Nursing Forum
RNID Excellence Ireland Network
RNLD Wales Network
Learning and Intellectual Disability Nursing Academic Network (LIDNAN)
LDNurseChat
Positive Commitment
Promote Learning Disability Nursing
LDNurse.com
LD Nurse Research
Twitter:
@WeLDNurses
@PCCConf
@lidnan
@RcnLDForum
@ldnursepodcast

WeLDNs (a twitter group) organises regular Twitter chats in which a topic of interest to learning disability nurses is chosen, a blog relating to this topic is posted online and at a specified time an online discussion regarding this topic is facilitated live on Twitter. Questions are posed by a facilitator, and anyone can respond/contribute by including the hashtag #weldns. Following the Twitter chat a transcript of the discussion (all the comments posted) is uploaded to the website, and it is also possible to access transcripts of all previous chats should you wish to. The website details can be found in the Resources section.

If you are not familiar with using social media for professional networking then support is available. For example, the WeCommunities (of which WeLDNS is a part) have a section of their website dedicated to supporting healthcare professionals to understand how to use Twitter. Details on how to access their 'Twitterversity' can be found in the Resources section at the end of this chapter. It is also essential that you remember that you are using social media as a professional and that it is important to always uphold

Professional Standards. The NMC therefore provides guidance in relation to using social media; a weblink has been provided in the Resources section.

Critical reflection 12.3

- Map out your existing professional networks. You should include both individuals and organisations, in person and online.

- What do you bring to these relationships and what do you gain from them?

- Are there any gaps you can see and how might you fill these gaps?

Finding a mentor

Earlier in this chapter the importance of preceptorship for newly registered nurses was explored. However, as you progress through your career it can be helpful to identify mentors who will help you to develop along your chosen career path. As Bryce and Redick (2016) observe, everyone can benefit from the support of a mentor *'no matter how junior or senior'*.

Rolfe (2021, p 12) provides the following definition:

A mentor enables the mentee to move towards their chosen goals with the benefit of their own insight and (possibly) advice or input based on the mentor's experience.

Commenting on this definition she notes that there are two keywords, namely 'enables' and 'insight': these highlight how the mentor both enables the mentee to do the required work themselves and challenges them to reflect and draw upon their own knowledge and experience (Rolfe, 2021). A mentor may provide you with support and opportunities for development (Bryce and Reddick, 2016). They may introduce you to key people, but they may also challenge you to move out of your comfort zone (Fowler, 2011) and in doing so enable you to grow professionally.

Some organisations provide formal mentorship schemes or, alternatively, mentoring relationships can develop organically (Bryce and Reddick, 2016). However, it may be that you need to personally take responsibility for seeking mentorship if you feel that this would assist you in your development (remembering what was mentioned above in terms of everyone being able to benefit from mentorship!).

Rolfe (2021) observes that there is no one way to 'do' mentoring since the needs and circumstances of individuals vary. For example, what meets your needs as a newly registered nurse may not be appropriate as you progress through your career. However, some people do have the support of one key mentor throughout their professional career. Bryce and Reddick (2016) suggest that the starting point is to assess what you want from a mentoring relationship and what your goals are. This may mean that you need to identify different mentors to support you with different aspects of your professional development. For example, if you are aiming to move into a leadership role in a particular clinical setting you may want to seek the support of a mentor who has extensive leadership experience and another that is a clinical expert in the field. Working with different mentors, and possibly even mentors outside of your direct area of work, will enable you to be exposed to a wider range of views and experiences (Bryce and Reddick, 2016).

Mentoring can take place face to face but, as communication has moved online over recent years, this has opened the possibility of mentorship from those who are at a geographical distance from you. Fowler (2011) advises that you seek out a mentor who is someone you have respect for, is (professionally) where you want to be and who is willing to invest their time and energy in your professional development. This latter point is important to remember since most mentors give of their time without any direct reward other than the satisfaction of supporting the professional development of another. Many people are more than willing to do this as they feel that they are paying forward the time and effort their mentors invested in them. Nonetheless, it is important to respect their time and be willing to engage in discussion actively and honestly with them. It is therefore important that you agree, with your mentor, how you will work together in terms of (for example) frequency of contact and whether it will be a formal or informal relationship.

As you progress through your career you will find that you are also sought out as a mentor. This can even happen while you are a student when a student who is earlier on in their studies seeks out your support. You will need, therefore, to consider not only what you might be seeking from a mentor but also what you might contribute and share with others as a mentor.

Critical reflection 12.4

Think about what your current professional goals are and how a mentor might assist you with achieving these.

- Can you identify someone who you might approach to be your mentor? Think also about what you might contribute as a mentor to other people.

- What would you bring to such a relationship, and is there anything you would need to do to develop your skills as a mentor?

Continuous professional development

CPD is viewed as essential if nurses are to deliver care and support that is person-centred, safe and effective (King et al, 2020). Accordingly, as noted earlier in this chapter, the NMC requires that all nurses provide evidence of 35 hours of CPD relevant to your sphere of practice, within each three-year period of revalidation. However, despite this professional requirement, King et al (2020) suggest there has been a reduction in access to CPD for nurses arguing that this gives rise to three key concerns, namely the ability of practitioners to meet their revalidation requirements, the impact on the capacity of practitioners to adequately supervise students and the impact on nursing recruitment and retention. As a learning disability nurse, it is therefore important that you recognise your professional responsibility for your own CPD, and that you seek out and take opportunities.

The NMC does not prescribe any form of CPD other than that the 35 hours must comprise at least 20 hours participatory learning (defined as any learning where you interact directly with other professionals, and which can include online interaction). The remaining 15 hours can comprise activities such as reading professional journals or writing for publication. This does, therefore, provide a wide range of potential opportunities for completing your minimum 35 hours.

The key thing to remember is that your CPD must be clearly linked to your sphere of practice. This is important since evidence suggests that nurses are more motivated to undertake CPD, and that it is more effective and impactful, if they can see direct relevance to their day-to-day work (King et al, 2020). If it is relevant to practice, then it is also more likely to secure organisational support in terms of funding (if required) and time.

Within your role as a learning disability nurse, you will be required to undertake a range of mandatory training such as health and safety and fire training. However, the NMC (2019) indicates that such training should only be included in your 35 hours if it is directly relevant to your scope of practice. Therefore, while you should not include fire training (since this is an element of all healthcare roles) you might, as a learning disability nurse, include mandatory updating in (for example) positive behavioural support if you work with service users whose behaviour may be viewed as challenging.

If you are undertaking a formal course of study, and this is directly related to your current role, then this may be included in your 35 hours. For example, you might be working with older people with learning disabilities and undertaking a master's course relating to dementia. You might be working with people with complex epilepsy and are undertaking a postgraduate epilepsy diploma. However, short courses and conference attendance can also provide opportunities to undertake relevant CPD.

While the above approaches to CPD have financial implications there are also alternatives that can be accessed freely. For example, there are often professional webinars that are free to access and many also record the presentations so that they can be accessed at a time that is convenient to you. Another alternative is participation in an activity such as the Twitter chats mentioned in the previous section. You can even extend your knowledge and skills by activities such as arranging to attend a key meeting outside of your usual practice or through arranging to shadow a colleague.

There are, however, a few things to remember. If you are intending to use a CPD activity as part of the process of revalidation it is important that you record the required information, namely:

- *the CPD method;*
- *a description of the topic and how it relates to your practice;*
- *the dates on which the activity was undertaken;*
- *the number of hours (including the number of participatory hours);*
- *the identification of the part of the Code most relevant to the activity;*
- *evidence that you undertook the CPD activity.*

(NMC, 2019c)

The NMC provides a template to assist with this recording and this can be accessed online (www.nmc.org.uk/revalidation/resources/forms-and-templates). They also provide examples of activities and acceptable forms of evidence.

The other important thing to remember in relation to CPD is that the 35 hours required by the NMC is a minimum and that as a registered learning disability nurse you should identify your learning needs and take all opportunities to extend your knowledge and skills.

Personal development planning

Whatever your current career stage you will probably have an idea of where you want to be in one, three and five-years' time. Previous sections of this chapter have highlighted some strategies that can be used to support your professional development but if you want to ensure that you achieve your goals you need to develop a plan of how you will get there. A personal development plan will provide you with a framework for this.

NHS Health Careers (nd) suggest that a personal development plan involves identifying and setting goals in relation to where you want to be educationally and professionally. They argue that this is a 'must' for healthcare practitioners since it is about thinking about your 'ideal future' and motivating yourself to translate this into reality. It is also important to remember that, by setting yourself a clear development plan, you will also be contributing to better care and support for people with learning disabilities since you will be ensuring that you constantly work to update and extend your knowledge and skills.

NHS Health Careers (nd) suggest that the starting point for a plan is to identify your personal strengths and learning style. Taking such an approach should be familiar to you as a learning disability nurse as the support you provide for people with learning disabilities should be strengths based. This is an opportunity to apply the same approach to your personal learning and development. When identifying your goals, it is helpful to refer to the SMART acronym (see Table 12.3) so that you are clear both as to what your goals are and how you will identify that they have been met.

Table 12.3 The key elements of SMART goals

Specific	Have you clearly identified what it is that you want to achieve and how you intend to achieve it?
Measurable	Will you be able to measure whether there has been progress/improvement?
Achievable	Is it a goal that you can achieve given your resources (time, finance, current knowledge/skill level)?
Relevant	Is the goal relevant to where you want to be personally/professionally? Will it support your development as a learning disability nurse?
Time bound	What timescale have you set for achieving your goal?

A goal that does not apply the SMART structure might read:

I will work to gain a position in a specialist behavioural support team.

In contrast a SMART version would be:

I will commence my Masters in positive behavioural support in September 2022 so that I have the knowledge and skills to gain a Band 6 post in a specialist behavioural support team by 2024.

When assessing whether a goal is achievable it is important to consider whether you have the required resources. These might include whether you have available the time that will be needed (eg study). Funding may be an issue both in terms of course fees and travel expenses. It may also be important that you assess whether there are any pre-requisites such as possessing any specific qualifications, professional experience or living in a particular geographical area.

A personal development plan can be something that you develop for your personal use to support your personal and professional development. However, some organisations use this approach as part of the annual appraisal/performance and development review process. Even where this is not a requirement of your employer you might choose to share your plan to seek organisational support to achieve your goals.

Finally, while it is important to have a clear plan it is also important to be open to adjustments and change. Sometimes circumstances will mean that it is no longer possible to achieve a particular goal and therefore regularly reviewing your progress is helpful to determine whether it is necessary to adjust either the goal or the method of achievement. However, new opportunities that had not been anticipated can also arise. For example, a position may arise in a new service that you wish to apply for or a new course may be offered that interests you and which will put you in a good position to apply for a key role. Again, it is ok to review, reassess and revise your plan.

Critical reflection 12.5

Try to write your own personal development plan.

- Consider where you want to be professionally in one year's time, three years' time and five years' time.

- What do you need to do to achieve this?

- What are your goals and how might you achieve them?

BRINGING IT ALL TOGETHER AND ADVANCING THE PROFESSION

Chapter 1 in this book explored the history of learning disability nursing and highlighted how, over the years, many challenges have been faced and addressed by the profession. Indeed, on several occasions the continued future of the profession has been questioned and it has been argued that (as with most other countries) initial nurse education should be generalist rather than having four fields of practice as we currently do in the UK. Throughout history, however, the learning disability nursing profession has responded to such challenges by adapting and developing to ensure continued relevance to the needs of people with learning disabilities.

The present time brings its own challenges and the RCN (2021) has highlighted several currently facing learning disability nursing. These include concerns regarding the overall numbers of learning disability nurses and the need to address this through a focus on both recruitment and retention. It is important that action is taken since learning disability nurses have a key role to play in addressing key challenges experienced by people with learning disabilities such as health inequities, supporting those whose behaviours are viewed as challenging, those who commit offences, those with profound and multiple disabilities and ensuring that human rights are upheld. It is thus stated that

> *Learning disability nursing in the UK is at a critical phase in terms of workforce development, leadership and education.*
>
> (RCN, 2021)

It is therefore crucial that, as a profession, learning disability nursing continues to develop and this requires that all learning disability nurses take responsibility for ensuring that this happens.

Thus far this chapter has focused on how you, as a learning disability nurse, can develop your knowledge, skills and your career. Through doing this you will be contributing to the development of the learning disability nursing profession. However, it is also important to consider what actions are required at a professional level to ensure continued development. Two key areas will, therefore, be considered – the importance of developing political awareness and a framework provided to bring together the various themes explored in this book as a basis for future development.

Developing political awareness and skill

While speaking at a global level, and encompassing all the nursing profession, the International Council of Nurses (2021) stresses the need for nurses to be at the centre of decision-making to effect positive change:

> *Having nurses in positions of influence and power leads to more people centred and integrated approaches to healthcare and helps to achieve the ultimate goals of more positive outcomes for the people and communities that nurses serve.*

The necessity of this within the context of learning disability nursing is particularly important given the health inequities that people with learning disabilities experience. Learning disability nurses are well positioned to make a positive difference through highlighting barriers to health and well-being, advocating for change and being a key part of the solution. To take on this role in an effective manner learning disability nurses need to ensure that they develop political awareness and the skills to use these effectively. However, while advocacy is widely recognised as a key element of the learning disability nursing role the importance of political awareness is not always acknowledged as a key to effective leadership and professional development in learning disability nursing.

This issue is not confined to learning disability nurses since, more widely, nurses often feel relatively powerless in relation to policy and politics. Policy tends to be viewed as something which is made by other (more powerful people) and which shapes the context within which nurses work, rather than something which they can shape. They may feel that they are implementers of policy rather than influencers. Given that the nursing workforce is the largest within healthcare it is interesting to note this self-perception which seems at odds with the view that there is usually strength in numbers.

One study examined student nurses' views of nurses' political power and awareness in the context of the Covid-19 pandemic and several barriers to political awareness were identified (Catiker, 2021). One key theme to emerge was 'depolititisation' which related to a sense of powerlessness (nurses feeling powerless despite their numbers), political ignorance (a lack of awareness leading nurses to distance themselves from political issues) and gender (nurses are often female and females within wider society are often viewed as being excluded from politics). However, another theme also focused on how nurses could be supported to become more political through education, organisation and political participation. While the study undertaken by Catiker (2021) involved a small sample of generic nursing students, in a different country, and a particular context, the themes that emerged reflect wider discussions and debates regarding political awareness in nursing and highlight some useful areas for consideration.

For learning disability nurses there may be specific challenges in becoming politically active given that, within the nursing workforce, we are numerically the smallest field of practice, and our field of practice is not internationally recognised. Nonetheless, given the inequities that people with learning disabilities often face it is a professional responsibility of learning disability nurses to develop political awareness and to take on a leadership role in advocating for change.

Political awareness requires an understanding of how power and influence operate at a range of levels – within teams, within organisations, between organisations, at a local, national and international levels. Healthcare services, and learning disability services more broadly, are shaped by a range of legal and policy instruments which govern which services and support we provide, how they are resourced and their strategic direction. These will impact directly on the context within which you work but, more importantly, on the lives of those you support. As a learning disability nurse, you are well placed to understand the impact of such policies, to highlight where there are negative consequences and the need to change. However, to do this it is important that you understand how policy is made, by whom, how to raise issues and influence in an effective manner.

Opportunities to influence might include, for example, bringing issues of concern to the attention of organisational managers, policymakers or professional organisations. It might also include putting yourself forward for membership of key committees or providing comments when new policies are being consulted on. You may feel that engaging in such activities may not bring about the desired result – however, if you fail to engage then a failure to effect change can be guaranteed and you cannot assume that someone else will take the action required. Having developed the awareness of the need for change as a leader it is then necessary to ensure that you develop the political skills required to be effective.

Political skill has been defined as *'the ability to effectively understand others at work and to use such knowledge to influence others to act in ways that enhance personal and/ or organisational goals'* and it is identified as one of the most critical competencies for nursing leaders (Montalvo, 2015). There are several strategies that can be helpful in developing this area of competence as a learning disability nurse particularly:

○ effective goal setting;

○ effective alliances;

○ effective communication.

When seeking to effect change and influence others it is important to be clear about what it is you are seeking to achieve. This might seem obvious but often we set out with a vague sense of wanting to effect change rather than a precise sense of what we are trying to achieve, and this can lead to either inaction or failure. Being clear about your goals and how you intend to achieve them helps to keep focus and enables you to be able to both monitor progress and to determine whether you have succeeded. When setting goals, however, it is important to consider factors such as appropriateness (are you targeting the right issue), priorities (both for you and others affected), feasibility (do you have the right resources) and timing (is this the right time to focus on this). You might find it helpful to refer to the SMART framework discussed earlier in this chapter (Table 12.3).

Alongside consideration of goals, you also need to consider whether working in partnership with others to achieve these might be helpful. Earlier in this section it was noted that despite being the largest workforce in healthcare nurses often feel powerless and this may, in part, be due to failing to develop effective alliances and to use the strength that can be gained from numbers. As well as increasing numbers, forming and using effective alliances can also mean that other perspectives are brought to bear on the issue. Consider, for example, if as a learning disability nurse, you are seeking to secure resources within your organisation to develop a new service. Working together with people with learning disabilities and their families to present the case and ensuring that their views and experiences are part of this case alongside presenting other evidence for change (see Chapter 4) is likely to ensure a stronger and better-informed argument for change.

Effective communication is essential when seeking to exert influence. Here, it is important to be clear about the message you want to communicate (another reason to be clear about your goals). However, it is also important to consider your audience and make sure that you present it in a format that is appropriate to them. For example, you may feel that you want to provide extensive information running to many pages but if you are wanting to present the information to a policymaker or senior manager, they are unlikely to have the time to read such a large document. In this instance two pages that present the key points such as the issue, what is being proposed and resources required is likely to be more effective in the first instance. If this gets their attention, then more detailed information can be provided at a later stage. As a learning disability nurse, it is also important to ensure that where you need to present information to people with a learning disability that you do so in ways that meet their communication needs (such as an Easy Read) format. A further consideration when considering communication is timing since there may be times when other priorities mean that the cause you are seeking to progress is more or less likely to get the attention of others.

Critical reflection 12.6

Think about some of the key challenges that are currently facing people with learning disabilities and learning disability nursing.

- Identify how, as a learning nurse, you might work with others to try and influence decision-making to enhance health and well-being for people with learning disabilities and their families.

- Who might you need to work with?

- What strategies might need to be used?

- How would you know if you had been effective?

'Change it'

Throughout this book the focus has been on supporting you to develop your role as a learning disability nurse and, through this, to enable you to play your part in developing the learning disability nursing profession so that it can make a positive impact on the lives of people with a learning disability both now and in the future. To assist you with bringing the various themes explored together the mnemonic 'CHANGE IT' is offered as a framework.

- **C**hallenge and communicate effectively.
- **H**old on to your values.
- **A**dvocate.
- **N**etwork effectively and collaborate.
- **G**enerate opportunities.
- **E**ncourage and support.
- **I**nfiltrate, inspire and innovate.
- **T**hink critically.

To ensure that learning disability nursing remains relevant to the needs of those we support we need to be able to recognise and **challenge** policies and practices that do not support the health and well-being of people with learning disabilities. This means that, as a profession, we need to be able to **communicate** effectively and challenge in a constructive and effective manner. The importance of these aspects of the learning disability nursing role were highlighted earlier in this chapter in relation to political awareness.

In Chapter 2, the importance of the **values** that underpin learning disability nursing was stressed. As a profession it is essential that these values are shared, their implications for practice understood and that they inform our practice. Where these values are challenged, and it is difficult to uphold them (eg where limited resources negatively impact on the environment of care) then we have a professional duty to raise concerns regarding this. This means that we need to be able to **advocate** for those we support and for the policies and resources that will make a positive impact on their quality of life, health, and well-being and to support people with learning disabilities to advocate for themselves. We also need to advocate for the learning disability nursing profession but not as an end in itself but rather from the perspective that learning disability nurses have the knowledge and skills to identify and address the inequalities and inequities often experienced by people with learning disabilities and their families. This requires that a range of clinical knowledge and skills are marshalled (see earlier chapters) and that we present an evidence-based case (Chapter 4).

All of this requires that learning disability nurses **network** effectively and collaborate with others to promote best practice and take a proactive approach to **generate opportunities** rather than simply waiting for them to happen. We need to **encourage** and support people with learning disabilities, their families and carers, other professionals and other learning disability nurses since through working together we can effect change.

You might be surprised to see that the need to **infiltrate** is mentioned along with inspiring and innovating. Infiltration is often viewed as a negative concept and brings with it the suggestion of perhaps being underhand and deceitful. This is not what is intended here. Instead, it is included to challenge the idea that learning disability nurses and the learning disability nursing profession only belong in arenas that carry the label of 'learning disability'. An important role of learning disability nurses is to ensure they are in positions in which they can challenge others to recognise, understand and respond appropriately to the needs of people with learning disabilities. For example, learning disability nurses know about the health inequities that people with learning disabilities experience but if we only talk to each other about this then our power to effect change is limited. Instead, if learning disability nurses are present in broader discussions regarding health inequities, then they can ensure that people with learning disabilities are considered in wider policies and service developments. Similarly, by contributing to broader research projects they can ensure that people with learning disabilities can participate if they so wish.

As a learning disability nurse by putting yourself forward to participate in activities such as committees and projects (infiltrating into areas perhaps learning disability nurses haven't traditionally operated in) it is then possible to **inspire** others to include a focus on the needs of people with learning disabilities and to work together to **innovate**. Through such innovation change and development can be achieved.

Finally, to achieve all the other elements of 'CHANGE IT' it is essential that learning disability nurses are **think critically**. It is important here not to confuse 'critical' with 'criticism' since it is not about just looking for faults (although it is important to identify these). Critical thinking is concerned with looking at situations, policies and practices from a range of perspectives, identifying strengths and weaknesses, posing questions and arriving at a reasoned and balanced position. It is about recognising what works and why it works, but also what needs to change and how such change might be achieved. It is fundamental to developing both as individuals and as a profession and essential if, as a profession, learning disability nursing is to remain relevant to the needs of people with learning disabilities.

Chapter summary

This chapter has sought to provide you with a toolkit you can use to develop yourself as a learning disability nurse. However, it has also recognised the need for the profession of learning disability nursing to continue to develop to ensure that it meets the needs of people with learning disabilities and their families. Of course, these two elements are related: if you ensure your continued professional development as a learning disability nurse then you will be contributing to the overall development of the profession.

This chapter has also sought to bring together several of the recurring themes and threads that have been explored in this book. In doing so it is hoped that it has enabled you to see how the various areas considered are all interdependent and essential for professional development. Whatever your current career stage and your future career plans, we hope that the material we have covered has, and will, support you to provide quality, person-centred care and support across the lifespan and across a range of settings.

FURTHER READING

Delves-Yates, C (2021) *Beginner's Guide to Reflective Practice in Nursing*. London: Sage.

This book will provide you with a broader understanding of reflective practice to support your professional development.

Price, B (2021) *Critical Thinking and Writing in Nursing*, 5th edition. London: Sage.

This book will assist you to further develop your skills in critical thinking which will support development of both your practice and your writing.

Salvage, J (1985) *The Politics of Nursing*. London: Heinemann Nursing.

While this book was published over 35 years ago it was one of the first books exploring politics and nursing and remains a key text.

RESOURCES

WeCommunities #WeLDNs Chat: www.wecommunities.org/tweet-chats/chat-details/5726 (accessed 21 June 2022).

This website hosts transcripts of questions and responses asked and answered on Twitter to topics of interest to learning disability nurses.

#WeLearnToTweet: www.wecommunities.org/blogs/3503 (accessed 21 June 2022).

This website hosts a 'Twitterversity' to assist healthcare professionals in engaging via Twitter.

Guidance on Using Social Media Responsibly: www.nmc.org.uk/globalassets/sitedocuments/ nmc-publications/social-media-guidance.pdf (accessed 21 June 2022).

This resource provides guidance on using social media professionally.

Nursing and Midwifery Council Revalidation: www.nmc.org.uk/revalidation/requirements/ (accessed 21 June 2022).

This link contains details regarding requirements for revalidation, guidance on fulfilling these requirements and templates to assist with recording.

Eight Ways to Improve Your Reflection: www.rcn.org.uk/professional-development/revalida tion/eight-ways-to-improve-your-reflection (accessed 21 June 2022).

This link takes you to an RCN page which provides advice and support in relation to reflective practice accounts. They also provide information regarding models of reflection via this link: www.rcn.org.uk/professional-development/revalidation/reflection-and-reflective-dis cussion.

A Guide to Planning Your CPD Nursing Training: www.nurses.co.uk/blog/a-guide-to-planning- your-cpd-nursing-training/ (accessed 21 June 2022).

This link takes you to a blog that provides support and guidance regarding continuous professional development.

References

Abdulla, S, Marsden, D, Wilson, S and Parker, M (2013) Networking Opportunities for Learning Disability Nurses. *Learning Disability Practice*, 16(5): 30–2.

Acheson, D (1988) *Public Health in England: The Report of the Committee of Inquiry into the Future Development to the Public Health Function*. London: DHSS.

Adair, J (2010) *Develop Your Leadership Skills*. London: Kogan Page.

Adam, E, Sleeman, K, Brearley, S, Hunt, K and Tuffrey-Wijne, I (2020) The Palliative Care Needs of Adults with Intellectual Disabilities and Their Access to Palliative Care Services: A Systematic Review. *Palliative Medicine*, 34(8): 1006–18.

Adlington, K, Smith, J, Crabtree, J, Win, S, Rennie, J, Khodatars, K, Rosser, E and Hall, I (2018) Improving Access to Genetic Testing for Adults with Intellectual Disability: A Literature Review and Lessons from a Quality Improvement Project in East London. *American Journal of Medical Genetics*. [online] Available at: https://qi.elft.nhs.uk/wp-content/uploads/2019/05/FinalArticle-pdf.pdf (accessed 16 June 2021).

Aguilar, F J (1967) *Scanning the Business Environment*. New York: Macmillan.

Ali, M (2018) Communication Skills 3: Non-verbal Communication. *Nursing Times*, 114(2): 41–2.

Aras Attracta Swinford Review Group (2016) *Key Messages*. Dublin: Aras Attracta Swinford Review Group.

Association of Directors of Adult Social Services (ADASS) (2018) Guidance and Principles for Aftercare Services Under Section 117. [online] Available at: http://londonadass.org.uk/wp-content/uploads/2018/01/Section-117-Protocol-reviewed-Dec-2018.pdf (accessed 13 January 2022).

Atkinson, D et al (2013) *The Health Equalities Framework (HEF): An Outcomes Framework Based on the Determinants of Health Inequalities*. [online] Available at: www.ndti.org.uk/assets/files/The_Health_Equality_Framework_final_word.pdf (accessed 22 November 2021).

Atkinson, D, Boulter, P, Hebron, C and Moulster, G (2015) HEF+: Health Equalities Framework – The Complete Practitioners Guide. [online] Available at: www.ndti.org.uk/assets/files/HEF2B_manual_plus_final.pdf (accessed 30 November 2021).

Audit Commission (1986) *Making a Reality of Community Care*. London: HMSO.

Avery, G (2013) *Law and Ethics in Nursing and Healthcare. An Introduction*. London: Sage.

Aveyard, H and Sharp, P (2017) *A Beginner's Guide to Evidence Based Practice in Health and Social Care*, 3rd edition. London: Open University Press.

Bandura, A (1977) *Social Learning Theory*. New Jersey: Prentice-Hall.

Bank-Mikkelson, N (1980) Denmark. In Flynn, R J and Nitsch, K E (eds) *Normalization, Social Integration and Community Services* (pp 51–70). University Park Press: Baltimore.

Barker, P (ed) (2013) *Mental Health Ethics. The Human Context*. London: Routledge.

Barr, J and Dowding, L (2016) *Leadership in Health Care*, 3rd edition. London: Sage.

Barr, J and Dowding, L (2019) *Leadership in Health Care*, 4th edition. Los Angeles: Sage.

BBC (2020) Woman with Learning Disability Can Have Teeth Removed, Court Rules. *BBC News*. [online] Available at: www.bbc.co.uk/news/uk-england-lincolnshire-52774498 (accessed 6 May 2022).

Beauchamp, T L and Childress, J F (2019) *Principles of Biomedical Ethics*, 8th edition. Oxford: Oxford University Press.

Beighton, C and Wills, J (2017) Are Parents Identifying Positive Aspects to Parenting Their Child with an Intellectual Disability or Are They just Coping? A Qualitative Exploration. *Journal of Intellectual Disabilities*, 21(4): 325–45.

Binger, N (2020) Don't Say 'I'm Sorry' When a Baby Has Down Syndrome. *The Mighty*. [online] Available at: https://themighty.com/2020/07/baby-down-syndrome-not-sorry/ (accessed 16 June 2021).

Blair, J, Busk, M, Goleniowska, H, Hawtrey-Woore, S, Morris, S, Newbold, Y and Nimmo, S (2016) Through Our Eyes: What Parents Want for Their Children from Health Professionals. In Chaplin, H, Woodward, P and Hardy, S (eds) *Supporting the Physical Health Needs of People with Learning Disabilities: A Handbook for Professionals, Support Staff and Families* (pp 197–212). London: Pavilion.

Blunden, R and Allen, D (1987) *Facing the Challenge: An Ordinary Life for People with Learning Difficulties and Challenging Behaviour*. Kings Fund Paper No 74. Kings Fund Centre, London.

Boardman, L, Bernal, J and Hollins, S (2014) Communicating with People with Intellectual Disabilities: A Guide for General Psychiatrists. *Advances in Psychiatric Treatment*, 20(1): 27–36.

Booth, A (2006) Clear and Present Questions: Formulating Questions for Evidence-based Practice. *Library Hi Tech*, 24(3): 355–68.

Bornman, J and Murphy, J (2006) Using the ICF in Goal Setting: Clinical Application Using Talking Mats. *Disability and Rehabilitation: Assistive Technology*, 1(3): 145–54.

Bowlby, J (1988) *A Secure Base: Parent–Child Attachment and Healthy Human Development*. New York: Basic Books.

Bradshaw, J (1972) The Taxonomy of Social Need. In Cookson, R Sainsbury, R and Glendenning, C (eds) *Jonathan Bradshaw on Social Policy. Selected Writings 1972–2011* (pp 1–12). York: York Publishing Services.

Bradshaw, P L (2000) Fitness for Practice. *Journal of Nursing Management*, 8: 1–2.

The British Psychological Society (2018) *Positive Behaviour Support (PBS): Committee and Working Group Position Statement*. [online] Available at: www.bps.org.uk/sites/www.bps.org.uk/files/Member%20Networks/Divisions/DCP/Positive%20Behaviour%20Support.pdf (accessed 21 November 2021).

Brown, B (2021) *Atlas of the Heart*. New York: Random House Penguin.

Brown, J (1992) The Residential Setting in Mental Handicap; An Overview of Selected Policy Initiatives 1971–1989. In Thompson, T Mathias, P (eds) *Standards and Mental Handicap. Keys to Competence* (pp 106–22). London: Balliere Tindall.

Bryce, S. and Redick, J (2016) Mentoring Is the Secret to Career Advancement. *Women Lawyers' Journal*, 101(1): 18–21.

Bryson, T (2017) Leadership and Inter-professional Practice. In Taylor, R and Webster-Henderson, B (eds) *The Essentials of Nursing Leadership* (pp 65–77). London: Sage.

Bush, T (2019) PESTLE Analysis of the NHS. [Online] Available at: https://pestleanalysis.com/nhs-pestle-analysis/ (accessed 30 January 2022).

Byatt, K (2008) Holistic Care. In Mason-Whitehead, E, Mcintosh, A, Bryan, A and Mason, T (eds) *Key Concepts in Nursing. Sage Key Concepts* (pp 168–73). London. Sage.

Caldwell, J (2010) Leadership Development of Individuals with Developmental Disabilities in the Self-Advocacy Movement. *Journal of Intellectual Disability Research*, 54(11): 1004–14.

CALL Scotland (nd) Personal Communication Passports. [online] Available at: www.communicationpassports.org.uk/home/ (accessed 8 June 2022).

Care Quality Commission (CQC) (2020) Identifying and Responding to Closed Cultures. Supporting Information for CQC Staff. [online] Available at: www.cqc.org.uk/sites/default/files/20191104_closedcultures_supportinginformation_full.pdf (accessed 4 March 2021).

Care Quality Commission (CQC) (2021) Protect, Respect, Connect – Decisions about Living and Dying Well during COVID-19. [online] Available at: www.cqc.org.uk/publications/themed-work/protect-respect-connect-decisions-about-living-dying-well-during-covid-19 (accessed 18 April 2022).

Carey, I M, Hosking, F J, Harris, T, DeWilde, S, Beighton, C, Shah, S M and Cook, D G (2016) Do Health Checks for Adults with Intellectual Disability Reduce Emergency Hospital Admissions? Evaluation of a Natural Experiment. *Journal of Epidemiological Community Health*, 71(1): 1–7. doi:10.1136/jech-2016-207557

Catiker, A (2021) Political Power and Awareness of Nursing during the COVID-19 Pandemic from the Views of Senior Nursing Students. *World Medicine and Health Policy*. doi:10.1002/wmh3.475 (accessed 11 February 2022).

The Challenging Behaviour Foundation (CBF) and Positive and Active Behaviour Support Scotland (PABSS) (2019) *Reducing Restrictive Intervention of Children and Young People Update Report.* [online] Available at: www.challengingbehaviour.org.uk/wp-content/uploads/2019/01/rireportfinal.pdf (accessed 29 December 2021).

Clawson, R, Patterson, A, Fyson, R and McCarthy, M (2020) The Demographics of Forced Marriage of People with Learning Disabilities: Findings from a National Database. *Journal of Adult Protection*, 22(2): 59–74.

Cole, M, John-Steiner, J, Scribner, S and Souberman, E (eds) (1978) *L.S. Vygotsky: Mind in Society: The Development of Higher Psychological Processes*. London: Harvard University Press.

Conolly, M, Perryman, J, McKenna, Y, Orford, J, Thomson, L, Shuttleworth, J and Cocksedge, S (2010) SAGE & THYME: A Model for Training Health and Social Care Professionals in Patient-focused Support. *Patient Education and Counselling*, 79(1): 87–93.

Coppus, A M W (2013) People with Intellectual Disability: What Do We Know about Adulthood and Life Expectancy? *Developmental Disabilities Reviews*, 18: 6–16.

Craig, J and Dowding, D A (eds) (2020) *Evidence-based Practice in Nursing* (4th ed). Edinburgh: Elsevier.

Critical Skills Appraisal Programme (CASP) (nda) CASP Checklists. [online] Available at: https://casp-uk.net/casp-tools-checklists/ (accessed 8 June 2022).

Critical Skills Appraisal Programme (CASP) (ndb) Glossary. [online] Available at: https://casp-uk.net/glossary (accessed 8 June 2022).

Crombie, A and Garland, G (2017) Nursing Leadership in Organisations. Theory and Practice. In Taylor, R and Webster-Henderson, B (eds) *The Essentials of Nursing Leadership* (pp 31–45). London: Sage.

Cullen, C (1991) *Caring for People. Community Care in the Next Decade and Beyond – Mental Handicap Nursing*. London: Department of Health.

Curtis, E A (2021) Nurturing, Implementing and Sustaining Distributed Leadership. In Curtis, E A, Beirne, M, Cullen, J G, Northway, R and Corrigan, S M (eds) *Distributed Leadership in Nursing and Healthcare. Theory, Evidence and Development* (pp 218–42). London: Open University Press.

de Winter, C F, Jansen, A A and Evenhuis, H M (2011) Physical Conditions and Challenging Behaviour in People with Intellectual Disability: A Systematic Review. *Journal of Intellectual Disability Research*, 55(7): 675–98.

Delaffon, V, Anwar, Z, Noushad, F, Ahmed, A and Brugha, T (2012) Use of Health of the Nation Outcome Scales in psychiatry. *Advances in Psychiatric Treatment,* 18(3): 173–9.

Department of Health (1983) Mental Health Act 1983: Code of Practice. [online] Available at: www.gov.uk/government/publications/code-of-practice-mental-health-act-1983 (accessed 8 June 2022).

Department of Health (1989a) *Caring for People: Community Care in the Next Decade and Beyond,* CM849. London: HMSO.

Department of Health (1989b) *Working for Patients. The Health Service – Caring for the 1990s,* CM555. London: HMSO.

Department of Health (1995) *Learning Disability: Meeting Needs through Targeting Skills*. London: Department of Health.

Department of Health (2012) Transforming Care: A National Response to Winterbourne View Hospital. [online] Available at: https://assets.publishing.service.gov.uk/government/uploads/system/uploads/attachment_data/file/213215/final-report.pdf (accessed 8 June 2022).

Department of Health (2013) Learning Disabilities Good Practice Project. [online] Available at: https://assets.publishing.service.gov.uk/government/uploads/system/uploads/attachment_data/file/261896/Learning_Diasbilities_Good_Practice_Project__Novemeber_2013_.pdf (accessed 28 January 2022).

Department of Health and Social Care (DHSC) (2021) Reforming the Mental Health Act: Joint Foreword from the Secretary of State for Health and Social Care and the Secretary of State for Justice and Lord Chancellor. [online] Available at: www.gov.uk/government/consultations/reforming-the-mental-health-act/reforming-the-mental-health-act (accessed 8 June 2022).

Department of Health and Social Services (1969) *Report of the Committee of Inquiry into Allegations of Ill-treatment of Patients and Other Irregularities at the Ely Hospital, Cardiff,* Cmnd 3975. London: HMSO.

Department of Health and Social Services (1971) *Better Services for the Mentally Handicapped,* Cmnd 4693. London: HMSO.

Department of Health and Social Services (1979) *Report of the Committee of Enquiry into Mental Handicap Nursing Care,* (The Jay Report) Cmnd 74681 (I) and (II). London: HMSO.

Desroches, M, Fisher, K, Ailey, S, Stych, J, McMillan, S, Horan, P, Marsden, D, Trip, H and Wilson, N (2022) Supporting the Needs of People with Intellectual and Developmental Disabilities 1 Year into the COVID-19 Pandemic: An International, Mixed Methods Study of Nurses' Perspective. *Journal of Policy and Practice in Intellectual Disabilities*, 19: 48–63.

Deveau, R and McGill, P (2019) Staff Experiences Working in Community-based Services for People with Learning Disabilities Who Show Behaviour Described as Challenging: The Role of Management Support. *British Journal of Learning Disabilities*, 47: 201–7.

Developmental Disabilities Nurses Association (2020) *Practice Standards for Developmental Disability Nursing* (3rd ed). [online] Available at: https://ddna.org/education/practice-standards/ (accessed 18 June 2022).

Donaldson, J and Sabin, M (2017) Preparation for Transition to Leadership in Qualified Practice. In Taylor, R and Webster-Henderson, B (eds) *The Essentials of Nursing Leadership* (pp 144–58). London: Sage.

Doody, O, Slevin, E and Taggart, L (2012) Intellectual Disability Nursing in Ireland: Identifying Its Development and Future. *Journal of Intellectual Disabilities*, 16(1): 7–16.

Dowding, D (2020) Using Research Evidence in Making Clinical Decisions with Individual Patients. In Craig, J and Dowding, D A (eds) *Evidence-based Practice in Nursing* (pp 143–60), 4th edition. Edinburgh: Elsevier.

Drake, K (2017) The Power of Networking. *Nursing Management*, 48(9): 56.

Drake, K (2020) Change Is Inevitable. *Nursing Management*, 51(7): 56.

Duff, H (2018) An Evaluation of the Health Equality Framework in South East Scotland. *Learning Disability Practice*. doi:10.7748/ldp.2018.e1898

Ellis, P (2020) *Understanding Ethics for Nursing Students*, 3rd edition. London: Sage.

Ellis, P (2022) *Leadership, Management and Team Working in Nursing*. London: Sage.

Emerson, E (2001) *Challenging Behaviour: Analysis and Intervention in People with Learning Disabilities*, 2nd edition. Cambridge: Cambridge University Press.

Emerson, E (2015) The Challenging Behaviour Foundation and Council for disabled Children Paving the Way: How to Develop Effective Local Services for Children with Learning Disabilities Whose Behaviours Challenge. [online] Available at: www.challengingbehaviour.org.uk/wp-content/uploads/2021/02/Paving-the-Way.pdf (accessed 21 December 2021).

Emerson, E and Einfeld, S (eds) (2011) *Challenging Behaviour*, 3rd edition. Cambridge: Cambridge University Press.

Emerson, E and Robertson, J (eds) (2011) *People with Learning Disabilities and Visual Impairment*. RNIB and SeeAbility Learning Disabilities Observatory. [online] Available at: www.seeability.org/sites/default/files/2021-06/Estimated%20prevalence%20of%20visual%20impairment%20among%20people%20with%20learning%20disabilities%20in%20the%20UK_0.pdf (accessed 8 June 2022).

Equality and Human Rights Commission (2018) The Human Rights Act. [online] Available at: www.equalityhumanrights.com/en/human-rights/human-rights-act (accessed 8 June 2022).

Esmaelzadeh, F, Abbaszadeh, A, Borhani, F and Peyrovi, H (2017) Ethical Sensitivity in Nursing Ethical Leadership: A Content Analysis of Iranian Nurses' Experiences. *The Open Nursing Journal*, 11: 1–13.

Evans, D, Coutsaki, D and Fathers, C P (2017) *Health Promotion and Public Health for Nursing Students*, 3rd edition. London: Sage.

Fabstuff (nd) A Social Movement for Sharing Health & Social Care Ideas, Services and Solutions That Work. [online] Available at: https://fabnhsstuff.net/ (accessed 9 June 2022).

Flood, B (2016) Medication Use in Residential Care for Older People with Intellectual Disabilities. *Learning Disability Practice*, 19(7): 24–9.

Flynn, M (2012) *Winterbourne View Hospital. A Serious Case Review*. South Gloucs: South Gloucestershire Safeguarding Adults Board. [online] Available at: https://hosted.southglos.gov.uk/wv/report.pdf (accessed 18 April 2022).

Folch, A, Salvador-Curulla, L, Vicens, P, Cortes, M J, Irazabal, M, Munoz, S, Rovira, L, Orejula, C, Gonzalez, J A and Martinez-Leal, R (2017) Health Indicators in Intellectual Developmental Disorders: The Key Findings of the POMONA-ESP Project. *Journal of Applied Research in Intellectual Disability*, 32: 23–34.

Foo, B, Wiese, M, Curryer, B, Stancliffe, R J, Wilson, N J and Clayton, J M (2021) Specialist Palliative Care Staff's Varying Experiences of Talking with People with Intellectual Disability about Their Dying and Death: A Thematic Analysis of In-depth Interviews. *Palliative Medicine*, 35(4): 738–49.

Foster, A, Titheradge, H and Morton, J (2015) Genetics of Learning Disability. *Paediatrics and Child Health*, 25(10): 450–7.

Fowler, J (2011) Supporting Self and Others: From Staff Nurse to Nurse Consultant: Part 4 Mentoring. *British Journal of Nursing*, 20(12): 765.

Francis, R (2010) Independent Inquiry into Care Provided by Mid Staffordshire NHS Foundation Trust January 2005–March 2009. Volume 1. [online] Available at: https://assets.publishing.service.gov.uk/government/uploads/system/uploads/attachment_data/file/279109/0375_i.pdf (accessed 26 January 2022).

Francis, R (2013) Report of the Mid-Staffordshire NHS Foundation Trust Public Inquiry. [online] Available at: www.gov.uk/government/publications/report-of-the-mid-staffordshire-nhs-foundation-trust-public-inquiry (accessed 8 February 2022).

Frankena, T, Naaldenberg, J, Cardol, M, Garcia-Iriarte, E, Buchner, T, Brooker, K, Embregts, P, Joosa, E, Crowther, F, Fudge Schormans, S, Schippers, A, Walmsley, J, O'Brien, P, Linehan, C, Northway, R, van Schrojenstein Lantman-de Walk, H and Leusink, G (2019) A Consensus Statement on How to Conduct Inclusive Health Research. *Journal of Intellectual Disability Research*, 63(1): 1–11.

Gates, B (2011) The Valued People Project: User Views of Learning Disability Nursing. *British Journal of Nursing*, 19(22): 1396–403.

Gates, B and Atherton, H (2001) The Challenge of Evidence-based Practice for Learning Disabilities. *British Journal of Nursing*, 10(8): 517–22.

Gates, B, Fearns, D and Welch, J (2015) *Learning Disability Nursing at a Glance*. Oxford: Wiley.

General Nursing Council for England and Wales (1970) *Syllabus of Subjects for Examination and Record of Practical Instruction and Experience for the Certificate of Nursing the Mentally Subnormal*. London: GNC.

Glover, G, Williams, R, Tompkins, G and Oyinlola, J (2019) An Observational Study of the Use of Acute Hospital Care by People with Intellectual Disabilities in England. *Journal of Intellectual Disability Research*, 63(2): 85–99.

Goleman, G (2020) *Emotional Intelligence: Why It Can Matter more than IQ.* 25th Anniversary Edition. London: Bloomsbury Publishing.

Gopee, N and Galloway, J (2017) *Leadership and Management in Healthcare*, 3rd edition. London: Sage.

Gould, S and Dodd, K (2013) Normal People Can Have a Child but Disability Can't: The Experiences of Mothers with Mild Learning Disabilities Who Have Had Their Children Removed. *British Journal of Learning Disabilities*, 42(1): 25–35.

Gov.uk (1989) *Children Act 1989.* [online] www.legislation.gov.uk/ukpga/1989/41 (accessed 18 April 2022).

Gov.uk (2005) *Mental Capacity Act 2005* [online] Available at: www.legislation.gov.uk/ukpga/2005/9/pdfs/ukpga_20050009_en.pdf (accessed 16 February 2022).

Gov.uk (2010) *Equality Act 2010.* [online] Available at: www.legislation.gov.uk/ukpga/2010/15/contents (accessed 30 November 2021).

Graham, Y N H, Wilson, R, Hayes, C, Stephenson, L, Wanless, A and Baker, L (2020) The Role of Learning Disability Nurses in Providing End-of-Life Care. *Nursing Times*, 116(12): 18–20. [online] Available at: http://search.ebscohost.com/login.aspx?direct=true&db=rzh&AN=147569462&site=ehost-live (accessed 3 May 2021).

Gray, J (2015) Strengthening Leadership in Learning Disability Nursing. *Learning Disability Practice*, 18(5): 34–8.

Gray, C A and Garand, J D (1993) Social Stories: Improving Responses of Students with Autism with Accurate Social Information. *Journal of Autism and Developmental Disorders*, 8(1): 1–10.

Greene, R W (2005) *The Explosive Child: A New Approach for Understanding and Parenting Easily Frustrated and Chronically Inflexible Children*, 6th edition. New York: HarperCollins.

Griffith, R and Tengnah, C (2020) *Law and Professional Issues in Nursing*, 5th edition, London: Sage.

Griffiths, D, Hingsburger, D, Hoath, J and Ioannou, S (2013). Counterfeit Deviance' Revisited. *Journal of Advanced Research in Intellectual Disabilities*, 26: 471–80.

Griffiths, P, Bennett, J and Smith, E (2009) The Size, Extent and Nature of the Learning Disability Nursing Research Base: A Systematic Scoping Review. *International Journal of Nursing Studies*, 46: 490–507.

Grundy, L (2001) Pathways to Fitness for Practice: National Vocational Qualifications as a Foundation of Competence in Nurse Education. *Nurse Education Today*, 21: 260–5.

Gwellent Cymru/Improvement Cymru (nd) Darparu Gofal Iechyd i Bobl ag Anableddau Dysgu/Delivering Healthcare to People with Learning Disabilities. [online] Available at: https://padlet.com/ImprovementCymru/DeliveringHealthcareLD (accessed 9 June 2022).

Ham, K and Davies, B (2017) 'Just Look at My Face': Co-production of a Positive Behavioural Support Plan. *Learning Disability Practice*, 21(2): 32–6.

Hartnett, L and McNamara, M (2021) Covid-19: Intellectual Disability Nurses and the Role of Networking During a Pandemic. *Learning Disability Practice*. doi:10.7748/ldp.2021.e2154

Hatton, C, Emerson, E, Robertson, J and Baines, S (eds) (2017) The Mental Health of British Adults with Intellectual Impairments Living in General Households. *Journal of Applied Research in Intellectual Disabilities*, 30: 188–97.

Hatton, C, Glover, G, Emerson, E and Brown, I (2016) People with Learning Disabilities in England 2015: Main Report. [online] Available at: https://assets.publishing.service.gov.uk/government/uploads/system/uploads/attachment_data/file/613182/PWLDIE_2015_main_report_NB090 517.pdf (accessed 8 December 2021).

Health Foundation (2015a) *Using Communication Approaches to Spread Improvement*. London: The Health Foundation.

Health Foundation (2015b) *Evaluation: What to Consider*. London: The Health Foundation.

Henderson, V (1966) *The Nature of Nursing: A Definition and Its Implications for Practice, Research, and Education*. New York: Macmillan Publishing.

Hermans, H and Evenhuis, H (2014) Multimorbidity in Older Adults with Intellectual Disabilities. *Research in Developmental Disabilities*, 35: 776–83.

Heslop, P, Blair, P, Fleming, P, Hoghton, M, Marriott, A and Russ, L (2013) *Confidential Inquiry into Premature Deaths of People with Learning Disabilities*. Bristol: Norah Fry Research Centre, University of Bristol.

Hirst, R and Irvine, J (2020) Role of a Learning Disability Nursing Network in Developing Students' Skills. *Learning Disability Practice*. doi:10.7748/ldp.2020.e1991

HM Government (2005) *Mental Capacity Act 2005*. London: The Stationary Office.

Hollins, S, Horrocks, C and Sinason, V (2009) *I Can Get through It*. London: RCPsych Publications/ St George's University.

Hollins, S W and Banks, R (2015) *How Good Is My Care?* London: Beyond Words.

Hopes, P (2016) Talking about Death and Dying. *Learning Disability Practice*, 19(8): 12.

Horan, P (2004) Exploring Orem's Self-care Deficit Nursing Theory in Learning Disability Nursing: Philosophical Parity Paper: Part 1. *Learning Disability Practice*, 7(4): 28–33.

House of Lords and House of Commons Joint Committee on Human Rights (2008) *A Life Like Any Other? Human Rights of Adults with Learning Disabilities*. [online] Available at: https://publications.parliament.uk/pa/jt200708/jtselect/jtrights/40/40i.pdf (accessed 4 March 2021).

Humphreys, L, Bigby, C and Iacono, T (2020) Dimensions of Group Home Culture as Predictors of Quality of Life Outcomes. *Journal of Applied Research in Intellectual Disabilities*, 33: 1284–95.

Hutchinson, N and Bodicoat, A (2015) The Effectiveness of Intensive Interaction: A Systematic Literature Review. *Journal of Applied Research in Intellectual Disabilities*, 28(6): 437–54.

Iacono, T and Carling-Jenkins, R (2012) The Human Rights Context for Ethical Requirements for Involving People with Intellectual Disability in Medical Research. *Journal of Intellectual Disability Research*, 56(11): 1122–32.

Ingham-Broomfield, B (2020) A Nurses' Guide to Using Models of Reflection, *Australian Journal of Nursing*, 38(4): 62–7.

International Council of Nurses (2021) *Nurses a Voice to Lead. A Vision for Future Healthcare*. [online] Available at: www.icn.ch/system/files/2021-07/ICN%20Toolkit_2021_ENG_Final.pdf (accessed 10 February 2022).

Iorizzo, J and Ames, S (2019) Planning, Implementing and Evaluating Reflective Nursing Care. In Moulster, G, Iorizzo, J, Ames, S and Kernohan, J (eds) *The Moulster and Griffiths Learning Disability Nursing Model: A Framework for Practice* (pp 55–66). London: Jessica Kingsley Publishers.

Jain, A G, Renu, G, D'Souza, P and Shukri, R (2011) Personal and Professional Networking: A Way Forward in Achieving Quality Nursing Care. *International Journal of Nursing Education,* 3(1): 1–3.

Joanna Briggs Institute (JBI) (nd) Critical Appraisal Tools. [online] Available at: jbi.global/critical-appraisal-tools (accessed 8 June 2022).

Johnson, D (2017) A Best Fit Model of Trauma-informed Care for Young People in Residential and Secure Services: Findings from a 2016 Winston Churchill Memorial Trust Fellowship. Mental Health Foundation. [online] Available at: www.kibble.org/wp-content/uploads/2017/08/best-fit-model-trauma-informed-care.pdf (accessed 25 June 2021).

Jolley, J (2020) *Introducing Research and Evidence-based Practice for Nursing and Healthcare Professionals* (3rd ed). Abingdon: Routledge.

Jones, B, Horton, T and Warburton, W (2019) *The Improvement Journey.* London: The Health Foundation.

Jones, K (1972) Better Services for the Mentally Handicapped. In Jones, K (ed) *The Year Book of Social Policy in Britain 1971* (pp 187–203). London: Routledge and Kegan Paul.

Jukes, M and Aspinall, S L (2015) Leadership and Learning Disability Nursing. *British Journal of Nursing,* 24(18): 912–16.

Kalseth, J and Halvorsen, T (2020) Health and Care Service Utilisation and Cost over the Life-Span: A Descriptive Analysis of Population Data. *BMC Health Services Research,* 20(1): 435.

Karas, M and Laud, J (2015) The Communication Needs of People with Profound and Multiple Learning Disabilities. *Optometry in Practice,* 16: 2.

Kay, B (1994) People with Learning Disabilities. In Tschudin, V (ed) *Ethics. Nursing People with Special Needs Part 2* (pp 1–43). London: Scutari Press.

Kay, B (1995) Grasping the Research Nettle in Learning Disabilities Nursing. *British Journal of Nursing,* 4(2): 96–8.

Kennedy, P and Huntley, D (2021) Nine Former Hospital Staff to Stand Trial in 2023 Over Abuse Allegations. *Teesside News.* [online] Available at: www.gazettelive.co.uk/news/teesside-news/whorlton-hall-staff-face-trial-22393272 (accessed 8 June 2022).

King, R D, Raynes, N and Tizard, J (1971) *Patterns of Residential Care. Sociological Studies in Institutions for Handicapped Children.* London: Routledge and Kegan Paul.

King, R, Taylor, B, Talpur, A, Jackson, C, Manley, K, Ashby, N, Tod, A, Ryan, T, Wood, E, Senek, M and Robertson, S (2020) Factors that Optimise the Impact of Continuing Professional Development in Nursing: A Rapid Evidence Review. *Nurse Education Today,* 98. doi:10.1016/j.nedt.2020.104652

King's Fund (2011) *The Future of Leadership and Management in the NHS: No More Heroes.* London: King's Fund.

King's Fund (2013) *Patient Centred Leadership. Rediscovering our Purpose.* [online] Available at: www.kingsfund.org.uk/sites/default/files/field/field_publication_file/patient-centred-leadership-rediscovering-our-purpose-may13.pdf (accessed 12 February 2022).

Kolyva, K, Butt, N and Eames, J (2018) *Fostering Student Leadership.* [online] Available at: www.councilofdeans.org.uk/wp-content/uploads/2018/12/COD.Student.leadership.programme_2-002-1.pdf (accessed 12 February 2022).

Kotter, J P (2014) *Accelerate: Building Strategic Agility for a Faster-Moving World.* Boston: Harvard Business Review Press.

Krahn, G and Fox, M H (2014) Health Disparities of Adults with Intellectual Disabilities: What Do We Know? What Do We Do? *Journal of Applied Research in Intellectual Disabilities,* 27: 431–46.

Krahn, G L (2019) A Call for Better Data on Prevalence and Health Surveillance of People with Intellectual and Developmental Disabilities. *Intellectual and Developmental Disabilities,* 57(5): 357–75.

Krahn, G L and Havercamp, S M (2019) From Invisible to Visible to Valued: Improving Population Health of People with Intellectual and Developmental Disabilities. *Intellectual and Developmental Disabilities,* 57(5): 476–81.

Kurt, S (2021) Theory X and Theory Y, Douglas McGregor. [online] Available at: https://educationlibrary.org/theory-x-and-theory-y-douglas-mcgregor/ (accessed 31 January 2022).

Laming, W H (2003) *The Victoria Climbie Inquiry: Report of an Inquiry by Lord Laming (Cm. 5730).* London: The Stationery Office.

Lancaster, G A and McCray, G (2020) Using Evidence from Quantitative Studies. In Craig, J and Dowding, D A (eds) *Evidence-based Practice in Nursing,* 4th edition (pp 72–94). Edinburgh: Elsevier.

Learning Disabilities Mortality Review (LeDeR), The LeDer Programme (2019) University of Bristol, Norah Fry Research Centre for Disability Studies, Annual Report. [online] Available at: www.england.nhs.uk/wp-content/uploads/2019/05/action-from-learning.pdf?msclkid=b1d5e694bf1111ec89d4d0c23195fc3a (accessed 25 June 2021).

Learning Disability Senate (2020) Top 10 Tips for Trauma Informed Approaches. [online] Available at: www.bild.org.uk/wp-content/uploads/2020/03/Top-10-tips-re-trauma-informed-care.pdf (accessed 25 September 2021).

Ledderer, L, Kjær, M, Madsen, E K, Busch, J, and Fage-Butler, A (2020) Nudging in Public Health Lifestyle Interventions: A Systematic Literature Review and Metasynthesis. *Health Education Behaviour,* 47(5): 749–64.

LeDeR (2021a) *Annual Report 2020.* [online] Available at: http://www.bristol.ac.uk/media-library/sites/sps/leder/LeDeR%20programme%20annual%20report%2013.05.2021%20FINAL.pdf (accessed 8 December 2021).

LeDeR (2021b) *Learning from Lives and Deaths – People with a Learning Disability and Autistic People.* [online] Available at: www.england.nhs.uk/learning-disabilities/improving-health/mortality-review/ (accessed 8 June 2022).

Lewin, K (1951) *Field Theory in Social Science.* New York: Harper and Row.

Liao, P, Vajdic, C, Troller, J and Reppermund, S (2021) Prevalence and Incidence of Physical Health Conditions in People with Intellectual Disability – A Systematic Review. *PLoS ONE,* 16(8): e0256294. https://doi.org/10.1371/journal.pone.0256294

Local Government Association (2013) Changing Behaviours in Public Health: To nudge or to shove? [online] Available at: https://pas.gov.uk/sites/default/files/documents/changing-behaviours-publi-6c6.pdf (accessed 25 June 2022).

Lord, M (2002) Making a Difference: The Implications for Nurse Education. *Nursing Times,* 98(20): 38.

Lovaas, O (1981) *Teaching Developmentally Disabled Children: The Me Book.* Austin, TX: Pro-Ed, Inc.

Lynne, P (2020) How I Make the Emergency Department Less Daunting: Lauren Johnston Describes Her Work as a Newly Qualified Learning Disability Nurse in a Pioneering Nursing Role. *Emergency Nurse*, 28(5): 14.

Mafuba, K and Gates, B (2013) An Investigation into the Public Health Roles of Community Learning Disability Nurses. *British Journal of Learning Disabilities*, 43(1): 1–7.

Magana, S, Parish, S, Morales, M A, Li, H and Fujiura, G (2016) Racial and Ethnic Health Disparities Among People with Intellectual and Developmental Disabilities. *Intellectual and Developmental Disabilities*, 54(3): 161–72.

Maguire, R, Wilson, A and Jahoda, A (2018) Talking About Learning Disability: Promoting Positive Perceptions of People with Intellectual Disabilities in Scottish Schools. *International Journal of Developmental Disabilities*, 65(4): 257–64. [online] Available at: https://pureportal.strath.ac.uk/files/81370538/Maguire_etal_IJDD_2018_Talking_about_learning_disability_promoting_positive_perceptions.pdf (accessed 25 June 2021).

Malcomess, K (ed) (2015) The Care Aims Intended Outcomes Framework. Collaborative Decision-making for Well-being. [online] Available at: https://careaims.com/wp/wp-content/uploads/2015/06/Care-Aims-Intended-Outcome-Framework-Summary-updated-2015.pdf (accessed 30 November 2021).

Mansel, B and Einon, A (2019) 'It's the Relationship You Develop with Them': Emotional Intelligence in Nurse Leadership. A Qualitative Study. *British Journal of Nursing*, 28(21): 1400–8.

Marks, L, Hunter, D J and Alderslade, R (2011) *Strengthening Public Health Capacity in Europe. A Concept Paper.* [online] Available at: www.euro.who.int/__data/assets/pdf_file/0007/152683/e95877.pdf (accessed 7 December 2021).

Marmot, M, Allen, J, Boyce, T, Goldblatt, P and Morrison, J (2020) *Health Equity in England: The Marmot Review Ten Years On*. London: Institute of Health Equity. [online] Available at: www.health.org.uk/sites/default/files/2020-03/Health%20Equity%20in%0England_The%20Marmot%20Review%2010%20Years%20On_executive%20summary_web.pdf (accessed 7 December 2021).

Marmot, M, Allen, J, Goldblatt, P, Boyce, T, McNeish, D, Grady, M and Geddes, I (2010) *Fair Society Healthy Lives. The Marmot Review*. [online] Available at: www.instituteofhealthequity.org/resources-reports/fair-society-healthy-lives-the-marmot-review/fair-society-healthy-lives-full-report-pdf.pdf (accessed 7 December 2021).

Marshall-Tate, K, Chaplin, E, Ali, S and Hardy, S (2019) Learning Disabilities: Supporting People in the Criminal Justice System. *Nursing Times*, 115(7): 22–6. [online] Available at: https://cdn.ps.emap.com/wp-content/uploads/sites/3/2019/06/190619-Learning-disabilities-supporting-people-in-the-criminal-justice-system.pdf?msclkid=fd56d58cbf0c11ec8d81c17f25129b10 (accessed 14 April 2022).

Maslin-Prothero, S and Finney, A (2011) Long-Term Conditions. In Linsley, P, Kane, R and Owen, S (eds) *Nursing for Public Health. Promotion, Principles and Practice* (pp 260–70). Oxford: Oxford University Press.

Maslow, A H (1954) *Motivation And Personality*. New York: Harper and Row.

Maulik, P K, Mascarenhas, M N, Mathers, C D, Dua, T and Saxena, S (2011) Prevalence of Intellectual Disability: A Meta-Analysis of Population-based Studies. *Research in Developmental Disabilities*, 32: 419–36.

Maushe, E (2020) Blog: Caring for women with learning disabilities. Nursing and Midwifery Council. [online] Available at: www.nmc.org.uk/news/news-and-updates/blog-caring-for-women-with-learning-disabilities/ (accessed 8 June 2022).

May, R (2021) *Making Research Matter. Chief Nursing Officer for England's Strategic Plan for Research*. [online] Available at: www.england.nhs.uk/publication/making-research-matter-chief-nursing-officer-for-englands-strategic-plan-for-research/ (accessed 18 January 2022).

Mazza, M G, Rossetti, A, Crespi, G and Clerici, M (2019) Prevalence of Co-occurring Psychiatric Disorders in Adults and Adolescents with Intellectual Disability: A Systematic Review and Meta-Analysis. *Journal of Applied Research in Intellectual Disabilities*, 33: 126–38.

McCarron, M, McCallion, P, Reilly, E and Mulryan, N (2014) A Prospective 14-Year Longitudinal Follow-Up of Dementia in Persons with Down Syndrome. *Journal of Intellectual Disability Research*, 58(1): 61–70.

McCarron, M, Sheerin, F, Roche, L, Ryan, A M, Griffiths, C, Keenan, P, Doody, O, D'Eath, M, Burke, E and McCallion, P (2018) *Shaping the Future of Intellectual Disability Nursing in Ireland*. Ireland: Health Services Executive. [online] Available at: https://healthservice.hse.ie/filelibrary/onmsd/shaping-the-future-of-intellectual-disability-nursing-in-ireland-2018.pdf (accessed 17 April 2022).

McClimens, A, Brennan, S and Hargreaves, P (2015) Hearing Problems in the Learning Disability Population: Is Anybody Listening? *British Journal of Learning Disabilities*, 43(3): 153–60.

McDaniels, B and Fleming, A (2016) Sexuality Education and Intellectual Disability: Time to Address the Challenge. *Sexuality and Disability*, 34: 215–25.

McGill, P (2021) Information Sheet Understanding Challenging Behaviour: Part 1. The Challenging Behaviour Foundation. [online] Available at: www.challengingbehaviour.org.uk/wp-content/uploads/2021/02/001-Understanding-Challenging-Behaviour-Part-1.pdf (accessed 21 November 2021).

McGill, P, Bradshaw, J, Smyth, G, Hurman, M and Roy, A (2020) Capable Environments. *Tizard Learning Disability Review*, 25(3): 109–16.

McGrath, A and Yeowart, C (2009) Rights of Passage: Supporting Disabled Young People through the transition to Adulthood. New Philanthropy Capital. [online] Available at: www.thinknpc.org/wp-content/uploads/2018/07/Rights-of-passage-1.pdf (accessed 16 June 2021).

McMahon, A and Hoong Sin, C (2013) Introduction to Economic Assessment. *Nursing Management*, 20(7): 32–8.

Medway Council v A & Ors (Learning Disability; Foster Placement) (2015) EWFC B66. [online] Available at: www.bailii.org/ew/cases/EWFC/OJ/2015/B66.html (accessed 18 April 2022).

Mee, S (2012) *Valuing People with a Learning Disability*. Penrith: M&K Publishing.

Mencap (2015) Communicating with People with Profound and Multiple Learning Disabilities (PMLD). [online] Available at: www.jpaget.nhs.uk/media/104336/Communicating_with_people_with_PMLD__a_guide__1_.pdf (accessed 10 April 2021).

Mental Welfare Commission for Scotland (2019) *Person Centred Care Plans: Good Practice Guide*. [online] Available at: www.mwcscot.org.uk/sites/default/files/2019-11/PersonCentredCarePlans_GoodPracticeGuide_August2019_6.pdf (accessed 20 January 2022).

Millar, E (2021) Leadership Principles for Health and Social Care in Wales. [online] Available at: https://leadershipportal.heiw.wales/repository/discovery/resource/604d8589-498a-48ae-a2cd-637613078929/en?sort=recommended&strict=0 (accessed 22 June 2022).

Mitchell, D (2000) Parallel Stigma? Nurses and People with Learning Disabilities. *British Journal of Learning Disabilities*, 28: 78–81.

Mitchell, D (2001) Nursing and Social Policy in the 1930s: A Discussion of Mental Deficiency Nursing. *International History of Nursing Journal*, 6(1): 56–61.

Mitchell, D (2003) A Chapter in the History of Nurse Education: Learning Disability Nursing and the Jay Report. *Nurse Education Today*, 23: 350–6.

Mitchell, D (2004) Learning Disability Nursing. *British Journal of Learning Disabilities*, 32: 115–18.

Mitchell, D (2019) A Century of Learning Disability Nursing. *Learning Disability Practice*, 22(1): 11–13.

Mitchell, D and Smith, P (2003) Learning from the Past: Emotional Labour and Learning Disability Nursing. *Journal of Intellectual Disabilities*, 7(2): 109–17.

Montalvo, W (2015) Political Skill and Its Relevance to Nursing. *Journal of Nursing Administration*, 45(7/8): 377–83.

Mooney, D, Hartley, K, McAnespie, L, Crocker, A, Mander, C, Elliot, A, Burnett, C A, Hazel, G, Bayliss, R, Beazley, S and Tucker, S (2016) Inclusive Communication and the Role of Speech and Language Therapy Royal College of Speech and Language Therapists Position Paper. [online] Available at: www.rcslt.org/wp-content/uploads/2021/02/20162209_InclusiveComms_final.pdf (accessed 7 April 2021).

Moore, C (2020) Nurse Leadership During a Crisis: Ideas to Support You and Your Team. *Nursing Times*, 116(12): 34–7. [online] Available at: www.nursingtimes.net/clinical-archive/leadership/nurse-leadership-during-a-crisis-ideas-to-support-you-and-your-team-16-11-2020/ (accessed 18 April 2022).

Morris, P (1969) *Put Away*. London: Routledge and Kegan Paul.

Moulster, G, Ames, S, Iorizzo, J and Kernohan, J (2019) A Flexible Model to Support Person-Centred Learning Disability Nursing. *Nursing Times*, 115(6): 56–9. [online] Available at: www.nursingtimes.net/roles/learning-disability-nurses/a-flexible-model-to-support-person-centred-learning-disability-nursing-13-05-2019/?msclkid=30ec9b24bf0511ecb5a79b4acedeb897 (accessed 14 April 2022).

Moulster, G and Atkinson, D (2019) Effective Outcome Measurement: A Complex Challenge for Learning Disability Nurses. In Moulster, G, Iorizzo, J, Ames, S and Kernohan (eds) *The Moulster and Griffiths Learning Disability Nursing Model: A Framework for Practice* (pp 75–82). London: Jessica Kingsley Publishers.

Mughal, A F (2014) Understanding and Using the Mental Capacity Act. *Nursing Times*, 110(21): 16–18.

National Audit Office (1992) *Nursing Education: Implementation of Project 2000 in England*. [online] Available at: www.nao.org.uk/pubsarchive/wp-content/uploads/sites/14/2018/11/Nursing-Education-Implementation-of-Project-2000-in-England.pdf (accessed 9 April 2022).

National Boards for England and Wales (1985) *Syllabus of Training Professional Register – Part 5. Registered Nurses for the Mentally Handicapped 1982*. London: English National Board for Nursing.

National Collaborating Centre for Determinants of Health (2015) *Let's Talk: Advocacy and Health Equity*. [online] Available at: https://nccdh.ca/images/uploads/comments/Advocacy_EN.pdf (accessed 8 December 2021).

National Institute for Health and Care Excellence (NICE) (2015) *Challenging Behaviour and Learning Disabilities: Prevention and Interventions for People with Learning Disabilities Whose Behaviour Challenges* (NICE guideline 11). [online] Available at: www.nice.org.uk/guidance/ng11 (accessed 8 June 2022).

National Institute for Health and Care Excellence (NICE) (2018) *Learning Disabilities and Behaviour that Challenges: Service Design and Delivery* (NICE guideline 93). [online] Available at: www.nice.org.uk/guidance/ng93/resources/learning-disabilities-and-behaviour-that-challenges-service-design-and-delivery-pdf-1837753480645 (accessed 8 June 2022).

National Institute for Health and Care Excellence (NICE) (2020) *Covid-19 Rapid Guideline: Critical Care in Adults*. [online] Available at: www.nice.org.uk/guidance/ng159/resources/covid19-rapid-guideline-critical-care-in-adults-pdf-66141848681413 (accessed 6 March 2021).

Naylor, C, Das, P, Ross S, Honeyman, M, Thonpson, J and Gilburt, H (2016) Bringing Together Physical and Mental Health: A New Frontier for Integrated Care. [online] Available at: www.kingsfund.org.uk/sites/default/files/field/field_publication_file/Bringing-together-Kings-Fund-March-2016_1.pdf (accessed 25 June 2022).

Ndadzungira, C (2016) People with Learning Disabilities Want to Find Love Too. The Conversation. [online] Available at: https://theconversation.com/people-with-learning-disabilities-want-to-find-love-too-54444 (accessed 3 May 2021).

The NHS Confederation (2020) What We Have Learned so far Best Practice and Innovation During COVID-19. [online] Available at: www.nhsconfed.org/sites/default/files/media/NHS%20Reset_Best%20practice%20and_innovation_FNL.pdf (accessed 31 January 2022).

NHS Digital (2021) Health and Care of People with Learning Disabilities Experimental Statistics 2019 to 2020. [online] Available at: https://digital.nhs.uk/data-and-information/publications/statistical/health-and-care-of-people-with-learning-disabilities/experimental-statistics-2019-to-2020 (accessed 20 November 2021).

NHS England (2016a) Accessible Information Standard. [online] Available at: www.england.nhs.uk/wp-content/uploads/2017/08/accessilbe-info-specification-v1-1.pdf (accessed 25 January 2021).

NHS England (2016b). *Stop the Over Medication of People with a Learning Disability (STOMPwLD)*. London: NHS England.

NHS England (2017) The Fifteen Step Challenge: Quality from a Patient's Perspective; An Inpatient Toolkit. [online] Available at: www.england.nhs.uk/wp-content/uploads/2017/11/15-steps-inpatient.pdf (accessed 1 February 2022).

NHS England (2018) STOMP – Stopping the Over Medication of People with a Learning Disability, Autism or Both. [online] Available at: www.england.nhs.uk/publication/stomp-stopping-the-over-medication-of-people-with-a-learning-disability-autism-or-both/ (accessed 21 June 2021).

NHS England (2020) Learning Disability and Autism, Dementia and Mental Health: Patient, Carer and Family Engagement and Communication During the Coronavirus (COVID-19) Pandemic. [online] Available at: HYPERLINK "http://www.england.nhs.uk/coronavirus/wp-content/uploads/sites/52/2020/03/C0590-Patient-carer-and-family-engagement-and-communication-during-the-coronavirus-COVID-19-pandemic.pdf" www.england.nhs.uk/coronavirus/wp-content/uploads/sites/52/2020/03/C0590-Patient-carer-and-family-engagement-and-communication-during-the-coronavirus-COVID-19-pandemic.pdf (accessed 25 June 2022).

NHS Health Careers (nd) *Personal Development Planning*. [online] Available at: www.healthcareers.nhs.uk/career-planning/developing-your-health-career/developing-your-health-career/personal-development-planning/personal-development-planning (accessed 20 February 2022).

NHS Improvement (2015) Five Whys. [online] Available at: www.england.nhs.uk/improvement-hub/wp-content/uploads/sites/44/2015/08/learning-handbook-five-whys.pdf (accessed 3 April 2022).

NHS Improvement (2018) Plan, Do, Study, Act (PDSA) Cycles and the Model for Improvement. [online] Available at: https://improvement.nhs.uk/resources/pdsa-cycles (accessed 3 April 2022).

NHS Leadership Academy (2013) *Healthcare Leadership Model. The Nine Dimensions of Leadership Behaviour.* [online] Available at: www.leadershipacademy.nhs.uk/resources/healthcare-leadership-model/nine-leadership-dimensions/ (accessed 9 February 2022).

NHS Wales (2015) Health and Care Standards. [online] Available at: www.wales.nhs.uk/sitesplus/documents/1064/24729_Health%20Standards%20Framework_2015_E1.pdf (accessed 25 June 2022).

NHS Wales and Social Care Wales (2021) *Compassionate Leadership Principles for Health and Social Care in Wales.* [online] Available at: https://leadershipportal.heiw.wales/api/stor age/2362a9e9-4682-495c-abb4-bd5eab47b133/Leadership%20Principles%20for%20Hea lth%20and%20Social%20Care%20in%20Wales.pdf?preview=true (accessed 29 January 2022).

NHSE/NHSI (2021) *Care Programme Approach NHS England and NHS Improvement Position Statement.* [online] Available at: www.england.nhs.uk/wp-content/uploads/2021/07/Care-Progra mme-Approach-Position-Statement_FINAL_2021.pdf?fbclid=IwAR2K9vEkOVHKWUpfMcFAlg6V1na O76AdVFl3Mi42BO2_9ieOPRb8Rs-G6qw (accessed 20 January 2022).

NICE (2018a) Learning Disabilities and Behaviour that Challenges: Service Design and Delivery. [online] Available at: www.nice.org.uk/guidance/ng93 (accessed 21 June 2021).

NICE (2018b) Overview | Care and Support of People Growing Older with Learning Disabilities. [online] Available at: www.nice.org.uk/guidance/ng96 (accessed 21 June 2021).

NICE (2019) Learning Disability: Care and Support of People Growing Older [QS187]. [online] Available at: www.nice.org.uk/guidance/qs187 (accessed 21 June 2021).

NICE (2020) NICE Updates Rapid COVID-19 Guideline on Critical Care. [online] Available at: www. nice.org.uk/news/article/nice-updates-rapid-covid-19-guideline-on-critical-care (accessed 21 June 2021).

NICE (2021) Shared Decision Making. [online] Available at: www.nice.org.uk/guidance/ng197? fbclid=IwAROJTWG71KrV2FLI9js-1QyA2AneFgY8_XtKuW5jNPEB8_TUqWfTIjSTxwc (accessed 8 June 2022).

NICE Guideline [NG197], (2021) https://www.nice.org.uk/guidance/ng197?fbclid=I wAROJTWG71KrV2FLI9js-1QyA2AneFgY8_XtKuW5jNPEB8_TUqWfTIjSTxwc

Nicol, J S and Dosser, I (2016) Understanding Reflective Practice. *Nursing Standard*, 30(36): 34–40.

Nirje, B (1980) The Normalization Principle. In Flynn, R J and Nitsch, K E (eds) *Normalization, Social Integration and Community Services* (pp 31–49). Baltimore: University Park Press.

Northouse, P G (2019) *Leadership Theory and Practice*, 8th edition. London: Sage.

Northway, R (2019) Moving Models: Leading Through Constant Change. In Sheerin, F and Curtis, E A (eds) *Leadership in Intellectual Disability Service. Motivating Change and Improvement* (pp 23– 43). Abingdon: Routledge.

Northway, R, Hurley, K, O'Connor, C, Thomas, H, Howarth, J, Langley, E and Bale, S (2014a) Deciding What to Research: An Overview of a Participatory Workshop. *British Journal of Learning Disabilities*, 42(4): 323–7.

Northway, R, Howarth, J and Evans, L (2014b) Participatory Research, People with Intellectual Disabilities and Ethical Approval: Making Reasonable Adjustments to Enable Participation. *Journal of Clinical Nursing*, 24: 573–81.

Nunkoosing, K (2011) The Social Construction of Learning Disability. In Atherton, H L and Crickmore, D J (eds) *Learning Disabilities Toward Inclusion*, 6th edition. Croydon: Churchill Livingstone. Elsevier.

Nursing and Midwifery Council (NMC) (2003) *Memorandum*. [online] Available at: https://publications.parliament.uk/pa/ld200304/ldselect/ldconst/68/68we53.htm#:~:text=2.,who lly%20appointed%20by%20the%20government (accessed 11 April 2022).

Nursing and Midwifery Council (NMC) (2018a) *Standards of Proficiency for Registered Nurses*. [online] Available at: www.nmc.org.uk/standards/standards-for-nurses/standards-of-proficiency-for-registered-nurses/ (accessed 30 April 2022).

Nursing and Midwifery Council (NMC) (2018b) *The Code Professional Standards of Practice and Behaviour for Nurses, Midwives and Nursing Associates*. [online] Available at: www.nmc.org.uk/globalassets/sitedocuments/nmc-publications/nmc-code.pdff

Nursing and Midwifery Council (NMC) (2019a) *How to Revalidate with the NMC. Requirements for Renewing Your Registration*. [online] Available at: www.nmc.org.uk/globalassets/sitedocuments/revalidation/how-to-revalidate-booklet.pdf#page=23 (accessed 7 March 2022).

Nursing and Midwifery Council (NMC) (2019b) *How to Revalidate with the NMC: Requirements for Renewing Your Registration*. [online] Available at: www.nmc.org.uk/globalassets/sitedocuments/revalidation/how-to-revalidate-booklet.pdf (accessed 18 April 2022).

Nursing and Midwifery Council (NMC) (2019c) *Guidance on Using Social Media Responsibly*. London: Nursing and Midwifery Council.

Nursing and Midwifery Council (NMC) (2020) *Principles for Preceptorship*. [online] Available at: www.nmc.org.uk/globalassets/sitedocuments/nmc-publications/nmc-principles-for-preceptorship-a5.pdf (accessed 7 March 2022).

O'Leary, L, Cooper, S A and Hughes-McCormack, L (2018) Early Death and Causes of Death of People with Intellectual Disabilities: A Systematic Review. *Journal of Applied Research in Intellectual Disabilities*, 31: 325–42.

Open University (2022) *Timeline of Learning Disability History*. [online] Available at: www.open.ac.uk/health-and-social-care/research/shld/timeline-learning-disability-history (accessed 18 April 2022).

Orem, D E (1991) *Nursing: Concepts of Practice*, 4th edition. St. Louis: Mosby Year Book Inc.

Orenstein, G A and Lewis, L (2020) Eriksons Stages of Psychosocial Development. [online] Available at: www.ncbi.nlm.nih.gov/books/NBK556096/ (accessed 18 April 2022).

Owenson, W (2018) For Whom We Serve. *Learning Disability Practice*, 21(2): 15.

Parahoo, K, Barr, O and McCaughan, E (2000) Research Utilization and Attitudes Towards Research Among Learning Disability Nurses in Northern Ireland. *Journal of Advanced Nursing*, 31(3): 607–13.

Parrish, A and Sines, D (1997) Future Directions for Learning Disability Nursing. *British Journal of Nursing*, 6(19): 1122–4.

Perry, B D and Winfrey, O (2021) *What Happened to You? Conversations on Trauma, Resilience, and Healing*. London: Flatiron Books.

Piaget, J and Cook, M T (1952) *The Origins of Intelligence in Children.* New York: International University Press.

Plomin, J (2019) Whorlton Hall Hospital Abuse and How It Was Uncovered. *BBC Panorama* [online] Available at: www.bbc.co.uk/news/health-48369500 (accessed 8 June 2022).

Pollard, C L (2015) What Is the Right Thing to Do: Use of a Relational Ethic Framework to Guide Clinical Decision-Making. *International Journal of Caring Sciences*, 8(2): 362–8.

Positive Behavioural Support (PBS) Coalition UK (2015) Positive Behavioural Support: A Competence Framework. [online] Available at: http://pbsacademy.org.uk/wp-content/uploads/2016/11/Positive-Behavioural-Support-Competence-Framework-May-2015.pdf (accessed 26 November 2021).

Powell, M (2019) Inquiries into the British National Health Service. *The Political Quarterly,* 90(2): 180–4.

Professional Association of Nurses in Developmental Disabilities Australia (PANDDA) (2020) *Standards for Nursing Practice 2nd Edition.* [online] Available at: www.pandda.net/files/PANDDA-2020-Standards.pdf

Public Health England (2016) *Making Every Contact Count Consensus Statement.* [online] Available at: https://assets.publishing.service.gov.uk/government/uploads/system/uploads/attachment_data/file/769486/Making_Every_Contact_Count_Consensus_Statement.pdf (accessed 21 November 2021).

Public Health England (2020) Deaths of People Identified as Having Learning Disabilities with COVID-19 in England in the Spring of 2020. [online] https://assets.publishing.service.gov.uk/government/uploads/system/uploads/attachment_data/file/933612/COVID-19__learning_disabilities_mortality_report.pdf (accessed 30 November 2021).

R(J) v Caerphilly County Borough Council (2005) 2 FLR 860. [online] Available at: www.casemine.com/judgement/uk/5a8ff73060d03e7f57ea954a (accessed 24 January 2022).

Regnard, C, Reynolds, J, Watson, B, Matthews, D, Gibson, L and Clarke, C (2007) Understanding Distress in People with Severe Communication Difficulties: Developing and Assessing the Disability Distress Assessment Tool (DisDAT). *Journal of Intellectual Disability Research*, 51(4): 277–92.

Reppermund, S, Srasuebkul, P and Dean, K (2020) Factors Associated with Death in People with Intellectual Disability. *Journal of Applied Research in Intellectual Disability*, 33: 420–9.

Robertson, J, Hatton, C, Emerson, E and Baines, S (2014) The Impact of Health Checks for People with Intellectual Disabilities: An Updated Systematic Review of Evidence. *Research in Developmental Disabilities*, 35: 2450–62.

Rolfe, A (2021) *Mentoring Mindset, Skills and Tools*, 4th edition. Great Britain: Mentoring Works.

Roper, N, Logan, W W and Tierney, A J (1990) *The Elements of Nursing*, 3rd edition. Churchill, Edinburgh: Livingstone.

Rose, S (2021) The Journey to the Promised Land. [online] Available at: https://learningdisabilitynurse.co.uk/learning-disability-resources?rq=rose (accessed 18 April 2022).

Roy, A, Matthews, H, Clifford, P, Fowler, V and Martin, D M (2002) Health of the Nation Outcome Scales for People with Learning Disabilities (HoNOS-LD). Glossary for HoNOS-LD Score Sheet. *British Journal of Psychiatry*, 180: 67–70.

Royal College of General Practitioners (2021) *Health Checks for People with Learning Disabilities Toolkit.* [online] Available at: www.rcgp.org.uk/clinical-and-research/resources/toolkits/health-check-toolkit.aspx (accessed 8 December 2021).

Royal College of Nursing (RCN) (2014) Mental Health in Children and Young People: An RCN Toolkit for Nurses Who Are Not Mental Health Specialists. [online] Available at: www.rcn.org.uk/-/media/Royal-College-Of-Nursing/Documents/Publications/2014/October/PUB-003311.pdf (accessed 25 June 2022).

Royal College of Nursing (RCN) (2018) *RCN Demonstrating Value: Applying the Principles of Economic Assessment in Practice*. London: RCN.

Royal College of Nursing (RCN) (2021) *Connecting for Change; For the Future of Learning Disability Nursing*. London: RCN. [online] Available at: www.rcn.org.uk/professional-development/publications/connecting-for-change-uk-pub-009-467 (accessed 9 February 2022).

Royal College of Nursing Community Nursing Forum for People with a Learning Disability (1992) *The Role and Function of the Domiciliary Nurse for People with a Learning Disability*. London: RCN.

Royal College of Psychiatrists and the British Psychological Society (2016) *Challenging Behaviour: A Unified Approach – Update Clinical and Service Guidelines for Supporting Children, Young People and Adults with Intellectual Disabilities Who Are at Risk of Receiving Abusive or Restrictive Practices. FR/ID/08.* [online] Available at: www.csp.org.uk/system/files/fr_id_08_challenging_behaviour_a_unified_approach_april_2016.pdf (accessed 26 November 2021).

Royal College of Speech and Language Therapists (2013) *Five Good Communication Standards*. London: RCSLT.

Ruiz, S, Giuriceo, K, Caldwell, J, Snyder L P and Putnam, M (2020) Care Coordination Models Improve Quality of Care for Adults Aging With Intellectual and Developmental Disabilities. *Journal of Disability Policy Studies*, 30(4): 191–201.

Ryan, J and Thomas, F (1987) *The Politics of Mental Handicap*. Revised edition, London: Free Association Books.

Sackett, D L, Richardson, W S, Rosenberg, W and Haynes, R B (1997) *Evidence-based Medicine. How to Practice and Teach EBM*. New York: Churchill Livingstone.

Saltmarsh, R, Taylor, C, Bamsey, M, North, G, Roberts, N and Davies K (2016) Developing an Outcome Measure and Feedback Tool for Children with Intellectual Disabilities. *Learning Disability Practice*, 19(7): 19–23.

Samuels, R and Stansfield, J (2011) The Effectiveness of Social Stories™ to Develop Social Interactions with Adults with Characteristics of Autism Spectrum Disorder. *British Journal of Learning Disabilities*, 40: 272–85.

Savarimuthu, D (2020) The Potential of Nurses in Leading Positive Behaviour Support. *British Journal of Nursing*, 29(7): 414–18.

Shalock, R L, Gomez, L E, Verdugo, M A and Claes, C (2017) Evidence and Evidence-based Practices: Are We There Yet? *Intellectual and Developmental Disabilities*, 55(2): 112–19.

Scheffler, J L, Stanley, I and Sachs-Ericsson, N (2020) Aces and Mental Health Outcomes. In Asmundson, G J G and Afifi, T O (eds) *Adverse Childhood Experiences: Using Evidence to Advance Research, Practice, Policy and Prevention* (pp 47–69). London: Elsevier.

Schmidt, E K, Hand, B N, Havercamp, S, Sommerich, C, Weaver, L and Darragh, A (2021) Sex Education Practices for People with Intellectual and Developmental Disabilities: A Qualitative Study. *American Journal of Occupational Therapy*, 75(3): 1–8.

Schwartz, A E, Kramer, J M, Cohn, E S and McDonald, K E (2020) 'That Felt Like Real Engagement': Fostering and Maintaining Inclusive Research Collaborations with Individuals with Intellectual Disability. *Qualitative Health Research*, 30(2): 236–49.

Scorer, D (2022) in Thomas, R (2022) Vulnerable People Denied Vaccines by 'Anti-Vaxxer' Carers and Families. *The Independent*. [online] Available at: www.independent.co.uk/news/health/vulnerable-people-vaccines-antivaxxer-b1990132.html (accessed 24 January 2022).

Scott, K (2017) *Radical Candour*. New York: Macmillan.

Scottish Government (2011) Principles of Inclusive Communication: An Information and Self-Assessment Tool for Public Authorities. [online] Available at: www.gov.scot/publications/principles-inclusive-communication-information-self-assessment-tool-public-authorities/pages/9/ (accessed 26 April 2021).

Scottish Government et al (2012) Strengthening the Commitment: The Report of the UK Modernising Learning Disabilities Nursing Review. [online] Available at: www.gov.scot/publications/strengthening-commitment-report-uk-modernising-learning-disabilities-nursing-review (accessed 14 May 2021).

Scottish Government et al (2015) *Strengthening the Commitment: Living the Commitment*. [online] Available at: www.gov.scot/publications/strengthening-commitment-living-commitment/ (accessed 30 April 2022).

Scottish Government et al (2018) *Sustaining the Commitment. Update Report*. [online] Available at: www.gov.scot/publications/sustaining-commitment/ (accessed 30 April 2022).

Seale, J, Nind, M and Simmons, B (2012) Transforming Positive Risk-taking Practices: The Possibilities for Creativity and Resilience in Learning Disability Contexts. *Scandinavian Journal of Disability Research*, 15(3): 233–48. [online] Available at: www.sjdr.se/articles/10.1080/15017419.2012.703967/ (accessed 21 June 2021).

Silver, S A, McQuillan, R, Harel, Z, Weizman, A V, Thomas, A, Nesrallah, G, Bell, C M, Chan, C T and Chertow, G M (2016) How to Sustain Change and Support Continuous Quality Improvement. *Clinical Journal of the American Society of Nephrology*, 11(5): 916–24. [online] Available at: www.ncbi.nlm.nih.gov/pmc/articles/PMC4858491/ (accessed 3 February 2022).

Sinclair, J, Unruh, D, Lindstrom, L and Scanlon, D (2015) Barriers to Sexuality for Individuals with Intellectual and Developmental Disabilities: A Literature Review. *Education and Training in Autism and Developmental Disabilities*, 50(1): 3–16.

Skills for Health (2014) *A Positive and Proactive Workforce*. London: Department of Health.

Skinner, B F (1953) *Science and Human Behavior*. New York: Free Press.

Smull, M, Sanderson, H and Allen, B (2004) *Essential Lifestyle Planning: A Handbook for Facilitators*. Belfast: North West Training and Development Team.

Solvoll, B A, Hall, E D C and Brinchmann, B S (2015) Ethical Challenges in Everyday Work with Adults with Learning Disabilities. *Nursing Ethics*, 22(4): 417–27.

Stans, S E A, Dalemans, R J P, de Witte, L P, Smeets, H W H and Beurskens, A J (2016) The Role of the Physical Environment in Conversations Between People Who Are Communication Vulnerable and Health-Care Professionals: A Scoping Review. *Disability and Rehabilitation*, 39: 25.

Stephenson, J (2019) A Brief History of Learning Disability Nursing in the UK. *Nursing Times*, 115(4): 11.

Stirton, F D and Heslop, P (2018) Medical Certificates of Cause of Death for People with Intellectual Disabilities: A Systematic Review. *Journal of Applied Research in Intellectual Disability*, 31: 659–68.

Strydom, A, Chan, T, King, M, Hassiotis, A and Livingstone, G (2013) Incidence of Dementia in Older Adults with Intellectual Disabilities. *Research in Developmental Disabilities*, 34: 1881–5.

Sullivan, E J (2012) *Effective Leadership and Management in Nursing*, 8th edition. New Jersey: Pearson.

Sweeney, J and Mitchell, D (2009) A Challenge to Nursing: An Historical Review of Intellectual Disability Nursing in the UK and Ireland. *Journal of Clinical Nursing*, 18: 2754–63.

Syed, M (2016) *Black Box Thinking*. London: John Murray Publishers.

Tee, S (2017) Leadership from the Perspective of the Public. In Taylor, R and Webster-Henderson, B (eds) *The Essentials of Nursing Leadership* (pp 78–93). London: Sage.

Tempest, E (2012) How to Draw up SMART Objectives that Will Work. *Nursing Times*. [online] Available at: www.nursingtimes.net/roles/nurse-managers/how-to-draw-up-smart-objectives-that-will-work-12-10-2012/?fbclid=IwAR2ObHT9XC8X5Ld2hQ9sf8DPwon6Tq1i3GuvXyFmN_OhkNmdnGYkG6W4Mas (accessed 24 January 2022).

Thomas, R (2022) Vulnerable People Denied Vaccines by 'Anti-vaxxer' Carers and Families. *Independent*, 12 January. [online] Available at: www.independent.co.uk/news/health/vulnerable-people-vaccines-antivaxxer-b1990132.html (accessed 21 June 2022).

Thomas-Gregory, A (2017) The Context of Leadership in Practice. In Taylor, R and Webster-Henderson, B (eds) *The Essentials of Nursing Leadership* (pp 17–30). London: Sage.

Thompson, C and Quinian, P (2020) How Can We Develop an Evidence-based Culture? In Craig, J and Dowding, D A (eds) *Evidence-based Practice in Nursing* (pp 161–80), 4th edition. Edinburgh: Elsevier.

Thompson, I E, Melia, K M and Boyd, K M (2006) *Nursing Ethics*. Edinburgh: Churchill Livingstone.

Tilly, L (2015) Being Researchers for the First Time: Reflections on the Development of an Inclusive Research Group. *British Journal of Learning Disabilities*, 43: 121–7.

Togher, L, Power, E, Tate, R, McDonald, S and Rietdijk, R (2010) Measuring the Social Interactions of People with Traumatic Brain Injury and Their Communication Partners: The Adapted Kagan Scales. *Aphasiology*, 24: 914–27.

Trueland, J (2021) How Nurses Can Tackle Taboos About Sexual Relationships with Adults with Learning Disabilities. Learning Disability Practice. [online] Available at: https://rcni.com/learning-disability-practice/features/how-nurses-can-tackle-taboos-about-sexual-relationships-adults-learning-disabilities-179256 (accessed 25 June 2022).

Tuffrey-Wijne, I (2012) *How to Break Bad News to People with Intellectual Disabilities: A Guide for Carers and Professionals*. London: Jessica Kingsley Publishers.

Tuffrey-Wijne, I, Bernaal, J and Hollins, S (2010) Disclosure and Understanding of Cancer Diagnosis and Prognosis for People with Intellectual Disabilities: Finding from an Ethnographic Study. *European Journal of Oncology Nursing*, 14(3): 224–30.

Tuffrey-Wijne, I and Butler, G (2009) Co-researching with People with Learning Disabilities: An Experience of Involvement in Qualitative Data Analysis. *Health Expectations*, 13: 174–84.

Turnbull-James, K (2011) *Leadership in Context: Lessons from New Leadership Theory and Current Leadership Development Practice.* [online] Available at: www.kingsfund.org.uk/sites/default/files/leadership-in-context-theory-current-leadership-development-practice-kim-turnbull-james-kings-fund-may-2011.pdf (accessed 8 February 2022).

United Kingdom Central Council for Nursing, Midwifery and Health Visiting (UKCC) (1984) *Code of Professional Conduct for the Nurse, Midwife and Health Visitor.* London: UKCC.

United Kingdom Central Council for Nursing, Midwifery and Health Visiting (UKCC) (1998) *Guidelines for Mental Health and Learning Disabilities Nursing.* London: UKCC.

United Kingdom Central Council for Nursing, Midwifery and Health Visiting (UKCC) (1999) *Fitness for Practice.* The UKCC Commission for Nursing and Midwifery Education. London: UKCC.

United Nations (2006) *Convention on the Rights of Persons with Disabilities.* [online] Available at: www.un.org/development/desa/disabilities/convention-on-the-rights-of-persons-with-disabilities.html (accessed 1 March 2021).

Wake, A, Davies, J, Drake, C, Rowbotham, M, Smith, N and Rossiter, R (2020) Keep Safe: Collaborative Practice Development and Research with People with Learning Disabilities. *Tizard Learning Disability Review*, 25(4): 173–80.

Waterworth, C, Willcocks, S G, Roddam, H and Selfe, J (2015) Implementing Care Aims in an Integrated Team. *British Journal of Health Care Management*, 21(1): 36–45.

Watkinson, S (2015) Ethics and Patients' Rights. In Buka, P (ed) *Patients' Rights, Law and Ethics for Nurses* (pp 27–48), 2nd edition. London: CRC Press.

Weberg, D (2012) Complexity Leadership: A Healthcare Imperative. *Nursing Forum*, 47(4): 268–77.

Welsh Government (2016) Nurse Staffing Levels (Wales) Act. [online] Available at: www.legislation.gov.uk/anaw/2016/5/enacted (accessed 3 February 2022).

Welsh Government (2020a) Transforming the Way We Deliver Outpatients in Wales: A Three Year Strategy and Action Plan 2020–2023. [online] Available at: https://gov.wales/sites/default/files/publications/2020-06/transforming-the-way-we-deliver-outpatients-in-wales–a-three-year-strategy-and-action-plan-2020-2023.pdf (accessed 28 January 2022).

Welsh Government (2020b) *Mental Health (Wales) Measure 2010: Quality report.* [online] Available at: https://gov.wales/sites/default/files/statistics-and-research/2020-11/mental-health-wales-measure-2010-quality-report.pdf (accessed 24 January 2022).

Welsh Government (2021a) Locked Out: Liberating Disabled People's Lives and Rights in Wales beyond COVID-19. [online] Available at: https://gov.wales/locked-out-liberating-disabled-peoples-lives-and-rights-wales-beyond-covid-19-html (accessed 20 June 2021).

Welsh Government (2021b). Reducing Restrictive Practice Framework. [online] Available at: https://gov.wales/reducing-restrictive-practices-framework (accessed 3 April 2022).

Welsh Office (1983) *The All Wales Strategy for the Development of Services for Mentally Handicapped People.* Cardiff: Welsh Office.

West, M, Eckert, R, Steward, K and Passmore, B (2014) *Developing Collective Leadership for Healthcare.* London: King's Fund.

West, M A (2021) *Compassionate Leadership: Sustaining Wisdom, Humanity and Presence in Health and Social Care.* UK: Swirling Leaf Press.

Whitehead, M (1991) The Concepts and Principles of Equity and Health. *Health Promotion International*, 6(3): 217–28.

Whitehouse, C et al (2021) Creating a Covid-19 Vaccination Clinic for People with Learning Disabilities. *Nursing Times*, 117(7): 236.

Willis, D (2020) Whorlton Hall, Winterbourne View and Ely Hospital: Learning from Failures. *Learning Disability Practice*, 23(6). doi:10.7748/ldp2020.e2049

Willott, S, Badger, W and Evans, V (2020) People with an Intellectual Disability: Under-reporting Sexual Violence. *Journal of Adult Protection*, 22(2): 75–86.

Wilson, N, Rees, S, Northway, R and Griffiths, P (2022) Toward Mainstream Nursing Roles Specialising in the Care of People with Intellectual and Developmental Disability. *Collegian*. doi. org/10.1016/j.colegn.2022.03.004

Wilson, S (2017) Mental Capacity Legislation in the United Kingdom: A Systematic Review of the Experiences of Adults Lacking Capacity and Their Carers. *British Journal of Psychiatry Bulletin*, 41(5): 260–6.

Wolfensberger, W (1984) A Reconceptualization of Normalisation as Social Role Valorisation. *Mental Retardation*, 34, 22–25.

World Health Organization (2015) Sexual Health, Human Rights and the Law. [online] Available at: http://apps.who.int/iris/bitstream/handle/10665/175556/9789241564984_eng.pdf; jsessionid=E310634FFE5DFB45E9FA277BCD4D86EC?sequence=1 (accessed 20 June 2021).

World Medical Association (2013) *Declaration of Helsinki – Ethical Principles for Medical Research Involving Human Subjects*. [online] Available at: www.wma.net/policies-post/wma-declaration-of-helsinki-ethical-principles-for-medical-research-involving-human-subjects/ (accessed 15 January 2022).

Young Minds (2018) *Addressing Adversity: Prioritising Adversity and Trauma-informed Care for Children and Young People in England*. London: The Young Minds Trust and Health Education England.

Young, C and McKinney, C J (2016) The Court of Protection. [online] Available at: https://fullfact.org/law/court-protection-explained/ (accessed 24 January 2022).

Yura, H and Walsh, M (1967) *The Nursing Process*. Norwalk, CT: Appleton-Century-Crofts.

Index

Note: Page numbers in italics and bold denote figures and tables, respectively.